Understanding and Preventing Harmful Interactions

Between Residents with Dementia

Understanding and Preventing Harmful Interactions
Between Residents with Dementia

Eilon Caspi, Ph.D.

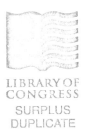

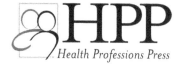

Baltimore • London • Sydney

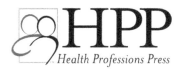

Health Professions Press, Inc.
Post Office Box 10624
Baltimore, Maryland 21285-0624

www.healthpropress.com

Cover and interior designs by Mindy Dunn.
Typeset and manufactured in the United States of America
by Integrated Books International, Dulles, Virginia.

The information provided in this book is in no way meant to substitute for the advice
or opinion of a medical, legal, or other professional or expert. This book is sold without
warranties of any kind, express or implied, and the publisher and authors disclaim any
liability, loss, or damage caused by the contents of this book.

The individuals described in this book are real people whose situations are masked;
all are based on the author's experiences and on the public record. In most instances,
names and identifying details have been changed to protect confidentiality.

Library of Congress Cataloging-in-Publication Data

Names: Caspi, Eilon, author.
Title: Understanding and preventing harmful interactions between residents
    with dementia / Eilon Caspi, Ph.D.
Identifiers: LCCN 2021023538 (print) | LCCN 2021023539 (ebook) |
    ISBN 9781938870521 (paperback) | ISBN 9781938870538 (ebook)
Subjects: LCSH: Long-term care facilities. | Dementia--Patients--Care. |
    BISAC: SOCIAL SCIENCE / Gerontology | MEDICAL / Long-Term Care
Classification: LCC RA997 .C35 2022 (print) | LCC RA997 (ebook) | DDC
    362.16--dc23
LC record available at https://lccn.loc.gov/2021023538
LC ebook record available at https://lccn.loc.gov/2021023539

British Library Cataloguing-in-Publication data are available from the British Library.

This book is dedicated to
all residents who have been
harmed during incidents with other residents
and
Elder Voice Family Advocates

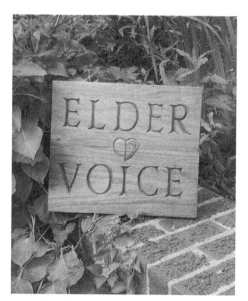

Wood carving created by the author

Author's Note

The suggestions and strategies described in this book must be carefully evaluated by interdisciplinary care teams and managers prior to implementation. No two elders living with dementia are the same. Cognitive abilities and losses vary greatly across individuals—and within an individual over time—and the circumstances surrounding each situation are often unique. The best clinical judgment of the care team and managers is paramount when considering the use of approaches and strategies described herein.

Contents

Downloadable Resources

The following collection of documents developed by the author, *Processes and Tools for Prevention of Distressing and Harmful Resident-to-Resident Interactions*, is available for download by purchasers of this book:

> **Introduction:** Conceptual Framework and Process for Assessment and Prevention of DHRRIs
> **Phase 1 Process:** Documenting and Assessing Behavioral Expressions
> **Phase 1 Tool:** Behavioral Expressions Log
> **Phase 2 Process:** Evaluation of Urgency of DHRRIs
> **Phase 2 Tool:** Evaluation of Urgency Form
> **Phase 3 Process:** Interdisciplinary Screening
> **Phase 3 Tool:** Interdisciplinary Screening Form
> **Phase 4 Process:** Behavioral Expressions Prevention Planning
> **Phase 4 Tool:** Behavioral Expressions Prevention Plan Form
> **Supplementary Resources**

To access and download these tools, go to:
https://www.healthpropress.com/downloadable-resources/caspi-downloads/
Password (case sensitive): V@C4rcC

About the Author

Born and educated in Israel, Eilon Caspi, Ph.D., is a gerontologist and dementia behavior specialist. He earned a doctoral degree in gerontology at the University of Massachusetts Boston, a master's degree in gerontology from University of Haifa, and a bachelor's in social work (aging concentration) from Tel Aviv University. He is the founder and director of Dementia Behavior Consulting, LLC, and a founding member, advisor, and board member of Elder Voice Family Advocates in Minnesota. He works as an assistant research professor at the Institute for Collaboration on Health, Intervention, and Policy, University of Connecticut. He is also a board member of the Long Term Care Community Coalition in New York City. His entire career has been devoted to the aging field, starting as a nurse aide in 1994 in a nursing home where his grandfather lived. Over time, he has worked as a social worker, consultant, applied researcher, educator, author, volunteer, and elder care advocate.

Starting in 2010, Caspi developed and implemented a comprehensive program for the prevention of resident-to-resident incidents in long-term care homes. He has spoken and trained on this topic for local, state, national, and international professional and scientific forums; nursing homes; long-term care trade associations; the Alzheimer's Association (United States and Canada); the U.S. Department of Veterans Affairs; Office of Ombudsman for Long-Term Care (Minnesota); state survey agencies; coroner offices; and the United Nations Open-ended Working Group on Ageing. He co-directed the first documentary film on injurious and fatal resident-to-resident incidents in dementia, entitled *Fighting for Dignity* (Terra Nova Films, 2020). His work has been featured in media outlets including *The Boston Globe*, *STAT*, *The Star Tribune*, KARE 11, FOX 9 KMSP, *CBC News Canada*, *The Canadian Press*, and *Stuff New Zealand*.

Other interests include research and advocacy surrounding the prevention of elder mistreatment such as healthcare neglect, abuse, financial exploitation, and theft of opioid pain medications in residential care homes. Professionally, Caspi is passionate about working to bridge academic/research activities and care practice/policy. In his free time, he enjoys woodcarving, including educational signs (below). He lives in West Harford, CT, with his wife, two daughters, and their border collie mix.

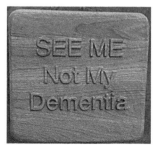

Wood carving created by the author

Acknowledgments

When I undertook my doctoral dissertation study in 2007, only a few studies were published on the phenomenon of resident-to-resident incidents in long-term care homes. As this book is publishing, over 40 studies, four reviews of the research literature, and a Government Accountability Office report examining various aspects of this public health problem are available. With each study, new insights and improved understanding of this phenomenon have emerged. I am deeply grateful for the dozens of researchers in the United States, Canada, Australia, and other countries who dedicated themselves to this line of inquiry. Many gaps in knowledge about this phenomenon remain, especially in assisted living residences but also in nursing homes. However, this growing body of empirical evidence, along with invaluable insights from decades of care practice, can now enable care homes to prevent the majority of these incidents and keep residents with dementia safe.

As with any project of this sort, many people played important parts in this book's years-long journey to publication. Without their encouragement, guidance, practical help, and patience, this project would have remained no more than an idea. Although it is not possible to recognize everyone, I endeavor in this limited space to thank those whose contributions were key to turning the idea into a book.

Heartfelt thanks to the residents, family members, care employees, and managers of the assisted living residence where I conducted my doctoral dissertation study, which planted the seeds for this book. You allowed me to learn from your lived experiences. My further thanks to the families of residents who were harmed during these incidents; you shared deeply painful stories in hopes that other residents will not experience the traumas your loved ones did.

Many of these injurious and deadly incidents would have never become public without investigative reporters who shed light on them, such as Chris Serres of *The Star Tribune* (USA) and Sandie Rinaldo of CTV's *W5* news program (Canada). The Geriatric and Long Term Care Review Committee in Ontario, Canada, should also be recognized for raising awareness about fatal resident-to-resident incidents through its annual reviews of these episodes. Applying the insights gleaned from these detailed reports can save lives.

Generous financial and other support by different organizations and individuals kept the flame of this book project alive. First and foremost was a postdoctoral fellowship from the Geriatrics and Extended Care Data Analysis Center (GECDAC) and the Ocean State Research Foundation of the Providence VA Medical Center. Special thanks to Orna Intrator of the University of Rochester, who is director of GECDAC, a national data analysis center for the VA Central Office of Geriatrics and Extended Care; she provided continued encouragement, and this project would not have been possible without her faith in its importance and my ability to carry it out. I also acknowledge Drs. Michele Karel, Christa Hojlo, Tom Edes, Richard Allman, and Kenneth Shay (VA Central Office) for their support. Notably, Dr. Hojlo provided helpful suggestions for improving an early version of the manuscript, encouraged me to expand and publish it as a book, and generously wrote one of the forewords in it.

Other organizations and people supported this book project, including Professor Christine A. Mueller and Dean Connie W. Delaney of the fabulous University of Minnesota School of Nursing. Amy Gorin, director of the Institute for Collaboration on Health, Intervention, and Policy, University of Connecticut, is another valued supporter.

Special thanks to Theresa Piccolo (Toronto, Canada), for her generosity and for her fierce advocacy aimed at ensuring that no other frail elder with dementia would experience the horrific traumas her late husband Frank did. She provided inspiration to me to stay focused on the prevention of this phenomenon.

I extend particular thanks to those who have been mentors and colleagues to me, beginning with the late Francis G. Caro, who provided outstanding guidance and advice during my doctoral dissertation study that led to the development of the book. Frank, a pioneering gerontologist, leading scholar, and beloved mentor by many, passed away unexpectedly not long before publication of the book. He is greatly missed by the people whose lives he touched, and his legacy will live on through the newly founded Frank Caro Scholarship for Social Justice in Aging.

Additional colleagues I wish to thank include other members of my dissertation committee: Donna Haig Friedman, for her friendship, for teaching me qualitative research methods, and for showing me the tremendous value these methods can have in improving understanding of unexplored phenomena; Jeff A. Burr, for his ongoing support and guidance during my years at the program and for leading the UMass Boston Gerontology Doctoral Program in graduating more Ph.D.s in Gerontology than any other academic institution; and Ann C. Hurley for her contributions during that early study. I also thank Ariela Lowenstein (Haifa University, Israel) and Nina M. Silverstein (UMass Boston) for their friendship and good advice over the years.

I am indebted to Dr. Paul Raia, former Vice President of Clinical Services, Alzheimer's Association–Massachusetts/New Hampshire Chapter, and the developer of Habilitation Therapy, for his years of mentorship, for reviewing and helping to improve an early version of the book, and for contributing one of the book's forewords. The Behavioral Expressions Prevention Plan Form, included in the downloadable materials accompanying this book, builds directly on Raia's Behavioral Analysis Protocol. The fingerprints of his wisdom and gentle guidance over the years are intertwined in many parts of the book.

A special thank you to Judy Berry, president, Dementia Specialist Consulting, for her extensive contributions during the writing of this book and for shining a light on a different path. A lot of people talk and write about person-directed care practices for elders living with dementia, but she actually did it, sacrificing greatly to develop her inspiring and effective Lakeview Ranch Model of Specialized Dementia Care™ for providing a safe and transformative home for residents deemed too dangerous to live in other care homes. Motivated by personal experience with her own mother, who was drugged, discharged, and labeled "aggressive," Judy pursued a more humane and dignified way to support and care for people with dementia who are often mistakenly labeled as "violent" and "abusive." I have been motivated by Judy's insistence that proactively identifying and meeting the emotional needs of people with dementia in care homes keeps people safe and reduces the vast majority of these episodes.

A big thank you to Lori La Bey, founder of Alzheimer's Speaks, for her friendship and for being a global leader in giving a public voice to people living with dementia. Through her, I have been introduced to many of these incredible human beings who serve as educators and advocates by teaching us about the lived experience of dementia and removing the stigma surrounding the disease.

Many thanks go to my friend and colleague Steven Orfield, President, Orfield Laboratories Inc. (Minneapolis, MN), for his wisdom and generosity of time in improving Chapter 5, Factors in the Physical Environment. His wealth of evidence-based knowledge and expertise in this area are unparalleled.

My profound gratitude goes to the many outstanding professionals at Health Professions Press. Special thanks to Mary Magnus, Director of Publications, for her ongoing guidance and assistance since the inception of the book. She has been patient, responsive, and flexible as well as committed to the book's purpose and key messages. Mary's insights and encouragement throughout this journey have been invaluable. Several other people who contributed meaning-ful support and direction for this project have moved on since the project began, namely As-sociate Editor Teresa Ingraham Iafolla and Editorial & Production Manager Cecilia González; each was instrumental in shaping early drafts. I am grateful to Kaitlin Konecke, Marketing Manager, for developing and leading a comprehensive plan for dissemination of the book. Her expertise and dedication to the success of this book project are greatly appreciated. I also want to thank Mindy Dunn, the designer responsible for the cover and interior of this book, as well as proofreader Janet Wehner.

I am deeply grateful to Linda Francis, the Editorial & Production Manager who shep-herded the book to its completion. Her rare combination of kindness, wisdom, determination, and organization skills made all the difference. I have no words to describe her generosity and editing skills with an author for whom English is not the first spoken and written language.

Thanks also to Jayne Clairmont, former owner and CEO of English Rose Suites; the late Sheri W. Sussman, former Executive Editor, Springer Publishing Company; and the anony-mous reviewers who examined early versions of the book and provided helpful suggestions for improvement, as well as David Dosa, M.D., author of the fascinating book *Making Rounds with Oscar,* for his advice on the publication process.

Last but not least, I am deeply grateful to my family. Caitlin, the love of my life, is an incredible human being, friend, wife, and mother. Your endless patience, understanding, wis-dom, practical help, and support throughout this long and sometimes painful journey enabled me to complete it. Many thanks to Grandma Ginny for being the best grandmother in the universe and for taking care of our young girls with unparalleled dedication, love, and wisdom during the years prior to and throughout the COVID-19 pandemic when this book was being completed; I could not have done it without you. Thank you, Grandpa Terry, for your endless love and support of our family and this project. Thanks also to my father Meir Caspi, whose love and support across the ocean and over the years have enabled me to realize my dreams in the aging field. Last but not least, my daughters Natalie and Eleanor were born during the writing process of this book. They bring boundless joy to our hearts and lives, brightening our days, and uplifting our spirits when we need it. You are loved beyond words.

Foreword

Knowledge depends largely on how you define what it is you investigate. The ancient astronomers, for example, saw humankind from their religious perspective to be preeminent, and thus placed Earth in the center of the universe. For centuries, astronomers then *saw* the sun and all the planets as revolving around the earth. Definition then, determines perception. Galileo reasoned a new and deferent definition of humankind, one where Earth was part of a larger celestial algorithm, and a whole new starscape opened to those who studied the heavens.

We are now beginning to redefine Alzheimer's disease in a new way that reveals options for treatment of symptoms. Previous definitions of Alzheimer's disease limited the options for symptom management.

From the time that humankind began to survive beyond the age of 50 years, dramatic changes in cognition and behavior in those who were older were observed and recorded but those changes were defined as a "normal" part of the human development. Thus, Shakespeare's *Seven Stages of Man* describes the last stage of life as a stage of mental confusion, lack of personal control, and dependence on others. To a certain extent, this view dominates the popular definition of Alzheimer's disease as not a disease at all, but rather a normal part of the aging process, and not a human state subject to change.

A second definition of Alzheimer's is that it is indeed a disease, but one for which there are no effective interventions. Therefore, the best that we can accomplish with those who are living and dying with Alzheimer's disease is to provide palliative care. Such care accepts the fact that the symptoms of the disease cannot be changed and that comfort care as the person declines is all that can be achieved.

Yet another definition, and perhaps the most dominant contemporary view, is that Alzheimer's is a disease that has limited opportunities for the treatment of cognitive and behavioral symptoms, so that all our resources should be placed in finding the magic elixir that will cure, mitigate, or prevent the symptoms associated with Alzheimer's disease. This definition has obscured our view of other options that might be available for the treatment of symptoms.

However, a new view of people living with Alzheimer's disease and other forms of dementia is emerging within the field of psychology that maintains that many of the symptoms associated with these diseases are potentially treatable using person-directed and behavioral methods. According to this school of thought, psychoactive medications might not be needed to improve how the person with Alzheimer's disease feels, interprets, and engages in the world.

For many years Eilon Caspi has been gathering data and building the case for the personalized, primarily psychosocial, approaches (often called nonpharmacological treatment by biomedical models of care) for the symptoms associated with Alzheimer's disease and other forms of dementia. He advocates for a vision of dementia that sees people as whole human beings, focusing on their emotional experiences and needs, and adopting a strength-based approach. This is in sharp contrast to biomedical approaches that focus primarily on people's functional *impairments,* cognitive *deficits,* and behavioral *symptoms.* When a person-directed, strength-based approach is used well, new, exciting, and humane opportunities for optimizing the psychological well-being of people with dementia and preserving their personhood open up, despite substantial cognitive disabilities.

Caspi is a pioneer in building the case for a psychology of dementia and the management of the symptoms characteristic of dementing illness. As articulated by the late Tom Kitwood in his groundbreaking book *Dementia Reconsidered: The Person Comes First,* overlooking the psychological needs of people living with dementia often causes these individuals to experience tremendous emotional suffering, which can lead to various forms of distressful and unsafe behavioral expressions.

In this book, Caspi makes the case that challenging or reactive behaviors associated with the middle and later stages of dementia is a form of communication telling us that something is awry in the person's sense of the world (when looking closely, it is usually something distressing and frustrating in the person's immediate social or physical environment). He lays out a systematic approach using a series of tools for identifying *triggers* that cause reactive behavioral expressions. Once triggers are identified, he offers simple useful protocols for implementing, charting, and assessing effective interventions. More than just a how-to book, this approach to understanding the inner "psychology of people living with dementia" changes the way we will "see" these individuals and dementia. It will also help shift the commonly held stigma about people with dementia as "aggressive," "violent," and "abusive" to seeing them as normal human beings attempting to cope as best they can using their remaining cognitive abilities. It will enable our society to view their behavioral expressions as attempts to preserve their dignity and personhood prior to and during distressing and frustrating daily situations. As with the ancient astronomers, *Understanding and Preventing Harmful Interactions Between Residents with Dementia* could open up a whole new starscape in the world of humane, holistic, and effective care for people living with dementia in long-term care homes.

Paul Raia, Ph.D.
Vice President for Professional Clinical Services
Alzheimer's Association, Massachusetts/New Hampshire Chapter
Developer of the Habilitation Therapy Approach in Dementia Care

Foreword

Dementia, a difficult and emotionally fraught diagnosis that affects millions of people in the United States, has no cure. It seemingly takes over all levels of function and leaves the person, family, friends, and care partners mystified as to how to help. The sadness and grief over the diagnosis is heartbreaking and raises questions about quality and quantity of life.

As an emeritus licensed nursing home administrator, clinician, and former national director of more than 130 U.S. Department of Veterans Affairs (VA) nursing homes (now referred to as Community Living Centers), I personally witnessed the various expressions of pain of family, residents, staff, and community agencies. I also witnessed the challenges regarding how to provide loving care for residents with dementia. The need for resources and support for all concerned is urgent.

One day, I was listening to a riveting presentation by Eilon Caspi and was moved by his compassion for these residents and his interest in a most challenging aspect of care for this population. Caspi had the courage and deep insight to address resident behavioral expressions. His presentation identified an array of expressions for which there were few to no tools readily available to assist care partners. I was mesmerized as he identified sets of behaviors, especially those that resulted in injury or harm to the individual resident, other residents, staff, or family. Most importantly, he identified underlying causes and described interventions that could result in successful outcomes. Afterward, we discussed the absence of a comprehensive, research-based manual or guide about this delicate and complex phenomenon. Thus, Caspi embarked on the journey that led to this book.

In his book, Caspi has thoughtfully and thoroughly aggregated a large body of research identifying how persons with dementia communicate needs along with approaches that care partners, especially those working in nursing homes and assisted living residences, can utilize to meet resident needs and prevent escalation of resident-to-resident incidents. He has creatively infused these pages with identification of physical, medical, environmental, interpersonal, social, and other factors that can affect an individual at a deep level. These factors can give rise to deep inner and unexpressed fear, anxiety, anger, rage, and discomfort. But, if recognized and addressed in time, they can also point the care partner toward ways of soothing or providing comfort and joy in the moment. Caspi offers approaches that can prevent harmful behavioral expressions of negative emotions, de-escalate incidents, and result in personal comfort and safety for the resident.

Any reader who has worked or lived with persons with dementia will be able to identify with the behavioral expressions described in this book. These can include restlessness, anxiety, crying, invasion of personal space, screaming, hitting, and loud or threatening verbal expressions, as well as physically aggressive acts. These expressions may be related to changes in an individual's physical health status, sensitivity to ambient temperature, noise that evokes uncomfortable memories, or even actions associated with combat. Approaches of the care partners—such as hands on the hips or an unhelpful tone of voice or attitude—can also be factors in these expressions, as can decisions such as seating arrangements in dining areas and roommate selection.

What is most captivating in the book are the useful and creative psychosocial strategies care partners can utilize to prevent or de-escalate these incidents and then soothe the resident and others directly and indirectly involved in the episode. This book reaches beyond identifying causes alone and presents successful approaches to compassionate and skilled care. Early chapters focus on the underlying causes and triggers of harmful behavioral expressions. Later chapters provide the tools and strategies for evaluating both the potential for and causes of harmful interactions between residents and, even more importantly, the care partner approaches that can be used to make a significant positive difference in resident outcomes. The respectful language used throughout the book reflects the compassion and dignity with which care partners can assess, plan, implement, and evaluate successful care outcomes for residents with dementia experiencing behavioral expressions.

The book can be read from cover to cover systematically or used as a reference for guidance in specific situations. Each chapter contains discussions of real-life examples and practical suggestions and approaches. Tables and charts are easy to read, use, and apply. The tools provided in this book—and those that accompany the book online—can help guide assessment, individualized care planning, and intervention.

I applaud this book for presenting a comprehensive, evidence-based discussion of the etiologies of resident-to-resident incidents and approaches to commonly known and observed resident situations that challenge traditional biomedical model interventions for the care and comfort of persons with dementia in long-term care settings. The extensive references are a goldmine of additional resources for addressing and further investigating this phenomenon.

The information provided in *Understanding and Preventing Harmful Interactions Between Residents with Dementia* could also be used to decrease the stresses on care partners and organizations in their daily attempts to serve persons with dementia experiencing behavioral expressions. They can learn from it how to provide loving, person-centered, and humane care while preventing the negative consequences of unmet needs. This book belongs in any library of essential resources on the care of residents living with dementia.

Christa M. Hojlo, Ph.D., R.N., NHA
Former National Director, VA Community Living Centers

Preface

*People with dementia may have something important to teach
the rest of humankind. If we make the venture one of genuine and
open engagement, we will learn a great deal about ourselves.*

Tom Kitwood

Alzheimer's disease doesn't take away people's dignity. We do.

Joanne Koenig Coste

My journey in the aging field started in Israel in 1994 shortly after I was discharged from my required 3-year army service. While searching for my first job, I was shown a list of organizations that were hiring. It included a local nursing home that coincidentally was where my grandfather, a Holocaust survivor, had lived during the last years of his life. I thought it was a sign and applied for the nurse aide position. Through my work at the nursing home, I discovered a fascinating world of elders—human beings who, like all of us, have hopes, dreams, joys, frustrations, and fears. They had unique and rich life histories and the same human needs we all share for love, dignity, respect, and safety. This experience sparked my interest in working with and on behalf of vulnerable and frail elders. I moved on to social work with low-income elders in the community, and later to another nursing home primarily serving elders living with dementia. These early experiences strengthened my interest in learning more about care of elders with dementia in long-term care (LTC) homes.

I pursued a master's degree in gerontology during which I interviewed 100 family members of community-dwelling elders with dementia about their perceptions of dementia and daily coping strategies. Then, I moved to the United States for doctoral studies in gerontology at the University of Massachusetts Boston. My dissertation study involved direct observation of elders with dementia in two specialized assisted living care homes. I witnessed distressing and harmful resident-to-resident interactions (DHRRIs) on a daily basis. Many of these episodes caused psychological distress and fear in a large number of residents. They also often placed residents at risk of physical harm.

Although the initial aim of my qualitative study was to focus on positive interactions between direct care partners and residents and strategies these care employees use for preventing distressing behavioral expressions, an early conversation I had with a resident encouraged me to dedicate increased attention to the phenomenon of DHRRIs. Specifically, a resident with early-stage Alzheimer's disease approached me one day and said, "Whatever you present at the end of the study, you have to be honest . . . you have to. You know that some interactions are not so positive. You have to be honest. You have to tell the whole story. People will not believe you if you don't tell the whole story."

Intense incidents between residents affect the care employees, too. One team leader said about a resident with Alzheimer's disease who frequently engaged in these episodes, "I am just afraid that he will hurt someone when we don't see it . . . especially someone frail who he can take down with one blow." Expressing her deep concern, another care employee said about the same resident, "He is going to kill someone one day." Seeing the effects of these frequent episodes on residents at all stages of dementia and care employees had a profound impact on me.

At the outset of my research, I found that only a very small number of studies were dedicated to the phenomenon of DHRRIs in nursing homes, and no study focused on it in secure dementia care homes operated within assisted living residences. Realizing a major gap existed in knowledge about this phenomenon encouraged me to dedicate a substantial portion of my exploratory study to examining it.

In subsequent years, I developed a comprehensive program aimed at improving understanding and prevention of these episodes in LTC homes. In devoting my attention to this poorly understood phenomenon, I have tracked deadly resident-to-resident incidents internationally, conducted the first study[3] on fatal incidents in the United States and Canada, provided staff training, and lectured on this subject for local, state, national, and international professional and scientific conferences. In 2020, I co-directed with my colleague Judy Berry the first documentary short film on the subject, *Fighting for Dignity* (https://terranova.org/film-catalog/fighting-for-dignity-a-film-on-injurious-and-fatal-resident-to-resident-incidents-in-long-term-care-homes/), which focuses on the emotional trauma and devastation experienced by family members of residents who were injured or died as a result of these incidents.

My review of hundreds of injurious and fatal DHRRIs in care homes in the United States, Canada, and Australia has revealed striking similarities in these occurrences across cultures and countries. In the vast majority of incidents, clear warning signs existed in the months, weeks, days, and hours prior to the injuries, and these harmful episodes could have been prevented. Each time I learn about another avoidable injury or death, my heart aches not only for the resident with dementia, but also for her or his family and the shock and emotional devastation they experience.

Giving Knowledge and Tools to Care Partners

Over the course of many years, I have realized that most direct care partners in LTC homes in the United States and other countries do not have the critical knowledge and skills necessary to adequately understand and prevent DHRRIs and keep residents with dementia safe. This book is a step toward filling this gap. I have assembled a user-friendly collection of available knowledge and research on DHRRIs and provide practical guidance on ways in which staff at all levels can effectively address them. It will be useful to direct care partners, nurses, social workers, psychologists, recreational therapists, physicians, managers, administrators, and owners of care homes. The book includes brief summaries of research findings, dozens of real-life stories of success and failure in addressing this phenomenon, and countless quotes of residents with dementia, their family members, care employees, researchers, and experts. It can inform the creation of specialized training content for new employee orientations or in-service education. And while there is much we still need to learn about effective strategies for prevention and de-escalation of these episodes in the context of residents with dementia, the book represents the most comprehensive effort to date on this front.

Through my work, I have learned that nearly everyone from direct care partners to CEOs has witnessed and struggled to address this phenomenon. For various understandable reasons, such as the potential for adverse publicity, sanctions by state survey agencies, or possible liability, they are often reluctant to discuss it in public. In this book, readers now can find information and tools to tackle the issue head on. They will gain an understanding of the many causes of these incidents and the array of strategies available to prevent them or, when they do happen, to de-escalate them quickly, skillfully, and safely. Readers can also access a collection of DHRRI–specific assessment tools made available online in connection with this book (see list on page viii). These can be used to strengthen the detection of the causes and contributing factors of these episodes and inform the development of individualized prevention plans. Using these new resources will allow LTC leaders and care professionals to provide residents with dementia with the basic human right to live in a safe environment. The same applies to the direct care partners, nurses, and all other care employees who come in regular contact with residents—and who often courageously put themselves at risk of psychological and physical harm while trying to protect residents' safety during serious episodes. These dedicated care workers can become more effective in preventing these episodes and, in turn, be safer at their workplace.

Calling Leaders in Long-Term Care to Action

Besides relieving the human suffering that results from these incidents, there is a strong business case to be made for owners and administrators of LTC homes to make every effort to understand their causes and proactively implement strong measures to prevent them. Preventable injuries and deaths of residents can lead to lawsuits and costly settlements, for example. Two such lawsuits settled in 2020—brought after fatal resident-to-resident incidents—resulted in $1.9 million and $1.2 million awards, respectively. Both of these tragic deaths occurred separately but in the same LTC chain. Would it not be wiser to proactively invest a small fraction of such settlements in preventive measures?

When owners, leaders in corporate offices, and administrators fully recognize the potential for serious psychological and physical harm experienced by residents with dementia during these episodes, they are more inclined to commit the resources necessary to prevent them. These measures include proper staffing levels, training, risk assessment, and care planning. A series of evidence-based changes in the physical environment may also be needed to make it safer and truly elder- and dementia-friendly.

To be clear, effectively addressing this prevalent but largely overlooked phenomenon cannot be accomplished using quick fixes or magic bullets. To be successful, it must be recognized as a continuous journey. Without full, attentive, and ongoing daily commitment to supporting this journey—at the highest levels of the care organization (owners and administrators)—prevention with lasting effects cannot be realized and residents living with dementia will continue to be needlessly harmed.

Fighting for Dignity

While this book stands on 12 foundational guiding principles (see Chapter 2), perhaps the most important insight I have gained about this phenomenon over the years—one I hope readers will take away after reading this book—could be summarized in these three words: *fighting for dignity*. My work experience in care homes, the thousands of hours of direct observations I spent in these care settings, my examination of hundreds of injurious and deadly incidents, and findings from more than 40 research studies published to date about this phenomenon have made it clear to me that in the vast majority of situations residents with dementia are "fighting" with each other in an effort to preserve their dignity and protect their safety. When people living with dementia feel their dignity threatened, and when their varied human needs (emotional, social, and physical/medical needs, as well as the need for meaningful engagement) are not being met by direct care partners who are all too often overworked, undertrained, and insufficiently supported, these episodes will continue to occur frequently and cause harm to residents. When these elders, who are living with a serious brain disease, experience situational frustrations and fears in their day-to-day interactions with other residents, they are bound to react in ways aimed at protecting themselves from real or perceived threats and to affirm their personhood, identity, and right to live with dignity. They are doing their best to cope using their remaining cognitive abilities in care environments they often perceive as distressing and frightening. It is the responsibility of the care providers to proactively, promptly, and skillfully address the unmet human needs underlying these frustrations to prevent them from escalating to serious consequences.

In sharp contrast to common beliefs, most elders with dementia are not *aggressive, violent,* or *abusive,* though, as noted earlier, the effects of some resident interactions can certainly be traumatic and tragic. To label the people involved in these incidents as "aggressive" implies a directed intention by the "aggressor" to do real harm, when in fact the behavioral expressions are often reflexive and *not* thought out. For this reason, I generally avoid use of these stigmatizing terms and instead refer simply to *interactions* or *harmful interactions.*

The goal is to acknowledge a harmful outcome but to remain neutral and free of judgment about the causes and situational triggers, and to see more clearly that these are not *behaviors* but rather understandable human expressions—deep yearnings for fulfillment of basic human needs for dignity, emotional security, and physical safety. Examined through this person-directed care lens, a fundamentally different story often emerges than the one conjured by labels of "aggression." It is a story of possibilities as opposed to a story of limits. It is a story of real opportunity for prevention, not one of "inevitable" incidents. These episodes often represent the best way a resident living with dementia can cope with frustrating situations in her or his immediate social and physical environment. When we fully recognize it, we see elders living with dementia as equal citizens with human rights we want to cherish and protect. Just as we expect to remain safe in our own homes, people with dementia who live in nursing homes and assisted living residences expect and deserve the same assurance.

Showing the Way

In *Understanding and Preventing Harmful Interactions Between Residents with Dementia,* I take a systematic, multilevel approach to proactively addressing the phenomenon of DHRRIs. A primary goal is improving understanding of the causes of these episodes. With this understanding, care employees are then ready to learn about the vast array of psychosocial prevention strategies they could use at different points in time, during unique situations, and at different levels of the care organization.

Does the book address every possible scenario of DHRRIs? Absolutely not; that would be impossible. It *does* give a working framework and a wide array of directions for direct care partners, other interdisciplinary care team members, managers, and owners to consider as they develop their care home–wide and individualized prevention efforts.

Successfully transforming the culture of care, policies, and operations to proactively meet each resident's seven domains of well-being (as described by The Eden Alternative, these are identity, connectedness, security, autonomy, meaning, growth, and joy) will likely result in substantial reduction of these episodes. While strong empirical evidence to substantiate this claim is needed, dozens of studies and outstanding care models and practices clearly point in this direction.

Ideally, all care homes for elders with dementia are aiming to enable their residents to experience the highest practicable psychological well-being (see G. Allen Power's excellent book entitled *Dementia Beyond Disease: Enhancing Well-Being*[65]), yet the reality is that many care homes have a long way to go on the culture change journey to get there. Many care homes are still largely stuck in biomedical and custodial models of care, focusing predominantly on meeting residents' physical and medical needs, with very little focus on fulfilling their emotional, psychological, social, and spiritual needs. Additionally, scores of care homes have not even made the commitment to transforming their culture of care. For now, we must "stop the bleeding." Thousands of older Americans living with dementia are physically injured during resident-to-resident incidents in care homes each year; a significant number of these individuals die as a result of the injuries. In other words, direct care partners desperately need specialized knowledge and psychosocial strategies for prevention and de-escalation of these incidents now; they can't wait several more years, a decade, or longer for their care homes to become culturally transformed. The basic premise underlying the book recognizes and reflects these facts.

Beyond my direct work experience and research in this field, my education in these matters has been profoundly influenced by the expertise and insight of fellow colleagues and leaders. We all stand on the shoulders of giants. The individuals that follow have inspired and transformed my thinking over the years about the human needs and person-directed care practices that can be provided successfully to elders living with dementia. They worked hard for many years to envision, develop, and hone enlightened, humane, relationship-based, life-affirming, and dignified care approaches to this underserved and stigmatized population. I will be forever grateful for their efforts, wisdom, and insights.

These pioneers and giants include Naomi Feil, developer of the Validation Method; the late professor Tom Kitwood, founder of Dementia Bradford Group and author of the groundbreaking book *Dementia Reconsidered: The Person Comes First*; G. Allen Power, developer of the Experiential Pathway to Well-Being and a leading thinker in the field who regularly charts our path forward, always pushing the limits of what *person-directed care* can be; Paul Raia, developer of Habilitation Therapy; Judy Berry, developer of the Lakeview Ranch Model of Specialized Dementia Care; Bill Thomas, founder of The Eden Alternative and the Green House Model; Jayne Clairmont, founder of English Rose Suites; and Lori La Bey, founder of Alzheimer's Speaks, to name a few.

Perhaps the most influential on my thinking are people living with dementia who are leading educators and advocates. These include, among others, Richard Taylor (deceased), Harry Urban, Michael Ellenbogen, Bob Savage, Laurie Scherrer, Paulan Gordon, Truthful Loving Kindness, Susan Suchan (deceased), Dr. Mary L. Radnofsky, Brian LeBlanc, Dena Dotson (deceased), Craig Hanke, Cate Lau-Booth, Dr. Jennifer Bute, and Kate Swaffer. We, professionals and researchers, can only imagine how it feels to live with a cognitive disability. They actually *know*, and we would all be wise to do our best to listen to them and to their advice. People living with dementia are the best teachers out there when it comes to *their* lived experience. As Power advises, "Ignore them at your peril!"

Finally, the late Meira Ekshtein (the legendary director of an adult day program for low-income elders with dementia in the city of Jaffa, Israel) was the first who taught me two decades ago, when I was a young social worker in a nursing home at Tzahalon Geriatric Center, the critical value of, first and foremost, being fully present, centered, and paying very close attention to and proactively meeting the emotional needs of this population. I will always be indebted to all these individuals who inspired me, showed me the way, and opened a path for my own journey in the aging field with the goal of realizing the basic human right of elders living with dementia to receive dignified and safe care.

I invite you to join me on this journey and hope that you will find this book useful in your efforts to preserve the dignity and improve the quality of care and safety of this population in nursing homes and assisted living residences. Feel free to contact me (eiloncaspi@gmail.com) if you have a question, comment, suggestion, or if you see a way in which we may be able to collaborate in addressing this phenomenon.

Eilon Caspi
September 2021

Introduction

Some of the most compassionate acts take place between residents in long-term care (LTC) homes. Many residents who are cognitively intact and those with early-stage dementia often teach us something important about empathy when they assist those with more advanced cognitive disability and advocate for protecting their right for dignified and safe care. It is also not uncommon to see residents with advanced stages of dementia compassionately trying to help others who are living with substantial cognitive impairment. Unfortunately, many interactions between people with dementia can also be emotionally stressful, and they can be psychologically and physically harmful.

This book addresses the prevalent but underrecognized and largely unaddressed phenomenon of distressing and harmful resident-to-resident interactions (DHRRIs) in LTC homes.[1] Dozens of research studies and hundreds of media reports have shed light on the psychological and physical harm experienced by residents, especially those living with dementia, during these episodes. Beyond the psychological impact—such as frustration, distress, anger, fear, and emotional trauma—thousands of residents in America's care homes sustain falls, broken bones (such as hip fractures), and brain injuries during these incidents each year. For many, these traumatic injuries lead to a further decline in physical and medical condition and even death. "Why can't we make our voice go through the walls of this building?" asked one resident with early-stage Alzheimer's disease who witnessed these episodes on a daily basis. We rarely hear the voices of residents with dementia impacted by DHRRIs.

Family members of these residents are frequently shocked to discover that their spouses and parents were injured or died as a result of these episodes. They have placed their loved ones in these care homes trusting that they will be safe there. Although many are devastated by the psychological harm and physical injuries experienced by their loved ones, their voices and hopes for systemic improvements in LTC homes are rarely heard in public. These family members ask that lessons be learned from the traumas experienced by their loved ones so that other vulnerable and frail elders will not be harmed in similar situations.[2,3,4]

Debbie Stultz-Giffin, daughter of 87-year-old Dorothy Stultz, who had Alzheimer's disease and who died after being pushed by another resident in a nursing home, said, "I think that my mother would be quite saddened that her death wasn't more openly discussed, that it wasn't looked at . . . under the microscope." She added, "They are our most vulnerable population, and we should do everything in our power to protect those people."[2] She said she hoped her mother's death would help prompt a deeper look at ways to prevent these incidents. "We do not want the death of our father to be in vain," said the son of an 87-year-old man with Alzheimer's disease who had been pushed by another resident with dementia. The push caused him to fall and hit his head on the floor, suffering blunt head trauma. He died four days later.[3] "We are out to find a solution. To make sure that our aging population is taken care of. I want to see something done so this doesn't happen again." The wife of an 85-year-old man with Alzheimer's disease who was severely injured inside his bedroom by another resident around 2 a.m. on a Saturday said she "feels sickened by what he has to endure at the end of his life." His daughter said, "If this happened to a child at Sick Kids hospital, people wouldn't stand for it."[4]

Direct care partners often consider the occurrence of these incidents to be the most distressing and challenging to address effectively and safely, despite their efforts at prevention. These dedicated, compassionate, and hardworking people often work in care homes that are understaffed—often dangerously so—with little specialized training in understanding, preventing, and de-escalating these episodes, and without sufficient emotional support from managers. Although they are extremely concerned about the safety of the residents with dementia under their care, many are also concerned about their own safety as they often selflessly and courageously attempt to intervene and de-escalate these episodes. Their voices need to be heard as well.

This book represents the most comprehensive effort to date to ensure that the voices of these three key groups—residents with dementia, their family members, and direct care partners—are heard outside the walls of nursing homes and assisted living residences. Dozens of real-life stories appear throughout, as well as findings from a large number of research studies. The chapters that follow present an overview of this phenomenon, an in-depth description of the many causes and circumstances that lead to these incidents, and a broad array of the many psychosocial strategies and processes that organizations and direct care partners can use to prevent and address them.

Organization of This Book

Part I describes the scope of the issue—the common and disturbing manifestations, as well as the consequences (Chapter 1)—and 12 guiding principles (Chapter 2) that constitute the book's approach to this problem and serve as reminders for readers to cultivate their own awareness of the conditions that lead to the incidents and strategies they might use to prevent them.

Part II (Chapters 3–6) outlines dozens of causes and factors that contribute to these incidents. Understanding these factors can help direct care partners and administrators realize skillful prevention with lasting effects.

Actions that direct care partners can take before, during, and after episodes between residents with dementia are detailed in Part III (Chapters 7–10). These chapters present dozens of psychosocial strategies for prevention and de-escalation of these episodes, with the aim of keeping residents with dementia and their direct care partners safe.

A full commitment to the routine, proactive, and skilled detection and assessment of residents' unmet human needs and situational frustrations is essential for addressing these incidents and preventing them in the future. The downloadable materials accompanying this text provide tools and guidance for this process, to strengthen the ability of direct care partners and administrators to identify the factors underlying these episodes and enhance their ability to develop individually tailored care plans that work in preventing these episodes. For a list of these materials and instructions for accessing them, see p. viii.

Important Exclusions

While comprehensive, the book does not address certain aspects of this phenomenon. First, since the book focuses primarily on psychosocial strategies for prevention of DHRRIs, it dedicates only very limited attention to physical and medical factors contributing to these episodes (selected examples are addressed for illustration and focus on conditions such as pain, constipation, and delirium). Important as they are, due to scope limitations in combination with my expertise in psychosocial prevention strategies (not in medical causes and treatments), addressing the full spectrum of medical and physical causes of these episodes and their medical treatments should be the focus of a separate article or book.

Second, although sexual DHRRIs (for example, unwanted intrusive sexual advances, sexual attacks, and rape) cause profound trauma to residents with dementia, these incidents are quite varied in manifestation and severity and are often quite complex and challenging to address. Attempts to realize the right of residents with dementia for sexual expression at the same time with other residents' right to remain safe and free from abuse by others often proves to be a delicate balancing act. To do justice to this important, complex, and emotionally charged phenomenon that is often rife with myths and misconceptions, full attention is warranted elsewhere.

Third, although a subgroup of residents with serious mental illness (such as schizophrenia, antisocial personality disorder, and bipolar disorder) are often involved in these episodes, a unique combination of care work experience, knowledge, and skill set is needed to effectively address these episodes in this population. LTC homes could gain this specialized knowledge from experienced mental health professionals (such as registered nurses trained in psychiatry) who have dedicated their careers to caring for these individuals, meeting their varied needs, and preventing and de-escalating their distressing and harmful behavioral expressions. Integrating these specialized mental health services into the day-to-day care operations of care homes (in general and through the ongoing training of all care employees in direct regular contact with residents with serious mental illness) would likely result in a significant reduction in DHRRIs and a safer care environment for all.

Language Matters

A word about words: They matter, a lot. Words used to describe elders living with dementia reflect and shape the ways in which they are perceived by direct care partners, which profoundly influences the ways in which they are approached, cared for, and treated.

Elders with Dementia

When we describe elders living in LTC homes as "dementia patients," we stigmatize them and run the risk of reducing them to their brain disease. We are no longer in a position to see each whole human being with her or his unique and rich life history and remaining cognitive abilities. We will be more inclined to focus on the cognitive disabilities, which limits important opportunities for providing person-directed care that helps the elder realize his or her highest practical psychological well-being. To ensure that we focus on the person before her or his brain disease, I use the terms "residents" and "elders with dementia" throughout the book.

Long-Term Care *Home*

Biomedical terms such as "facility" can perpetuate a dangerous situation by overlooking the critical fact that the care setting is the residents' *home*—at least it is the home of residents who are there to receive long-term care (i.e., long-stay vs. short-stay residents). Using the word "home" encourages us to remember that direct care partners work in the home of residents with dementia. The term "facility" reminds me of a factory with an assembly line of physical objects, which is not the kind of humane model of care we aspire to. Similarly, when we describe a care home specializing in caring for elders living with dementia as "memory care unit" or "dementia care unit," we inadvertently perpetuate the biomedical perception that care is provided to impaired memories or brain diseases rather than to people—elders living with cognitive disabilities as well as their remaining cognitive abilities (it is important to keep in mind that memory functions represent only one of several domains of cognition).

Behavioral Expressions

"Words matter, and so the way in which behaviour is talked or written about is important, since this can define or label how the behaviour is construed," asserts dementia care expert Claire Surr. "All behaviours should be viewed, primarily, as attempts at communication, re-lated to need."[5] When we describe elders living with dementia or their behavioral expressions as "aggressive," "combative," "violent," or "abusive," or refer to them as "perpetrators," we are labeling, stigmatizing, and harming these individuals. These commonly used terms assume that elders with serious brain diseases are inherently aggressive, which could not be further from the truth with most individuals. Such labeling mistakenly assumes that the majority of these people intend to mistreat, psychologically harm, injure, or kill their fellow residents—a common misconception that has been demonstrated in the hundreds of injurious and fatal res-ident-to-resident incidents I have examined over the years. I myself used the term "aggressive behaviors" when I started studying this phenomenon. Besides the effect this type of language has on the care and treatment of elders, it is also not supported by a growing body of research studies on this phenomenon in the United States and abroad. That is why, whenever possible, the commonly used terms resident-to-resident "aggression," "abuse," "violence," and "elder mistreatment" will not be used in this book. My hope is that this book will contribute to on-going efforts aimed at reaching a tipping point on this grossly neglected front that has caused tremendous harm to scores of residents with dementia worldwide.

Once residents with dementia are labeled with these terms, direct care partners are less likely to try to identify the unmet needs and situational frustrations in the person's physical and social environment—intersecting with the cognitive disabilities—that lead to the majority of these understandable human expressions.

Even the term "behaviors" can be problematic, as it implies a negative judgment against the person who is living and coping with a serious brain disease. When was the last time you heard the term "behaviors" used in a positive context? I currently use the terms "behavioral expressions" and "distressing and harmful resident-to-resident interactions," while being aware that language used to describe this population is evolving and more person-directed care terms will likely emerge in the future.

Imagine that you and I are elders with dementia living in a care home. I invade your personal space 10 times over a period of 15 minutes. At first you respond politely by asking me to leave the area, but the invasions continue and gradually you lose your patience and be-come very angry. Direct care partners are not nearby to de-escalate the situation. Eventually, you reach a breaking point and push me strongly to the floor. Would it be accurate or fair to describe you as "aggressive"? Is defending one's personal space after reaching a "breaking point" really a "behavior"? Is there a real need for the nurse or physician to give you an anti-psychotic medication?

Again, these acts should largely be viewed as understandable human expressions by people with serious brain disease—reactions to care needs that are not met, interpersonal stressors, and situational frustrations that are not addressed skillfully and in time. In fact, these expres-sions can be perceived as gifts—among the most effective ways for elders living with dementia to telegraph that something is upsetting them, when their ability to express it in words fails them. I challenge you to try and see these expressions as precious assets for prevention and as sensitive barometers of the quality of care and approaches used in your care home.

The hard truth is that many injurious and deadly episodes are a direct result of neglect of care by the LTC home and/or its employees, managers, and owners. Often, the stigma created by the use of these terms leads to a slippery slope toward an inappropriate and excessive use of largely harmful antipsychotic drugs (the use of these drugs in elders with dementia has been shown to substantially increase their risk of experiencing stroke and death). Once the person with dementia is significantly sedated, the ability of direct care partners to identify and fulfill her or his unmet human needs is reduced substantially; meanwhile, side effects of these medications can introduce new problems, such as physical suffering and falls.

Exhibitors

As mentioned earlier, when discussing elders living with a serious brain disease, there is an urgent need to shift away from using terms borrowed from the elder abuse and mistreatment literature. In the vast majority of incidents, elders with middle- to late-stage dementia do not try to verbally, physically, or sexually abuse or injure other residents. Although the outcomes of these incidents can be as harmful and traumatic as in cases of staff-to-resident abuse, these two types of incidents are fundamentally different. Overlooking this distinction often exacerbates the stigma associated with elders living with dementia. That is why this book will not use the term "perpetrator" in the context of the vast majority of episodes where residents with middle- to late-stage dementia say or do something that causes psychological or physical harm to another resident (except when it is used within quotes published by other authors). This issue is explained by Mark Lachs as follows:[6]

> "Victim," "Perpetrator," or both may be "blameless" in many of these episodes, in that they are facilitated by brain disease and not volitional ill will. Indeed, even the label "elder mistreatment" suggests, often incorrectly, that malevolence is a motivator in these situations, although it may promulgate more work in this sorely ignored area.

For lack of a better word, the term "exhibitor" will be used throughout the book to describe residents with dementia whose verbal or physical expressions during interactions with another resident or a group of residents result in psychological distress and/or physical harm to these individuals. My hope is that more person-directed care terms will be developed and used in the coming years.

Residents Harmed

In line with the need to avoid using terms borrowed from the elder abuse and mistreatment literature, in the context of residents with dementia harmed during interactions with other residents with dementia, this book will not use the terms "victim" and "target." Although in some circumstances residents with dementia are being victimized and targeted by other residents, in the majority of situations when the exhibitor has dementia that is not the case. Again, while the consequences of these incidents can be as emotionally and physically devastating to the residents harmed, moving away from using mistreatment language will open up important opportunities for improved understanding of the contributing factors underlying these episodes, which is the basis for prevention.

In addition, despite common beliefs, when conducting continuous direct observations of these episodes—as I did in two secured care homes for elders with dementia in an assisted living residence—it is often not straightforward to determine who is really the exhibitor and who is the target. Picture two physically frail residents with advanced dementia who struggle to gain possession over a walker they find in the hallway, each believing it belongs to her- or himself. They pull it in opposite directions for a minute or two until one of them loses balance, falls, hits the floor, and sustains a hip fracture. Can we say with confidence who is the "perpetrator" and who is the "victim" in this incident when the resident who remained standing at the end of the episode could just as easily have been the one harmed?

Actually, the term *victim* may be appropriate in certain circumstances when considering an incident as a case of neglect by the care home: For example, when the frail resident with dementia seriously harmed during an episode was the victim of neglect of supervision by well-meaning, caring, and hardworking but overworked and undertrained direct care partners in understaffed care homes. This is very different from being considered a victim of abuse by another resident with dementia. And yes, some residents with dementia are verbally, physically, or sexually victimized by other residents who are not cognitively impaired, or only mildly so, and who have a history of violent behaviors. Although many of the prevention principles described in the book apply to this latter group of residents, the book focuses primarily on distressing and harmful interactions *between* residents with dementia.

Taken together, this book will use terms such as "resident harmed" to describe those negatively impacted—psychologically and/or physically—during interactions between residents with dementia. Using this term encourages us not to judge the behavioral expressions exhibited by residents with a serious brain disease in an overly categorical way. In reality, DHRRIs in the context of residents with dementia typically unfold in a much more dynamic and even reciprocal way than they are commonly portrayed in care practice, research, and the media. Avoiding terms such as "perpetrator" and "victim" from discussions about this phenomenon also enables us to see that, often, both residents involved could be harmed, even if to a different degree. Resorting too quickly to using rigid categorical classifications limits the ability of direct care partners to see most of these episodes for what they are, the best possible attempt of a vulnerable and frail person to cope with a cognitive disability and fulfill his or her emotional, psychological, social, physical, medical, and other basic human needs.

Direct Care Partners

When we use the term "caregiver," we convey the perception that interactions between care employees and residents with dementia are solely unidirectional, that is, one person giving the care and the other passively receiving it. This common biomedical trap also reflects and shapes day-to-day interactions between direct care partners and residents with dementia. The unidirectionality premise is often created when we inadvertently use a pathological rather than a holistic, person-directed care lens. Elders living with dementia have *a lot* to give to the people around them—direct care partners, family members, and other residents—well into the progression of their brain disease, if we look closely and proactively and we thoughtfully create the opportunities for them to do so successfully. As recognized at the outset, compassionate acts are frequently exhibited by residents with dementia toward other residents with dementia as well as toward direct care partners. If we ignore the potential contributions of the elders in our care, then we will miss important opportunities for building and nurturing an authentic partnership with them.

Reciprocity, collaboration, inclusivity, and basic respect, critically important to all human beings, is equally important to elders living with dementia. An authentic partnership allows us to develop and maintain close, reciprocal, and trusting relationships with residents with dementia, which allow direct care partners to recognize and meet the varied care needs of these individuals and work proactively to prevent their situational frustrations. We must see care staff not only as the most important employees in the care home (which they are) but also as real partners in care with residents with dementia. This is why I use the term "direct care partners" throughout the book.

It is important to recognize that language is evolving; many of the "person-centered" care terms used in this book may not be accepted a few years after its publication, which is a good thing. We should see change on this important but often overlooked front as a constant but healthy challenge we should welcome. As long as we strive to shift away from language that stigmatizes to language that reflects the basic humanity and needs of elders with dementia and the true origins and nature of their behavioral expressions, we will continue to move steadily in the right direction. We will increasingly be able to better interact with, emotionally support, and more effectively care for this population in dignified and safe ways. We will succeed in moving from *labeling* to *learning*.

A Hard Look in the Mirror

Although this book focuses primarily on equipping direct care partners, nurses, social workers, recreation therapists, and managers with the knowledge and skills necessary to address these incidents, we must not lose sight of systemic factors that limit our ability to study and improve understanding of risk and protective factors of these episodes. The phenomenon of DHRRIs has been well known by nurse aides, nurses, social workers, psychologists, managers, administrators, and owners of LTC homes for several decades. Reflecting on injurious and deadly resident-to-resident incidents, Miranda Ferrier, President, Ontario Personal Support Workers Association, stated[7] that the phenomenon of DHRRIs "is nothing new. It has been, in our opinion, hidden...In some places it is looked at as the norm."

Auguste Deter

The first person diagnosed with Alzheimer's disease, Auguste Deter, invaded other residents' personal space; these residents responded by hitting her. A note in her clinical record stated, "When walking about groped the faces of other patients, and was often struck by them in return."[8]

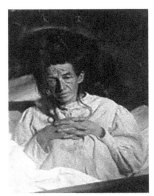

Auguste Deter. (Photograph dated November 1902)

This phenomenon was also identified using disturbing descriptions of injurious incidents in a government report two decades ago.[9] Despite these facts and studies demonstrating its injurious and deadly nature, it remains largely invisible. A recent investigative report by the U.S. Government Accountability Office (GAO)[10] found that these incidents are not currently being tracked by the Centers for Medicare & Medicaid Services (CMS), the federal regulatory agency overseeing approximately 15,000 U.S. nursing homes. The GAO report recommended that CMS should require that "abuse perpetrator type" incidents (including staff-to-resident abuse and resident-to-resident incidents) be submitted by state survey agencies in CMS's databases for deficiency, complaint, and nursing home-reported incident data, and that CMS systematically assess trends in these data. The U.S. Department of Health and Human Services concurred with the GAO recommendation but, as of this writing, CMS has yet to implement it.

The lack of centralized tracking of this phenomenon stands in sharp contrast to growing calls for its implementation. For example, a recent review of the research literature concluded, "The development of a population-based incident database is required to better understand the magnitude and etiology of resident-to-resident elder mistreatment in residential aged care services."[1]

A couple of years prior to the aforementioned GAO report, in an extensive journal article, I reported that the phenomenon of DHRRIs is not being tracked in the CMS F-tag coding system (F-tags are deficiency citations issued to nursing homes by state survey agencies across the country for violations of federal nursing home regulations).[11] In the article, I identified 20 problem areas caused by the chronic lack of tracking them. In addition, Minimum Data

Set 3.0, which is the largest federally mandated clinical dataset in U.S. nursing homes, does not capture the phenomenon (in the Behavior E Section).[12] It is also not adequately tracked in a centralized way in most assisted living residences, which represent the fastest growing residential care option for elders in the United States; a substantial portion of residents in this care setting have dementia (40%–50%), and the phenomenon has been shown to be prevalent in it.

Taken together, when a prevalent and harmful phenomenon is not being tracked in a centralized way by state and federal governments, for all practical purposes, it does not exist. The result is that meaningful, centralized, and well-coordinated policy action to address it remains grossly lacking. Without action by government agencies, vulnerable and frail elder residents with dementia will continue to be seriously harmed during these episodes when important and life-saving lessons could have otherwise been drawn from routine examination of data pertaining to the phenomenon (large-scale studies on various aspects of it such as risk and protective factors are sorely needed).

Indeed, Karl Pillemer, a prominent U.S. researcher who is a member of the Cornell University research group that conducted the largest number of studies on DHRRIs to date, recognized the urgent need to develop "a comprehensive and data-driven national action plan" to address this phenomenon. Pillemer's historic call followed his earlier assertion that this phenomenon represents "a highly significant public health problem. It deserves to be treated like a serious public health problem in long-term care." Woolford and colleagues concluded their review of 26 research studies on resident-to-resident incidents by asserting that prevention efforts "must become a public health priority."[1] In accordance, Lynn McDonald, University of Toronto, an accomplished researcher and a leading advocate for addressing the phenomenon in Canada, stated, "If we ever want to deal with this problem, we will need a national strategy." (McDonald, e-mail communication, June 28, 2021)

As part of this national action plan and strategy, we must also look hard in the mirror and fully recognize that without a commitment to adequate funding of safe staffing levels, at all times, of well-trained direct care partners in LTC homes, addressing this phenomenon effectively will remain largely unrealistic. We should ask ourselves why there are state-regulated and enforced minimum staffing levels in licensed childcare settings in many states but not in nursing homes and assisted living residences.

We need to continue to work hard to minimize widely held ageist perceptions in our society—perceptions that are incredibly effective in perpetuating the dangerous normalization of these episodes and serving as persistent barriers for advancement in reducing them. It is only when we are able to reduce ageism and dementism (discrimination against elders living with cognitive disabilities) in our local communities and care homes nationwide that we will be willing to allocate the necessary financial resources and take the measures necessary to enable them to realize their human and federal right to live in safe care environments. For that to happen, we must demonstrate our unwavering commitment to becoming an elder-friendly and dementia-friendly society—a place where vulnerable and frail elders and those living with dementia are cherished and seen as human beings with value and rights equal to those of all other citizens. It is only when we see the care provided to the most vulnerable people in our society as a sacred work that we will have real hope for keeping them safe and preserving their dignity. We will then be able to more clearly see largely untapped opportunities that can enable them to continue to grow and thrive emotionally, psychologically, socially, and spiritually in the final years of their lives. In the words of Gloria Gutman, Simon Fraser University, Canada,

> We have come to normalize distressing and harmful resident-resident incidents—to think that is just how it is, when older persons live together in a care environment. Doing so, however, is a reflection of ageism; of minimizing or trivializing its occurrence because the residents engaged in these incidents are old and one or both may have dementia. People

living with dementia have a right to feel and be safe in the place they live (Gloria Gutman, Ph.D., e-mail communication, April 7, 2019).

I am humbled and delighted to invite you to read this book. It is the product of several years of work. My hope is that you will find it helpful in improving your understanding of this concerning phenomenon and that the insights and psychosocial prevention strategies contained in it will assist you in your daily efforts aimed at transforming this vision of safe care homes into a reality.

Part I

Scope of DHRRIs
and Guiding Principles

The first part of this text discusses the broad scope of the problem of distressing and harmful resident-to-resident interactions (DHRRIs), as well as general principles for approaching and addressing these incidents. Chapter 1 presents examples of the many documented manifestations of the phenomenon and various negative consequences for all involved, from the residents to the larger society.

The principles outlined in Chapter 2 provide the foundation for the compassionate, person-directed care approach that is the basis of the entire book. This chapter is worth revisiting frequently, both as a helpful reminder of the needs of the people in our care and as a challenge to commonly accepted practices in the care of elders living with dementia.

1

Spectrum and Consequences of Distressing and Harmful Resident-to-Resident Interactions

This is a matter of serious concern.
It happens very often and will be fatal.

Resident with Alzheimer's disease[13]

Distressing and harmful resident-to-resident interactions (DHRRIs) are often referred to in the research literature as "resident-to-resident aggression" and defined as "negative and aggressive physical, sexual, or verbal interactions between long-term care (LTC) residents that in a community setting would likely be construed as unwelcome and have high potential to cause physical or psychological distress in the recipient."[14] As Lachs[15] reflected, "If someone would enter my office at Cornell University and say 'Mark, [blank] you,' I would have to lie down for two hours. Let alone if the person would lay a hand on me . . . If those events would happen in our homes and communities, we would be horrified." In homes and communities where people with dementia live, however, occurrences like these are often incorrectly accepted as normative, which is a persistent barrier to preventing them.

These types of interactions in care homes can result in injuries and deaths of residents and lead to psychological and physical consequences for others who are directly or indirectly involved. They also result in substantial healthcare costs for the residents, their families, the care home, and society at large.

Types of DHRRIs

As noted above, the spectrum of DHRRIs is broad and diverse. This section presents numerous examples of the verbal, relational, and physical forms of these episodes.

Resident-to-Resident Verbal Episodes

A comprehensive and rigorous study in 10 nursing homes in New York state has shown that negative verbal interactions between residents are more common than physical, intrusive (such as invasion of personal space), and sexual forms.[16] Although these resident-to-resident verbal episodes may range from minor to serious in severity, they are generally considered less harmful than the physical forms. However, they can and often do cause substantial distress, anxiety, and fear among residents directly involved, as well as those who witness them. The most common verbal manifestations during these episodes include using "bad words" toward another resident, screaming at another resident, trying to scare or threaten another resident with words, and "bossing"/telling another resident what to do.[17] In addition, DHRRIs commonly develop along a trajectory from negative body language and facial expressions (often accompanied by frustration, emotional distress, or anxiety) to negative verbal expressions that, if not promptly and skillfully addressed by direct care partners, may develop and escalate into potentially harmful physical episodes.

Following are examples of distressing and harmful resident-to-resident verbal episodes that have been reported in the research literature and media to have taken place in LTC homes:

- Verbal exchanges or arguments labeled by employees as "aggressive," such as an angry dispute about use of a television or radio

- Arguments and conflicts with a roommate about preferred ways for using a shared bedroom (for example, temperature control, lighting, having the window open or closed, use of the shared bathroom, noise level, or speaking loudly or repetitively)

- Name calling and use of foul language or "bad words"; embarrassing or humiliating another resident; making harassing remarks to another resident; loudly and publicly making insulting comments ("You're stupid"; "He's a wise guy"; "You're nuts"); making mean-spirited comments ("Why do you always seem to drop your fork?"), insults ("That's a fat head"; "You're ugly"), or unkind judgments ("He calls me 'fatso' and walks down the hall making oinking noises"; "Her face alone must weigh 200 pounds"; "She always makes mean comments about my thinning hair")

- Angrily telling a resident to shut up ("You don't even know what you're talking about, so keep your mouth shut" or "Shut up before I hit you")

- Ordering a resident to get up from his or her chair ("Get the hell out of my chair")

- Angrily yelling at a resident during recreational activities ("How dare you call out Bingo when you don't have a Bingo!" or "How dare you sing that hymn that way!")

- Angrily asserting social control over other residents by using imperative statements or commands, bossing others around, ordering a resident to leave a room, dictating who may sit where, demanding a resident do something he or she does not want to do, or dictating who may participate in an activity or use a shared space. One resident reported, "The first time I went to the recreation center, a man yelled at me, 'This is a private club. You aren't welcome here!' I don't even want to go out and make friends with people in this community anymore."[18]

- Screaming, yelling, shouting, or lashing out at a resident who is trying to move past in his wheelchair

- Making threatening remarks toward another resident; intimidating or trying to frighten a resident ("You say it one more time, and I'll drop you Goddamn dead"); threatening to poison the food of another resident; and threatening to throw an object at or kick, hit, injure, or kill another resident ("If you're going to burp, that plate is going to go in your face"; "One of these days, I'm going to smack you with a hammer"[19])

- Accusing a resident with dementia of stealing personal belongings, such as clothes, glasses, or a gift received from a family member

- A resident repeatedly walking after another accusing him of wanting to kill her (when no such threat was made)

- Making racist comments toward another resident; belittling a person because of her or his race; expressing racial or ethnic prejudices; or using slurs, insults, or malicious comments (for example, a resident accused a neighbor of theft "because he's Black," and another resident harassed someone in reaction to her accent)

Relational and Social Episodes

Relational aggression is often indirect, and it is sometimes hard to recognize the specific person manifesting it.[20] Hawker and Boulton[21] define relational aggression as "a manipulative, nonphysical form of aggression meant to negatively impact the development of friendships by social exclusion or harming the social status of a victim by spreading negative rumors or gossip." When an indirect aggression is delivered successfully, it can be effective in socially excluding or harming a resident.[22] This type of behavior may occur to the extent that the cognitive function of a resident enables him or her to strategically plan to inflict harm without being identified. It is therefore more likely to occur when the resident exhibiting it is not cognitively impaired or has mild cognitive impairment or early-stage dementia. As explained by Robin Bonifas,[23]

> Engaging in bullying and relational aggressive behaviors requires a certain level of cognitive and social skills. You have to be able to remember who it is that you don't like. You have to be able to plan how you're gonna get that person's goat. And the farther you move along in terms of cognitive impairment, the more difficult that is to do. So what that means is that senior environments where there are higher functioning residents, we tend to see the most bullying in those types of environments.

Examples of negative relational and social episodes that have been reported to occur between residents are the following:

- Excluding someone from activities, not allowing a resident to use a community clubhouse where residents gather for luncheons ("There is no room for you"), and refusing to allow a resident to sit at a card table ("It is saved for a friend"); even one attempt to exclude another resident can have devastating effects. Marsha Frankel[20] shares a sad story about an older woman who wanted to join a group activity but was told, "We don't want you here"; after hearing this, the resident never again returned to the activity area

- Shunning or persistently avoiding, ignoring, or rejecting a resident ("Some residents ask in an unfriendly manner why I live in the residence"), or turning away when the person is speaking

- Discouraging other residents from befriending a resident, encouraging them to stop having contact with a resident, or using other residents as a medium to socially ostracize another resident (for instance, having them spread malicious rumors or lies about another resident, such as that the resident had been evicted from a previous residential setting or had previously lived in a homeless shelter and that the care community will soon start admitting other people from these settings)

- Making fun of a resident behind his or her back, or using negative nonverbal body language (mimicking, making offensive gestures, rolling the eyes)[19]

- Teasing, jeering, or making sarcastic comments toward a resident, who, in turn, perceives it as hurtful; residents who are teased and hurt by a comment, joke, or gesture report lasting emotional distress[24]

- Bullying other residents and never apologizing ("It was only a joke. Can't you realize that?")[25]

Resident-to-Resident Physical Episodes

Although distressing and harmful resident-to-resident physical episodes in care homes are not as common as verbal forms, they do occur frequently.[16] These physical episodes may range from mild to serious in severity. Because of the cognitive impairment and frailty of many residents, more severe physical episodes may lead to falls, physical injuries, and deaths.[26,27] A single push of a frail resident can often lead to an injurious fall (resulting in a hip fracture or brain injury), decline in physical function, medical complications, and subsequent death.[27] In fact, three studies examining fatal resident-to-resident incidents (RRIs) have shown that "push–fall" incidents constitute 44% to 63% of these incidents.[28,29,30] It is important to recognize that pushing during resident-to-resident incidents can also have psychological consequences on the person being pushed such as anxiety and fear.[31]

Physical episodes typically consist of some type of direct physical contact (e.g., pushing or hitting someone) between the residents engaged in the episode, although not always. The physical contact may also be indirect, through use of an object in a potentially frightening or harmful way, such as threatening or actually hitting another resident with a cane. Examples of documented physical episodes between residents include the following:

- One resident physically threatening another, such as by making a threatening gesture with a fist

- An escalating argument between residents, which leads to hitting

- Angry verbal and/or physical reactions after reaching a "breaking point"; a resident may direct these reactions toward another resident after experiencing ongoing frustration with the other resident's verbal or behavioral expressions, such as screaming, crying, talking during sleep, unwanted touching, and repetitive questions or comments

- Invading a resident's personal space, for example, standing very close to another resident, repeatedly following another (in a way that is perceived as a threat), or reaching one's hand into another's personal space; invading a resident's personal space often triggers a negative physical response from the resident because he or she may perceive the intrusion as frustrating or threatening regardless of whether it was intentional

- Entering another resident's bedroom or apartment without invitation, which is often perceived by residents living in these spaces as a violation of their privacy, and thus is a common trigger of verbally and physically harmful interactions, when the resident tries to kick the uninvited person out

- Entering the bedroom of another and searching through drawers and closets or taking personal belongings

- Trying to, or actually getting into, the bed of another resident (whether or not the resident is in it), which can trigger a physical response by the resident whose bed has been invaded

- Pulling a resident out of her or his own bed

- Taking an object from another resident, such as food, drink, or a napkin during a meal; grabbing a resident's chair and shoving it back and forth; taking a resident's walker

- Competing for shared resources, including a preferred chair, a table in the dining room, television channels, or even care employees' attention; for example, when a resident always sits in the same chair, he or she may think, "That's my chair." If somebody else sits in the chair, the resident might ask the other person to get out of it and may react physically and harmfully if the other person does not want to move

- Scratching a resident with fingernails; pinching, biting, or slapping a resident; twisting or bending a resident's arm or hand backward; or pulling another resident's hair

- Spitting at a resident

- Pushing a resident (to the floor, down a flight of stairs), or dragging a resident on the floor

- Engaging in fisticuffs (throwing punches) with a resident

- Bumping deliberately into a resident, or trying to trip the resident such as by intentionally sticking out one's cane when another resident walks by

- Clearing the way through a congested space ("Hurry up, get out of my way, move!"), blocking a resident's path, knocking over residents who are in one's path, colliding and scuffling with fellow residents who are trying to move through a space at the same time

- Striking a resident from behind just for fun while walking along the hallway; this may be experienced as startling, frustrating, annoying, frightening, or painful

- Kicking another person in the stomach, kicking someone under the dining room table, or kicking a resident's walker or wheelchair, causing him or her to lose footing or balance

- Pulling hard on a resident's shirt

- Grabbing another resident's wrist, causing it to bruise; grabbing a resident's arm and squeezing it with fingers and nails; or grabbing or squeezing private parts such as testicles or breasts

- Forcibly removing another resident or hurling her or him from a chair or wheelchair, pulling a resident by the hair and causing her or him to fall to the floor, or slamming a resident into the wall

- Throwing an object, such as a walker, at a resident

- Dumping one's food onto a tablemate's lap, pouring liquid on another resident, or tossing a food tray or a bowl of gelatin at another resident

- Using any object in a harmful way against another resident, causing physical injury or death; examples are hitting with one's shoe, dishware, a metal ashtray, or activity board; beating a resident to death with a chair, wooden coat hanger, cane, umbrella, or towel bar; bumping someone with a walker or wheelchair or using a medication cart as a battering ram against a person; jabbing or stabbing a resident with a pair of scissors or dining utensil; and strangling a resident to death with a plastic bag

- Choking a resident, causing injury or death, suffocating a resident by holding his or her head under bedcovers or clothing or using a pillow to smother his or her face, and stuffing tissues into a roommate's mouth (after he was talking repeatedly and loudly in his sleep)

Consequences of Distressing and Harmful Resident-to-Resident Interactions

It is a fundamental right of every person in LTC homes, regardless of the degree of cognitive disability, to live in a safe care environment free of psychological and physical harm inflicted by others. The U.S. Federal Nursing Home regulations state, "The resident has a right to a safe, clean, comfortable and homelike environment, including but not limited to receiving treatment and supports for daily living safely."[32] The Centers for Medicare & Medicaid Services has also stated its expectation from nursing homes in the context of resident-to-resident incidents: "CMS expects long-term care facilities to take any necessary action to prevent resident-to-resident altercations to every extent possible."[33]

The consequences of DHRRIs are as diverse as the examples presented in the previous section and affect not only the residents immediately harmed, but also residents exhibiting these behavioral expressions, other residents witnessing these incidents, direct care partners, family members, the LTC home, and society at large. Consider the following statements:[34,13]

> "Some of them really get afraid of him, and I mean when I say get afraid . . . I mean get afraid. . . . When they see him coming, they don't want to sit in the dining room." (Certified nursing assistant)

> "I am just afraid that he will hurt someone when we don't see it . . . especially someone frail who he can take down with one blow." (Certified nursing assistant)

> "He is going to kill someone one day." (Certified nursing assistant)

> "The residents were trying to avert a huge disaster." (Resident with early-stage Alzheimer's disease after witnessing a tense episode)

> "I want to know that someone will be there for me if something will happen to me." (Resident with middle-stage Alzheimer's disease)

Consequences for Residents Harmed

Residents harmed by the verbal and behavioral expressions of other residents report a range of feelings, such as frustration, anger, anxiety, tension, worry, fear, emotional trauma, and depression. In some cases, a resident who was harmed during an episode may react forcefully, resulting later in feelings of guilt and shame; one resident who had pushed another, causing her to break her hip and subsequently die, apologized: "I didn't mean to push her so hard." Residents who have been harmed may be at risk of self-isolation from the care community. A resident may stay in her bedroom and avoid going to the dining room or participating in group activities, fearful of encountering the resident who had harmed her previously. Or, a resident may leave a group activity when an incident occurs. One resident shared, "When a problem starts to occur, I go to my apartment. I do not want to be caught up in the action." Residents who have been harmed may also experience declines in physical and functional abilities, well-being, sense of security and safety, and quality of life. Some residents have reportedly expressed a wish to move out of the LTC home,[35] and others have been so impacted by what they have experienced that they have thought about committing suicide.[36] As importantly, a study conducted in 249 nursing homes in ten states found that verbal, physical, psychological, and sexual incidents between residents contribute to an atmosphere of disrespect, mistrust, and fear among residents with dementia.[36]

The impact of these incidents on residents can go well beyond psychological and social effects. A groundbreaking study by Shinoda-Tagawa and colleagues (2004) found that physical resident-to-resident incidents can result in falls, dislocations, bruises or hematomas, reddened areas, fractures, lacerations, and abrasions; more than half of the injuries caused during the episodes were to the head, face, nose, or neck, and a quarter of the injuries were to the upper extremities.[26] Three recent studies examining the circumstances surrounding fatal resident-to-resident incidents yielded similar findings.[28,29,30]

Consequences for Residents Exhibiting These Behavioral Expressions

A resident who exhibits distressing and harmful behavioral expressions toward other residents may also experience some of the aforementioned consequences and others. The person's behavioral expressions may result in damaged relationships (he or she may be less likely to be chosen as a friend by other residents[37]), as well as reduced social support from other residents.[22] Other consequences may include being labeled and stigmatized as "problematic," "aggressive," "abusive," or "violent" and thus becoming ostracized and isolated from other residents.[38,39] Direct care partners may choose to deal with the behavioral expressions by not allowing the person to sit at a dining room table with other residents. Because of the hesitancy and fear experienced by certain direct care partners, the risk of compromised care may also increase, such as avoiding the resident, ignoring his or her questions or requests for help, reprimanding or punishing the resident, or responding in other ways that neglect, abuse, or otherwise mistreat the resident.[40,41] These residents may also experience negative consequences in the form of physical restraints or chemical restraints (i.e., being inappropriately and excessively prescribed "unnecessary drugs," such as psychotropic or antipsychotic medications aimed at reducing behavioral expressions labeled as aggressive).[38] The Centers for Medicare & Medicaid Services (CMS) defines "unnecessary drugs" as any drugs used in excessive dosage (including duplicate drug therapy), for excessive duration, without adequate monitoring, without adequate indications for its use, or in the presence of adverse consequences that indicate the dose should be reduced or discontinued—or any combination of the reasons stated above.[32]

Cohen-Mansfield and Jensen (2008) found that 69% of nursing home physicians believe that nursing staff request medication too quickly for residents who engage in behavioral expressions perceived as aggressive. Also, direct care partners' requests for medication were identified as one of the primary barriers to the use of personalized psychosocial approaches.[42] Research on people with dementia who received psychotropic medications revealed a range of effectiveness, from ineffective to only modestly effective, in reducing behavioral expressions classified as agitated or aggressive, and the positive effects were shown in only a small portion of these people.[43,44] Increasing dosages of these medications have been shown to cause serious side effects, including the following:

- Sedation

- Gait disturbance and falls[45]

- Hip fractures[46]

- Tardive dyskinesia (a disorder that involves involuntary movements such as facial grimacing, finger movement, jaw swinging, repetitive chewing, and tongue thrusting)

- Drowsiness

- Osteoporosis

- Diabetes mellitus

- Orthostatic hypotension (low blood pressure that happens when one stands up from sitting or lying down and that may cause dizziness)

- Myocardial infarction (heart attack)

- Venous thromboembolism (blood clots that break off and move through the bloodstream to the brain, lungs, or heart, leading to severe damage or death)

- Increased neurofibrillary tangles[47]

- Lethargy (lack of energy, abnormal drowsiness or sleepiness)

- Rigidity

- Constipation

- Weight gain

- Elevated blood sugar

- Increased risk of pneumonia[48]

- Accelerated cognitive decline

- Parkinsonism

- Edema

- Chest infections

- Increased risk of stroke

- Akthisia (a state of agitation, distress, and motor restlessness that is an occasional side effect of antipsychotic and antidepressant medications)[49]

- Death[43]

One of the major barriers to addressing the negative side effects described above is the fact that physicians often fail to recognize and respond to them or to respond in a timely manner.[50] Furthermore, a subgroup of nursing home residents with dementia reject or do not cooperate in taking these medications when they are offered to them.[51]

When a resident's behavioral expression poses a risk to others in the environment, he or she may be moved to another section of the LTC home or to a different care home altogether. This move may create an added challenge and frustration for the resident with dementia, who may not be able to understand or recall the reason for the relocation, may lose friends and other supportive peers, and may experience difficulty adapting to the new and unfamiliar care environment.[40] The resident may be sent to a more restrictive care setting such as a state hospital, psychiatric ward, or neurobehavioral unit for acute treatment to "control" the behavior through a combination of restraint and sedation, at times with limited or insufficient effort to identify the causes and unmet human needs underlying the behavioral expressions.[49,52] Finally, residents who exhibit behavioral expressions considered as aggressive or violent on a continual basis may be blacklisted and ultimately discharged from the LTC home, and their family members may find it difficult, if not impossible, to find another suitable LTC home near them that will accept their loved one.

Consequences for Family Members

Family members of residents involved in DHRRIs may feel worried, distressed, anxious, and fearful that their loved one may be unsafe living in the care environment. They may be frustrated and shocked to discover that their loved one's safety has been compromised and may feel guilt for having placed the person in the LTC home. The niece of an 85-year-old woman who died after being injured by a resident with dementia said, "I don't know how to describe the feeling. You just sort of feel sick." Family members of a resident who has harmed other residents may feel helpless, embarrassed, and ashamed, and are often also extremely concerned for the safety of other residents.[45]

When a relative engages in behavioral expressions that pose a safety risk to other residents, family members are often asked to visit the LTC home as soon as possible, to consult with the interdisciplinary care team, or to try and calm their relative. These visits often disrupt the daily routine of family members and may be costly, as when they require leaving in the middle of a workday, taking days off from work to come to the LTC home, or even traveling a significant distance to get there.

Consequences for Direct Care Partners

As a consequence of DHRRIs, direct care partners and other interdisciplinary care team members may experience stress, a sense of powerlessness, frustration, anger, or guilt (such as when they do not intervene or do so ineffectively). They may fear being physically attacked, and in fact they *are* at risk of being injured and hospitalized. These incidents may cause care employees to experience low morale and low job satisfaction, leading to high levels of burnout, absenteeism, use of sick leave (due to injury or stress), and turnover for the organization.

Direct care partners' overall productivity and ability to provide routine care and support to other residents are also impacted by these incidents. When direct care partners intervene, the time needed to address DHRRIs can quickly add up across multiple instances. For example, Souder and O'Sullivan (2003) recorded the nursing staff time across 21 shifts in LTC homes at nine U.S. Veterans Affairs medical centers.[53] They found that the time necessary to manage 36 types of behavioral expressions classified as disruptive among 153 older male residents (43% with dementia, 30% with psychiatric diagnosis, 27% with both) was, on average, 23 minutes. Some forms of behavioral expressions took longer to address, such as hitting (26 minutes), throwing objects (29 minutes), scratching others (33 minutes), and threatening harm (53 minutes). When owners of LTC homes invest adequately in shifting the balance from a mode of care that mostly *reacts* to these behavioral expressions to one that aims to *prevent* them by meeting each resident's varied needs proactively, they can save precious care employees' time and keep residents safer.

Consequences for the Care Home

The impact of these incidents on direct care partners is also felt by the LTC home as an organization, in the form of reduced time spent on providing routine care for residents as well as added costs due to loss of productivity, burnout, injury, absenteeism, and turnover. Recruiting and employing new care employees, retraining existing ones, and hiring external agency staff also create additional costs for care homes. The care community may also be faced with costs associated with property damage (e.g., a chair thrown by a resident through a large window), higher insurance premiums, and litigation. When psychotropic medications are used to address these incidents, considerable time and money are spent obtaining, administering, and monitoring their use—time that in most cases would be better spent in assessing and addressing the resident's unmet needs and situational frustrations and triggers that often lead to DHRRIs in the first place.

Care homes that neglect or fail to protect their residents from harmful behavioral expressions by other residents may incur federal and state fines, as well as progressive sanctions, based on the severity and scope of the violations. In its Federal Nursing Home Regulations, CMS defines neglect as "the failure of the facility, its employees or service providers to provide goods and services to a resident that are necessary to avoid physical harm, pain, mental anguish or emotional distress." Repeated and unaddressed DHRRIs may be considered neglect,[6,36] but even a single, serious incident could be considered neglect, when the factors leading to the incident posed a clear risk but were not addressed.

Federal sanctions may include civil monetary penalties, denial of payment for new admissions (for Medicare or Medicaid residents), and termination of participation in the Medicare or Medicaid programs. In addition, CMS may designate as a Special Focus Facility a nursing home that receives more frequent inspections because of its history of serious quality issues and violations of federal regulations. State sanctions may include fines, issuance of a conditional license, placement on a watch list, a 6-month survey cycle, a moratorium or "stop placement" order prohibiting any new admissions, appointment of new management, action to deny renewal of a license or to revoke a license, or an emergency suspension order necessitating the immediate relocation of all residents.[54]

Care homes, as well as direct care partners, supervisors, administrators, and owners, may become liable in civil or criminal lawsuits for neglecting and failing to protect residents harmed during these incidents.[55] These actions can result in substantial costs and, in turn, a diversion of resources from resident care.[56] The reputation of an LTC home may also suffer (because of negative media coverage), which could negatively affect marketing efforts.[57,35] In addition, police involvement and presence at the LTC home during and after a serious incident, which has been shown in a research study to be frequent,[6] can result in an erosion of trust on the part of residents, their families, and direct care partners; it is worth remembering that experts consider trust the single most important aspect of caring for elders living with dementia.[58,59]

Consequences for Society

These harmful resident-to-resident incidents also impact society at large, given the high Medicare and Medicaid costs related to preventable behavior-related emergency room visits and hospitalizations, emergency ambulance services, and the overprescribing of psychotropic medications and their associated serious side effects.[60] More broadly, though, DHRRIs that result in psychological and physical harm to all involved—residents and care employees—reflect badly on the society in which they occur. As Mohandas Gandhi said, "A nation's greatness is measured by how it treats its weakest members." Some of our society's weakest members are vulnerable and frail elders living with dementia, and we have a moral and legal obligation to improve policies and care practices aimed at understanding, recognizing, and proactively addressing their care needs in order to prevent DHRRIs and keep them safe and free from harm.

2

Twelve Principles for Approaching Distressing and Harmful Resident-to-Resident Interactions

Relationships are everything. Everything is possible
when there is mutual trust and respect.

Jitka Zgola[59]

The situational causes and triggers that lead to distressing and harmful resident-to-resident interactions (DHRRIs) are many and varied, as you will see throughout the book. Underlying both the events leading to these episodes and the psychosocial strategies necessary for addressing and preventing them effectively are the principles listed on the next page.

1. Dangerous Normalization Is a Major Barrier to Prevention

These incidents are chronically, and dangerously, normalized in many long-term care (LTC) homes. Direct care partners may say things like, "They have dementia . . . what do you expect?"; "It was always like that here. It's part of our job, and it will never change!"; or even "It happens frequently . . . but honestly I don't think that old people with dementia can cause serious harm to each other."

The truth is that the *vast majority* of these episodes are preventable. It is dangerous to consider them a normal part of life in LTC homes. When we consider these understandable human expressions as normal—that is, when we fall into the trap of using a biomedical lens as the main framework for viewing them—we mistakenly assume that their primary source can be traced back to a brain pathology. We are then more likely to think that they are simply inevitable and thus overlook the critical role that key factors in the physical and social environment commonly play in the development of these episodes. To become effective in preventing and skillfully responding to these episodes, a deep understanding and full adoption of personalized needs-based biopsychosocial approaches is needed. The chapters that follow will provide abundant support for this statement.

2. Words Matter

The words we use to describe these episodes—human expressions of unmet needs—among elders living with dementia matter a lot. The power of stigma, as created and conveyed by words, is still largely overlooked in a large number of LTC homes; this power must be fully understood and recognized if we are serious about preventing these incidents and keeping residents safe. Specifically, it is urgent that we continue the shift from using biomedical, labeling, and stigmatizing language to person-directed care language that aims to preserve the dignity

Principles for Approaching
Distressing and Harmful Resident-to-Resident Interactions

1. Dangerous normalization is a major barrier to prevention.

2. Words matter.

3. People with dementia have strong relational needs.

4. People with dementia have strong emotional and psychological needs.

5. It is essential to listen to people with dementia and validate their emotions and experiences.

6. People with dementia benefit tremendously from personally meaningful engagement.

7. A culture of empathy must be nurtured throughout the care community.

8. Pushing among residents can be injurious and deadly.

9. All care employees should be aware of the common risk and protective factors.

10. Care homes must provide safe people-to-people ratios of well-trained care employees at *all* times.

11. Family members of elders with dementia are key partners in addressing incidents.

12. It is the human right of elders with dementia to live in safe care homes.

and personhood of residents living with a serious brain disease. It is critical to ensure that all words used to describe DHRRIs in residents with dementia reflect their true nature and origins in the context of universal human needs.

After carefully examining hundreds of injurious and deadly resident-to-resident incidents in several countries, I can say that the real story in the vast majority of these incidents is a story of neglect (such as neglect of supervision) and/or gaps in care, such as the insufficient proactive fulfillment of residents' varied human needs and the lack of timely and skilled prevention and de-escalation of interpersonal situational frustrations. In most situations in the context of Alzheimer's disease and other forms of dementia, a close observation reveals that this is not a story of residents' "abuse" of and "violence" toward other residents. Some readers may be surprised to hear that in most situations in the context of residents with dementia, it is not even a story of "aggressive" behaviors.

The majority of residents with dementia do not intend to injure or kill other residents. Instead, many are forced to cope with substantial challenges caused by their serious brain disease as well as with living conditions and situations that are often very distressing, frustrating, and frightening, which threaten their dignity and sense of security. They respond to these situations to the best of their remaining physical and cognitive abilities. For us to use language that assumes intention on the part of the person with dementia lays the ground for labeling and confrontation (in other words, the resident versus others) rather than understanding (i.e., we all must work collaboratively to proactively meet the unmet needs that underlie the behavioral expression).

To take it even further, it is often not even a story of "behaviors." I want you to think for a moment, when was the last time you heard the word "behavior" used in a positive context? Using the word *behavior* implies misbehavior and even the need for punishment. It suggests acts that need to be *controlled* and *fixed*, diverting our attention away from the root causes of these episodes, which are the basis for their prevention. We have become accustomed to inadvertently labeling residents living with dementia using these largely unhelpful, stigmatizing, inaccurate, misleading, and harmful terms.

We do a tremendous service to elders with dementia if we fully recognize the need to avoid using terms such as resident-to-resident "mistreatment," "abuse," and "violence" (terms commonly used in practice, research, policy, guidelines, and federal and state regulations). Using these terms can also contribute to a "slippery slope" that leads to inappropriate, unnecessary, and excessive use of antipsychotic drugs. Once an elder with dementia is sedated, it is much more difficult to identify and therefore address the unmet human needs underlying his or her engagement in DHRRIs.

3. People with Dementia Have Strong Relational Needs

Building and maintaining close trusting relationships with residents with dementia is fundamental to detection and timely fulfillment of their varied human needs and early warning signs for DHRRIs, as well as to the skilled use of individualized prevention strategies. When direct care partners are provided with the resources and support needed to build and nurture positive relationships (such as safe people-to-people ratios [staffing levels]), they are in a much better position to recognize, prevent, and de-escalate DHRRIs.

As importantly, there is often a substantially higher level of cooperation by residents with dementia during these incidents when they have close trusting relationships with care employees trying to help. It is like a bank account. The more effort you put into developing a person's trust (during routine care as well as during episodes), the more trust you are able to "draw on" during tense situations leading up to and during incidents. Every interaction with a resident with dementia is an opportunity to build trust with her or him. It is worth considering why a resident will completely ignore one direct care partner but completely cooperate with another during the very same incident. Although there are exceptions to this rule (such as when a person with dementia perceives a care partner to be someone else from her or his past—a person she or he was scared of), my work and observations in care homes over the years have shown that trust and a skilled and respectful approach are key factors accounting for the difference.

One of the main tools direct care partners need in order to build this trust is thorough, extensive knowledge of the life history of the residents in their care. This tool is so critical that some care homes in the United Kingdom have developed a full-time position called a locksmith. An essential function of this position is identifying "pearls," or important information, from a resident's lifelong history. Direct care partners use these critical life background pieces of information proactively to enrich the resident's life (such as through personalized meaningful engagement) and to keep her or him safe.[61] There are many reasons why direct care partners would want to know the early life history of the residents with dementia; many of these are directly relevant to the ability to understand the true meaning and root causes underlying various forms of behavioral expressions in this population, including DHRRIs.[62]

Using these pearls from a resident's life often reveals remaining abilities and other untapped assets, such as preserved long-term memory of personally meaningful events and lifelong interests that could guide the development of a personally meaningful engagement program (a key strategy for prevention of DHRRIs). It can also help the care partner discover remote triggers from the person's distant past (such as life-threatening experiences and traumas) that can contribute to the development of DHRRIs. These triggers need to be known and avoided by care employees, or affirmed and validated by them when already activated and causing the resident to feel anxious and fearful. Direct care partners need to use these assets intentionally and in the spirit of a strength-based, rather than deficit-based, approach to improving the care and safety of residents with dementia.

4. People with Dementia Have Strong Emotional and Psychological Needs

One of the most important but often overlooked aspects of supporting and caring for elders living with dementia is the need to develop a deep understanding of their emotional and psychological needs, and proactively meet them. This domain of universal human needs in this population was originally identified by giants in our field such as Naomi Feil, who developed the Validation Method,[63] and Tom Kitwood, an early champion of person-centered care for people with dementia.[64]

In the decades-long efforts to meet residents' physical, medical, functional, and cognitive needs, their emotional and psychological needs have not received adequate attention in policies and care practices. This is exactly where the paradigm shift is urgently needed, as advocated by Al Power,[65] as well as by Judy Berry with her enlightened, effective, and safe Lakeview Ranch Model of Specialized Dementia Care™.[60]

In closely examining the sequence of events leading to DHRRIs, it becomes clear that overlooking residents' emotional and psychological needs is a persistent barrier in efforts aimed at preventing and de-escalating these episodes. In the majority of cases, people with dementia "fight" with each other in an effort to protect their dignity and enhance their emotional and psychological well-being when they feel that these are being threatened. Dignity is defined as "the quality or state of being worthy, honored, or esteemed."[66] Recognition of the strong relationship that exists between emotional/psychological well-being and dignity, both in general and in the context of DHRRIs among residents with dementia, is an essential first step in any prevention efforts that aim to bring about lasting effects.

5. It Is Essential to Listen to People with Dementia and Validate Their Emotions and Experiences

The fifth principle, a natural extension of the fourth, reminds us of the need to listen closely and validate the emotions of residents with dementia. I recommend using the communication techniques that are part of the Validation Method. Many care professionals not trained in the method mistakenly believe that validation is simply "going with the flow" with a resident with Alzheimer's disease. However, validation as practiced with the Validation Method goes much deeper than that, with its humanistic philosophy, series of emotion-based communication techniques, and rigorous guidance for their application with different elders with Alzheimer's disease (at different stages of the disease) and situations.

One important aspect of the Validation Method is to avoid arguing about facts with a resident who has Alzheimer's disease when the person is clearly unable to tolerate it. Instead, direct care partners need to be present and centered as much as possible so that they can listen and "tune in" to the person's internal and subjective reality in order to validate their underlying emotional states. You can never "win" an argument with an elder resident with middle- to late-stage Alzheimer's disease; if you try, both of you will likely become even more frustrated and angry.

Although older residents with Alzheimer's disease may look healthy physically, it is often easy to forget that they have a serious brain disease that limits their ability to recall and retain information as well to process and understand what is communicated to them in words. Remember that they will often respond to the underlying emotional state conveyed by the direct care partner (or other residents for that matter), no matter what is said in words. Many people with dementia are experts in recognizing our core emotions and, since this is what they are more likely to respond to, we would be wise to recognize it and focus our efforts on building strong relationships with them while using emotion-based approaches and communication techniques during routine care and DHRRIs.

As importantly, if we are committed to providing person-directed care, we must always do our best to seek out the thoughts, preferences, concerns, and suggestions of residents living with dementia about *their* care, life, and safety. People living with dementia are the best teachers out there about living with dementia! They actually know what it means to live with a cognitive disability due to a serious brain disease. We will be wise to listen to them. As people with dementia increasingly tell us, "Nothing about us without us."

6. People with Dementia Benefit Tremendously from Personally Meaningful Engagement

Personally meaningful engagement is one of the most effective means for enriching residents' lives, enabling them to have a purpose in life and to experience joy. It is also a critical, often-overlooked, and cost-effective strategy for preventing DHRRIs. Such engagement is "meaningful when it reflects a person's interests and lifestyle, [is] enjoyable to the person, help[s] the person feel useful, and provide[s] a sense of belonging."[67] It is appropriate "when it is meaningful for a person, and when it respects the person's age, beliefs, culture, values, and life experience."[67] Boredom among elders living with dementia (the normal human response to the absence of personally meaningful engagement) is a serious risk factor commonly contributing to DHRRIs.

7. A Culture of Empathy Must Be Nurtured Throughout the Care Community

One important asset for prevention and de-escalation of these episodes is a well-coordinated, community-wide effort to instill empathy and compassion between residents and, of course, between care employees and residents. This initiative should be implemented in a consistent way by all employees who come in direct regular contact with the residents. Staff and administrators can develop creative ways to publicly recognize and reward residents who regularly show acts of empathy and compassion toward other residents with dementia. As noted at the outset of this book, some of the most compassionate acts in LTC homes are performed by residents toward other residents. We would be wise to tap into this precious but free resource by seeking to learn from these inspiring acts and harness their power to strengthen the quality of relationships between residents. Doing so will likely contribute to creating a safer care environment for residents and direct care partners.

8. Pushing Among Residents Can Be Injurious and Deadly

A substantial portion of injurious and fatal resident-to-resident incidents can be character-ized as "push–fall" incidents, especially among residents with dementia who are physically frail. For these residents, a single push, such as in response to their having invaded another's personal space or bedroom, can result in a fall-related hip fracture and/or head trauma/brain injury. As noted earlier, it can also cause residents to experience tremendous fear. Residents with dementia are known to be at higher risk of falls compared to those without dementia, and these push–fall incidents put them at an even higher risk of experiencing a fall-related injury. When I speak with administrators and managers of LTC homes, they are often sur-prised to learn about the prevalence of push–fall events in deadly incidents. It is important for all care employees (direct and nondirect care partners) to be aware and sensitive to this danger, and to intervene promptly in triggering situations such as invasion of personal space and unwanted touch.

9. All Care Employees Should Be Aware of the Common Risk and Protective Factors

The ninth principle consists of a series of common risk factors for DHRRIs; many of these factors are described in detail in Part II. Two of these highly prevalent risk factors are briefly discussed here for illustration.

Bedroom Conflicts

It is important to remember that a resident's bedroom is his or her home and the last frontier of privacy. Conflicts that arise in this setting—either as a conflict between roommates or as a result of unwanted entry by one resident into another's room—can be especially triggering. Would we accept conflict and intrusion in our own homes without fighting back?

Evenings and Weekends

A substantial portion of injurious and deadly resident-to-resident incidents take place during the evening hours and weekends, and there are known, basic preventive measures that should be taken to mitigate the risks. Some examples of the risk factors for these time periods are lower people-to-people ratios, a reduced active presence of managers, a decrease in meaningful engagement programming, and an increase in "float" and external agency staff. In the evening hours, residents with dementia are much more tired and irritable and thus less likely to cope well with interpersonal situational frustrations and more likely to engage in DHRRIs. These risks have been well known for decades, but owners and administrators often invest inade-quately in protective measures aimed at keeping residents with dementia safe during these time periods.

10. Care Homes Must Provide Safe People-to-People Ratios of Well-Trained Care Employees at *All* Times

The 10th essential principle is full commitment on the part of owners and administrators to providing and maintaining adequate staffing levels (at *all* times) of well-trained, well-supported, and supervised direct care partners. This factor is one of the most important for preventing and addressing DHRRIs, but over the past several decades it has been commonly neglected in nursing homes and assisted living residences. A large-scale study in ten New York state nursing homes (2,011 residents) demonstrated what we already know in practice: A higher direct care partners' workload (total number of residents assigned each shift to a nurse aide) was associated with a higher rate of DHRRIs.[16] When residents are not adequately supervised, early warning signs of distress and anxiety between them are often missed, and harmful incidents are not detected and de-escalated in time. At least one-quarter of U.S. nursing homes are dangerously understaffed, and approximately half offer low staffing levels.[68] Ignoring the risk factor of low and poor staffing levels essentially gives a green light to thousands of additional traumatic injuries and tragic deaths of residents with and without dementia in LTC homes in the coming years. Such inhumane and dangerous staffing levels are a gross violation of residents' basic human and federal right to live in a safe LTC environment.

The need for a paradigm shift from a decades-long major risk factor to becoming a major protective factor is urgent not only as a critical strategy for protecting the safety of residents but also for protecting the care partners who wake up every day wishing they could provide dignified and safe care to these individuals. Low and poor staffing levels are cruel for residents as well as for dedicated, hardworking, and compassionate direct care partners. Ageist perceptions (toward residents) and sexist attitudes (toward the care partners, the vast majority of whom are women) must be fully acknowledged and addressed by all key stakeholders (including but not limited to care employees, care homes, and federal and state governments) if meaningful progress on this front is to be made. As asserted by Gloria Gutman (e-mail communication, April 7, 2019),

> We should have zero tolerance for the excuse "but we are short staffed" when it comes to a care home's responsibility for preventing distressing and harmful resident-to-resident incidents. To do otherwise is clearly and simply a reflection of ageism and our society's devaluation of elders who are vulnerable and frail.

It is important to emphasize that the majority of the situational causes and triggers of DHRRIs described in this book cannot be adequately addressed by direct care partners if staffing remains low. It is not realistic to expect care partners to prevent all DHRRIs no matter how caring and dedicated they are. It is time to demand humane and safe people-to-people ratios of well-trained direct care partners in all nursing homes and assisted living residences. Perhaps a first step necessary to make this a reality is to recognize that when we use the term "staffing levels," we mean people caring for people. Continuing to risk the former group with the provision of unsafe number of care employees will continue to place the latter group at serious risk of harm. Is this something our local communities and society are willing to accept for vulnerable and frail elders with dementia?

11. Family Members of Elders with Dementia Are Key Partners in Addressing Incidents

It is now widely recognized that "involving families can certainly lead to improved well-being for people with dementia in care settings."[69] Family members of elders with dementia are often key to care homes' efforts to provide adequate and safe care as well as to understand the origins of, prevent, and de-escalate DHRRIs. Their lifelong intimate knowledge of the individual as a whole person is frequently crucial in the development and implementation of psychosocial prevention strategies that work. They know what tends to upset and calm their loved one. They know the person's personality traits and coping style. They know her or his value system, lifelong routines, and preferences. They know what brings the person joy.

Although the standard of care of elders with dementia views family members as an integral part of the care team, unfortunately this precious asset remains untapped in many care homes. Care homes that cherish and deeply value ongoing collaborations with family members proactively seek to inform and consult with them about the care provided to their loved ones. They know that regularly listening to their input, concerns, and suggestions can often mean the difference between an injury sustained and one that is prevented. When trust and authentic partnership with family members is built and maintained, it can also mean the difference between a lawsuit filed or not filed against the care home when a resident is harmed under preventable circumstances. Owners and administrators of care homes need to make this commitment explicit in their mission statement and in their policies, procedures, and care practices.

As importantly, this commitment must also be fulfilled with residents who have early-stage dementia who are cognitively capable of meaningfully participating in decisions affecting *their* care and safety; the vast majority of these individuals are capable of such participation when elder-friendly and dementia-friendly conditions are created for them. Their lived experiences of the care provided to them and their knowledge gained through their direct and indirect involvement in DHRRIs must be viewed as an asset in all efforts aimed at preventing these episodes and keeping them safe and free from harm. Anything less would remain short of fulfilling the basic expectation inherent in the term "person-directed care" practices.

12. It Is the Human Right of Elders with Dementia to Live in Safe Care Homes

The last guiding principle is an overarching one. It underlies virtually all principles and messages contained in this book. It is where every discussion about this prevalent and harmful phenomenon should start and end. It comes full circle with the first principle outlined in this chapter; as such, it reinforces our commitment to minimizing the chronic and dangerous normalization of these incidents in LTC homes.

Moving into a care home does not strip elders living with dementia from their basic human, and federal, right for safety. We demand that our children be kept safe and protected from others in schools and childcare settings, and we must expect and demand the same for vulnerable and frail elders who live with a serious brain disease in nursing homes and assisted living residences. It is not only a matter of safety, justice, and accountability but also a matter of trust. Elders with dementia, whose voices are often not heard outside the walls of care homes, ask us: Will you step up and meet this challenge that lies at the heart of the legal, social, and moral contract with us?

Part II

Contributing Factors, Causes, and Triggers

A substantial proportion of behavior problems in dementia arise when care does not appropriately address the underlying causes.

Jiska Cohen-Mansfield and Jacobo E. Mintzer[70]

This section of the book presents dozens of factors, causes, and situational triggers that have been reported in the practice and research literature as contributing to the development of distressing and harmful resident-to-resident interactions (DHRRIs) in care homes. Chapters 3–6 correspond to four distinct domains of factors, including residents' personal history and background factors, situational causes and triggers, factors in the physical environment, and factors related to direct care partners. A fifth domain—medical, physiological, and functional factors significantly contributing to DHRRIs—receives only limited focus in the book because the primary focus of the book is on psychosocial factors and factors in the physical environment. These medical contributing factors, which are beyond my work and research expertise, deserve full attention elsewhere.

It should be emphasized that in the vast majority of situations, a single incident results from the cumulative effect of *multiple* interrelated factors, causes, unmet needs, and situational triggers, not one factor alone, operating at several levels of the care organization, as well as across the five domains. A comprehensive, holistic, proactive (anticipatory), and ongoing individualized assessment approach is therefore necessary for early identification of contributing factors, causes, and triggers and timely fulfillment of the residents' unmet needs.

Of course, key factors and agencies operating *outside* the care home also influence care providers' ability to address DHRRIs and keep residents with dementia and direct care partners safe. These include, among others, the following:

- Role of policy makers in addressing this public health problem (such as in a data-driven nationwide campaign)

- Helpful and unhelpful state and federal regulations

- Effectiveness of state survey agencies' oversight, such as mistreatment investigations and enforcement of standards of care

- Role of the Office of Ombudsman for Long-Term Care
- Adult Protective Services (in states where this agency has authority to investigate mistreatment in care homes and protect residents from mistreatment)
- Medical examiner's or coroner's office
- Law enforcement
- Medicaid fraud control units
- Emergency medical services
- Acute care hospitals
- Psychiatric hospitals
- Owners' and corporate offices' policies in LTC homes

As importantly, specialized DHRRI–specific training of all of these agencies as well as close collaboration among them in addressing this phenomenon is often crucial in a care home's ability (or lack of thereof) to prevent these incidents and keep residents safe.

In addition, inadequacy of federal reimbursement rates (such as for residents receiving care in nursing homes under the Medicaid program) has long been a barrier for improved care practices and safety. Furthermore, financial incentives for illness, physical dependency, and frailty (instead of a system of incentives or rewards for wellness) also limit, rather than enhance, care improvements in nursing homes nationwide. Finally, the lack of centralized tracking of the phenomenon of DHRRIs in the Minimum Data Set (MDS) 3.0 (the largest federally mandated clinical dataset in CMS–certified nursing homes)[12] and CMS's survey deficiency citation (F-tag) system[11,10] represents a chronic and persistent barrier for learning from these incidents (such as through research and other quality improvement initiatives) to inform large-scale prevention.

3

Resident's Personal History and Background Factors

Know the residents like you know the back of your hand.

Staff member caring for people with dementia[71]

Being aware of a resident's personal history and background and taking this information into consideration during preadmission and ongoing assessments increases the likelihood of early identification of residents at risk of engaging in distressing and harmful resident-to-resident interactions (DHRRIs). Individualized approaches and prevention strategies could, in turn, be developed and implemented in a proactive, anticipatory, and timely manner to meet these individuals' varied human and care needs.

The background factors presented in this chapter are grouped into two subcategories: nonmodifiable (◆) and partially modifiable (◈). Nonmodifiable factors are factors that cannot be changed but have been shown to contribute to the development of a resident's engagement in DHRRI. Although these factors cannot be changed, it is important for direct care partners to be aware of their potential role in the development of DHRRIs. Knowing these factors could assist, for example, during interdisciplinary care team (IDT) meetings in informing decisions about proactive and anticipatory provision of targeted risk assessment, supervision, and personally meaningful engagement of residents at risk of engaging in DHRRIs, as well as individualized prevention and de-escalation strategies. Partially modifiable factors have also been shown to contribute to the development of DHRRIs, but when individualized psychosocial approaches and strategies are used by direct care partners, it is often possible to reduce or eliminate their negative effects. This, in turn, can decrease the likelihood that a resident will engage in these episodes. Table 3.1 lists the factors discussed in this chapter.

Typically, only a small subgroup of residents in long-term care (LTC) homes in general and those with dementia in particular are involved as exhibitors in a large proportion of serious resident-to-resident incidents.[34,45,72,73,74] It is important to emphasize that many residents with dementia whose personal history and background include one or more of the factors and characteristics described in this chapter do *not* necessarily engage in DHRRIs. That said, a higher number of these factors generally increases the likelihood that a resident will engage in these episodes in general and as an exhibitor.

Demographics and Birth Order

In light of a large body of evidence, this section addresses the role of age and gender in the development of DHRRIs. In addition, a factor that so far has received only very limited attention in the practice and research literature is the potential role of birth order in a subset of

Table 3.1 Personal History and Background Factors That Increase the Risk of DHRRIs

Personal History and Background Factors	◆ Non-modifiable	◇ Partially Modifiable
Demographics and birth order		
Age	X	
Gender	X	
Birth order	X	
Prior occupation, personality, and cognitive status		
Prior occupation	X	
Premorbid personality traits	X	
Current personality traits	X	
Exhibitor's higher cognitive function	X	
Psychiatric and emotional status		
Loss of independence and autonomy		X
Depression		X
Posttraumatic stress disorder	X	
Addiction		
Past addiction to alcohol or drugs	X	
Current addiction and use of alcohol or drugs		X
Cigarette addiction		X
Past behavioral expressions and convictions		
Behavioral expressions reported as aggressive before admission	X	
Past convictions for violent acts	X	

DHRRIs. Awareness of these factors could assist direct care partners and IDTs in development of individualized psychosocial approaches and prevention strategies.

◆ Age

Previous studies examining fatal resident-to-resident incidents have found that exhibitors in DHRRIs are typically younger than residents who die as a result of these incidents (the range of age difference across these studies was 6–16 years).[28,29,30] Although exhibiting residents have been older than residents who died as a result of these incidents, the body of evidence to date suggests that, overall, this is less likely to be the case.

Although further research is needed to replicate, shed light on, and explain these findings, one possible explanation is that, in general, younger residents tend to be physically stronger and more medically healthy than older residents. They may also be more stable on their feet and less likely to fall and sustain an injury during falls. Younger residents are also more likely have higher cognitive function, that is, to be in earlier stages of dementia, relative to residents who are harmed, who tend to be in the later stages. The likelihood of being injured during these episodes increases as the cognitive function declines. Younger people are also less likely to sustain a fall during these incidents.[26]

Finally, even when injured, younger residents' overall better health status may enable them to recover more successfully from medical complications resulting from an injurious incident. Taken together, younger residents *generally* have a higher physical ability to cause injury to residents who are older than they are while avoiding an injury during these episodes or recovering from an injury once sustained. Direct care partners' awareness of the potential vulnerability of residents who are older, more physically frail, and more cognitively disabled should sensitize them to this risk in ways that inform their targeted and individualized prevention efforts.

◆ Gender

Studies on elders living with dementia in the community and LTC homes have shown that behavioral expressions classified as aggressive are substantially more common in men than women[75,76] and that male gender predicted engagement in these behavioral expressions.[77] In addition, a review of the research literature found that, among the eight studies that examined the role of gender in DHRRIs, the aggregated total of these studies showed that substantially more men than women (male, n = 425/511; 83.2%) were reported to be exhibitors in these episodes.[1] Furthermore, studies on fatal incidents have shown that the majority of exhibitors were men (ranging from 74% to 86%) in care homes in the United States, Canada, and Australia.[29,30,28] Although there are exceptions, of course—and older women certainly engage as exhibitors as well—the gender disparity should be considered as part of efforts to address this phenomenon and in preadmission assessment and decision making, individualized care assessment and planning, daily supervision, personally meaningful engagement, risk assessment, and use of assistive technology.

◆ Birth Order

Stephen Soreff[78] reports that being the oldest child and carrying over into the care home a bossy, "in-charge," and demanding personality may contribute to development of DHRRIs. It is important to emphasize that only a small subgroup of these residents have this inclination and often only during stressful, frustrating, and frightening situations that threaten their sense of control, privacy, identity, and dignity. In fact, many first-born elders often take leadership positions while living in care homes in positive, constructive, and helpful ways (for example, serving as resident representative on a resident council), as they have done throughout their lives. However, with the small subgroup of first-born residents who tend to make a negative impact on other residents and the life in the LTC home, it is important to develop approaches that on one hand maintain the resident's sense of control and identity while ensuring that these attempts at social control do not violate the rights and safety of other residents. Offering the resident appropriate opportunities to express his or her frustrations and validating the person's concerns by actively listening to him or her is essential. When the resident is calm, direct care partners can work with him or her on the development of a personalized psychosocial strategy that aims at avoiding and preventing similar situations in the future, to the extent that the resident's cognitive abilities allow him or her to do it meaningfully without causing him or her significant distress.

Marsha Frankel[79] shares the following challenge and creative solution. A resident was bullying other residents by controlling what was going on in group activities. The director of assisted living brought her into her office and asked her, "Mrs. Smith, do you remember what it was like when you had to move here a couple of years ago? Were you happy to leave your apartment and move into assisted living?" Mrs. Smith: "No, but I couldn't take care of the apartment anymore and I needed more help." Director: "That's right. And it was a really scary and stressful time for you, wasn't it?" Mrs. Smith concurred: "It was." Director: "Well, I really need your help. We are finding that other people are having a tough time when they move in, and I wonder if we could count on you to help them to settle in and adjust by letting them know that it gets better. I need an ambassador to welcome new people." The executive director gave Mrs. Smith a badge and monitored her bullying behavior. Frankel explains that the director helped Mrs. Smith to have some control by helping other people and by being given a meaningful role in the building. Doing so increased her level of empathy by reminding her what her experiences had been when she had moved in. The resident's bullying behavior decreased substantially because of this empowering role.

For residents who are leaders, find opportunities to let them lead[80] while adapting these opportunities to their current cognitive abilities, disabilities, and preferences. Examples include having the resident assist in leading or facilitating a group activity, having a key role in resident council meetings, or serving on a welcoming committee for newly admitted residents. That said, it is important to regularly observe, assess, and make sure that the resident is not using the leadership role to control and negatively affect other residents. Brainstorm creative ways to harness and fulfill the person's need for control in productive and safe ways. Such personalized psychosocial approaches can go a long way in reducing a resident's engagement in DHRRIs.

Prior Occupation, Personality, and Cognitive Status

Personality traits (past and current) and prior occupation are factors for direct care partners and IDTs to consider when assessing residents' risk of involvement in DHRRIs. In addition, research has also shown a common difference in cognitive function levels between exhibitors and residents who are harmed.

◆ Prior Occupation

Many residents with dementia held positions of authority, power, and prestige before they retired and developed dementia. Some worked as top executives, lawyers, military or police officers, and prison officers. The abundant opportunities for loss of control, choice, and privacy inherent in the daily life of many LTC homes (for example, rigid scheduling, limited shared resources, overcrowding, or being forced to live in close quarters with many strangers or to share a small bedroom with a roommate) often cause tremendous frustration to these and other residents. Although all residents with dementia are affected by stressful and frustrating living conditions, those who worked for many years in positions of power and authority often attempt to regain control over their life, care, privacy, dignity, and social environment (other people) and while trying to do so, they may engage in DHRRIs.

It could be helpful to acknowledge a resident's past career achievements, such as during one-on-one interactions, group activities, and special events. However, it is as important to ensure that any authoritative and controlling verbal or behavioral expressions that were a part of the person's experience in a prior occupation do not violate the rights, well-being, or safety of other residents in the care setting. For example, one resident with Alzheimer's disease frequently engaged in behavioral expressions perceived by other residents as aggressive and scary. After learning from direct care partners about his honorable service in the Navy decades before this, they became more empathetic and understanding of his cognitive disabilities and were willing to work with direct care partners on ways to meet his needs and prevent his frustrations and behavioral expressions. Although this approach did not always work, it did make a difference at times.

◆ Premorbid Personality Traits

Personality traits that existed before the onset of dementia can contribute to development of DHRRIs in care homes. In particular, traits such as neuroticism, negative mood, low agreeableness, arrogance, shortness of temper, bossiness, or a dominating or controlling nature are especially of concern. A study[81] of 213 community-dwelling people with dementia by Hamel and colleagues found a relationship between "premorbid aggression" and "aggression" after the onset of dementia. The researchers reported that some people with dementia who responded "aggressively" when confronted with frustrating situations were probably demonstrating long-standing patterns of response to frustration. Another study[82] among 208 community-dwelling people with Alzheimer's disease by Archer and colleagues found that lower premorbid personality agreeableness (during one's 40s) predicted irritability, agitation, apathy, and disinhibition after the onset of Alzheimer's disease.

By contrast, having a personality that could be described as agreeable can consist of the tendency toward cooperation and social harmony as well as being courteous, thoughtful, and considerate toward others. Although these individuals may play a role in defusing DHRRIs, some of these people may also end up being harmed while trying to resolve episodes between other residents. It is easy to see how a resident's attempt to de-escalate a tense episode, such as by trying to physically separate two residents, could result in her or him being hit by one of the residents involved in the episode.

It is important to recognize that, although personality characteristics may change in a subgroup of elders as their dementia progresses, lifelong personality traits continue in many individuals well into the disease. Naomi Feil, who developed the Validation Method, describes a subgroup of elders in the early stages of Alzheimer's disease who tend to blame, accuse, and complain about others (such as other residents, direct care partners, and family members) when things go wrong.[63] Blaming becomes their way of coping, a way to survive their personal, social, physical, and cognitive losses (present-day losses and fears that trigger vivid memories of past losses and similar fears). These people are often labeled or diagnosed with paranoid delusions and hallucinations. Feil describes these individuals as "maloriented" and explains that their distressing behavioral expressions "are a result of physical changes as they age and the psychological ways in which they have dealt with crises throughout their lives." These lifelong coping strategies often contribute to the development of DHRRIs in care homes.

Feil and de Klerk-Rubin[63] state that these individuals must express their feelings of psychological pain that were buried for a lifetime, and when these feelings are validated by a trusted and well-trained care partner, over time many experience relief and become less anxious. Feil reports, "After about 6 weeks of consistent validation (three 5- to 10-minute validating sessions a day) by direct care partners trained in the Validation Method, their accusing and whining lessen and often cease altogether."

In general, during distressing situations, avoid trying to reorient residents to facts or forcing them to confront reality. Avoid trying to give them insight into their behavioral expressions. Instead, actively listen, while affirming, acknowledging, and validating their underlying emotional experience (such as stress, shame, guilt, feelings of inadequacy, boredom, fear, anger, and loneliness). These people want to be heard, to have someone who can be fully present while genuinely listening with respect and empathic affirmation of feelings they may have never expressed or dealt with (e.g., trauma from having been abused during childhood, grief over the loss of a spouse or feeling terrified of becoming incontinent). They desperately need someone they can trust, and trust building with these elders takes time and *consistent* effort during routine times as well as before, during, and after DHRRIs develop.

◆ Current Personality Traits

The personalities of a significant portion of elders may change with the progression of dementia. Residents who were generally mild-mannered throughout their lives may now have traits that include a "short fuse," impulsiveness, impatience, inflexibility, and jealousy. They may now be prone to quarrelling, bullying, controlling, and being demanding of others and thus are at risk of instigating or otherwise becoming involved in DHRRIs.[78] Living in and sharing small and overcrowded spaces with a large number of other residents with dementia and severe mental illness (SMI) can give rise to significant and frequent situational distress (due to invasion of personal or private space, for example). The combination of the aforementioned personality traits and cognitive disabilities (such as problems with impulse control) makes some of these residents particularly likely to express their frustrations and anger verbally and physically during interactions with other residents.

It is important to work with the resident and, when appropriate, with his or her close family members to identify the situational triggers and unmet needs that commonly cause him or her to become frustrated, upset, and angry, and to develop an individualized care strategy aimed at proactively meeting these needs and eliminating these triggers. A social worker, for example, can conduct one-on-one weekly meetings with a resident in the early to middle stages of Alzheimer's disease to listen actively to the person's concerns, acknowledge his or her frustrations, validate these emotions, and develop a plan to minimize triggers and maximize positive engagement. A realistic goal in these sessions, and the general approach with most of these individuals, is not to try to change the person but rather to develop a better understanding of her or his perceived unmet needs and minimize the negative effects of the manifestations of her or his personality traits on other residents. Striving to connect with and tap into the inner reservoir of empathy in these people can sometimes also prove helpful in reducing their involvement in DHRRIs.

Another preventive strategy is to proactively assist these residents in finding ways to channel their frustrations and anger into constructive, appropriate, and personally meaningful group or one-on-one engagement. Make sure that the activities offered to the person match her or his current preferences and cognitive abilities and disabilities.

Volunteers could be recruited and trained to work as companions to residents with personality traits that give rise to DHRRIs. These companions can help enhance personally meaningful engagement, increase supervision during vulnerability time periods, and assist direct care partners in their efforts to prevent these incidents, such as by alerting them in real time to residents' early warning signs of distress and anxiety. The mere presence of a thoughtful, skilled, and trusted volunteer in close proximity to the resident a few times each week could go a long way in reducing her or his instigation and involvement in DHRRIs. The preventive value of this approach is self-evident, especially during periods when direct care partners are busy providing care and assistance to other residents in other parts of the care home.

◆ Exhibitor's Higher Cognitive Function

In a qualitative study conducted by Sifford-Snellgrove and colleagues, certified nursing assistants reported that residents who initiated physically, verbally, or emotionally "aggressive" behaviors had higher cognitive function levels than residents who were harmed during these episodes.[83] In addition, Shinoda-Tagawa and colleagues[26] (2004) found that a lower level of cognitive function was associated with a greater likelihood of being injured by another resident. Compared with cognitively intact residents, the likelihood of being injured was about five times higher for those with borderline or mildly impaired cognitive function levels, eight times higher for those who had moderate impairments, and 12 times higher for those who had severe impairments.

One common trigger of injurious resident-to-resident incidents occurs when a resident with more advanced dementia invades the personal space or bedroom of a resident in an earlier stage of dementia. The aforementioned study shows an association between a resident's tendency to walk around the care home in places and ways that interfere with other residents' space and activities and being hit and injured by these other residents.

It is important to recognize that there are exceptions to the trend by which the likelihood of being harmed and injured in these incidents increases as cognitive function declines. One preliminary report from a qualitative study has shown that certain residents with severe cognitive impairment may exhibit behavioral expressions perceived as aggressive toward other residents who had less severe impairments.[13] Remember that many people in advanced stages of dementia are ambulatory and physically strong, and even a single push, such as by a resident in late-stage dementia of a frail resident in mid-stage dementia, can result in serious injury and death of the resident on the receiving end, no matter their level of cognitive impairment.

Psychiatric and Emotional Status

One important factor contributing to many of these episodes is a resident's experience of a deep sense of loss in one or more domains of life, such as aging-related changes and loss of cognitive or physical function. Being depressed is also a major risk factor for residents exhibiting behavioral expressions labeled as aggressive in general as well as being involved in DHRRIs as exhibitors. Particularly challenging are the effects of posttraumatic stress disorder, which can impact a person decades after the initial trauma. Routine assessment of these emotional and psychiatric states should prompt the IDT to develop individualized psychosocial approaches and strategies as well as evidence-based pharmacological treatments (such as antidepressant medications that have been shown to reduce depression in elders with dementia) to alleviate their negative impact on the person. This, in turn, can reduce the likelihood that residents experiencing these emotional states will engage in DHRRIs.

◆ Loss of Independence and Autonomy

The experience of having lost independence and autonomy may lead to frequent frustrations and anger, which in turn could contribute to residents' involvement in DHRRIs.[78] Many elder residents with dementia have experienced a series of losses in various domains of their lives. Examples include losses in physical and cognitive functions, independence, loved ones or close friends, a home, a career, financial security, general control over their own lives and over important decisions affecting their lives and care, privacy, rights and dignity, and hopes and dreams for retirement.

Experiencing one or more of these losses may threaten these residents' sense of independence and autonomy and increase their levels of daily frustration and anger. Such profound experiences may, in turn, increase the likelihood that they will experience increased irritability and a lower threshold for annoyance when faced with verbal or behavioral expressions (such as repetitive questions or intrusion into personal space) by other residents. In general, a resident with dementia experiencing loss of independence and autonomy may be more likely to reach a "breaking point" and become involved in these DHRRIs in an effort to end frustrating situations that arise as they occur in their social and physical environment. When assisting residents with dementia in minimizing the negative effects caused by loss of independence and autonomy, consider the following approaches.

Develop personalized psychosocial approaches that aim to enhance residents' "sense of gain"[78] and accomplishment, and always work to proactively create the conditions for them to be as successful as possible in everything they do. Direct care partners should be trained to plan and assist residents with dementia *only* with those care-related tasks or parts of tasks they are no longer able to do on their own; for instance, a resident who is unable to wash his legs may be able to wash his face and chest with a washcloth. As Jennifer Brush and colleagues say, "When caregivers take over activities of daily living (ADLs) for a person with dementia, excessive disability and aggressive behaviors often result."[84] Lack of skilled, gentle, and timely assistance to residents with dementia in areas of care and life in which they clearly want to participate but struggle to be successful often sets them up for failure. This can have far-reaching negative consequences to their self-esteem, sense of independence and autonomy, and dignity. Therefore, work to raise direct care partners' awareness of the need to assess and identify each resident's optimum level of need for assistance in various daily and care tasks. Striking a good balance at the individual resident level will reduce those negative emotional states that often contribute to development of DHRRIs.

Depending on the level of cognitive function, it is a good idea to involve residents in small and large decisions and choices affecting their daily care, lives, and rights. The profound humiliation and deep frustration experienced by a resident with dementia who is unable to participate meaningfully in decisions that affect his or her life and care will thus be reduced (this is true in all stages of Alzheimer's disease), decreasing the likelihood that the resident will carry these negative experiences and "emotional buildups" into interactions with other residents.

❖ Depression

It is estimated that nearly half of nursing home residents with cognitive disorders experience depression.[85] Previous research found that nursing home residents with dementia who manifested "physical or verbal aggression" had a higher prevalence of depression than those not engaged in these behavioral expressions.[86] A study by Pillemer and colleagues[87] among 1,405 residents in nursing homes in New York found that experiencing depression was associated with being involved in DHRRIs.

The following suggestions may assist you in supporting residents with dementia who are depressed and thus reduce the likelihood that they will become involved in these incidents.

- First, identify residents with dementia experiencing depression. The IDT could use the Cornell Scale for Depression in Dementia for determining this. A 19-item clinician-administered instrument, this scale uses information from both the resident and a nursing direct care partner familiar with the resident; a score greater than 12 suggests probable depression.[88]

- Once depression has been identified, make sure that all direct and non-direct care partners (including float staff and external agency staff) are aware of this condition among these individuals and its potential for contributing to involvement in DHRRIs. Heightened awareness to this risk factor is a basic first step in prevention.

- Support the resident in connecting with personally meaningful sources of inspiration, realistic hope, rekindled or new meaning, and purpose in life. Think about ways to affirm their individuality, empower them, increase their sense of belonging to a group of people they care about, and enable them to do things that enrich their lives and make them feel useful to others.

- Encourage, nurture, and reward other residents' acts of empathy and compassion towards the person. Foster the resident's sense of belonging to a small group of people the person cares about or that he or she can grow over time to care about.

- Consider providing regular one-on-one support and counseling (from a social worker, psychologist, or chaplain) to residents in the earlier stages of dementia who can benefit from it. Many elders in the early stages of Alzheimer's disease can benefit tremendously from psychotherapy.[89] A study in the south of England examined the effects of six 10-week-long psychotherapy groups on 19 people with dementia (average *Mini-Mental State Examination* [MMSE] score of 23; all had MMSE scores of 18 or above; 13 had mild cognitive impairment and 6 had moderate cognitive impairment). The study found a significant treatment effect (measured using Cornell depression scale scores), which was maintained at follow-up 10 weeks after the end of the psychotherapy groups. The study shows that although group psychotherapy is not for every person with dementia, it could have a role to play in reducing levels of depression in people with mild and moderate dementia.[90]

- When possible, pay extra attention to these individuals. A simple recognition of the person's existence (such as by saying hello while walking in the hallway, asking how the person is doing today, or offering a hug when wanted) and affirmation of his or her individuality and humanity could provide a modest measure of support to residents with dementia who feel depressed. No acts of compassion are too small; in fact, they could be as important as a lifeline offered to a person who is drowning.

- Finally, consider whether the person may benefit from an antidepressant medication, with careful attention to striking a good balance between treatment effectiveness of depressive feelings and any adverse side effects.

◆ Posttraumatic Stress Disorder

Deeply traumatizing experiences with lifetime effects may put individuals at risk for developing posttraumatic stress disorder (PTSD).[91,92] These may include, among others, childhood neglect and physical, psychological, or sexual abuse; rape; combat experience (including being a prisoner of war); experiencing or witnessing a violent event or threat of death; violent prison environments; serious physical injury; a bad car accident; surviving a severe illness; sudden, unexpected death of a loved one; or being an affected civilian or first responder in a disaster such as an earthquake, volcanic eruption, flood, fire, bridge collapse, nuclear accident, terror attack, the Holocaust, or other genocidal or politically motivated violence.

Previous research found that older veterans with a diagnosis of PTSD had twice the odds of having a diagnosis of dementia as their counterparts without PTSD.[93,94] Having a diagnosis of PTSD among veterans of previous wars has been shown to be associated with an elevated risk of anger, hostility, and DHRRIs.[77] In addition, a case series by Mittal and colleagues[95] showed that PTSD symptoms (such as persistent and intrusive recall and re-experiencing of combat trauma, avoidance of stimuli associated with the war, difficulty falling or staying asleep, or increased intensity and frequency of nightmares related to combat) might be exacerbated by dementia. This report suggests that dormant PTSD symptoms may be disinhibited as a result of neurodegeneration of memory pathways. For example, combat-related PTSD symptoms, such as intrusive, distressing, and recurrent nightmares involving military service in World War I, were reported to be experienced by a veteran with Alzheimer's disease 75 years after the war.[96]

In one case, an 86-year-old woman with Alzheimer's disease insisted that she was 4 months pregnant and needed to be taken to the doctor immediately to have an abortion. When her daughter tried to reorient and convince her that she was not pregnant, she cursed, grabbed, and scratched her. A review of her early life using communication techniques of the Validation Method revealed that when she was young, a technician who came to her home to fix the radiator when her parents were away on vacation raped her. After getting pregnant, she desperately tried to undergo an abortion without informing her parents.[63] This early-life trauma "traveled" several decades with her into her older age but was not initially recognized by her daughter. Knowing the traumas experienced by residents with dementia in their early life is key to understanding the root cause of a subset of their distressing behavioral expressions (otherwise, these individuals tend to be mistakenly labeled as aggressive and violent). Skillfully validating the resident's verbal and emotional expressions in response to reliving these traumas is critical to alleviating their negative effects on these individuals and, in turn, on those around them.

Stephen Soreff[78] explains the role of PTSD in the context of DHRRIs as follows:

> There are three major categories of symptoms: re-experiencing, avoidance, and hyper-arousal. Any one of these three types of reactions can result in resident-to-resident aggression. In the first, the resident relives, often seeming in real time, the dreadful episode. This vivid recollection is a flashback. Suddenly, they are experiencing it in the present moment.

> A loud noise might lead one to believe he is in combat again. Nightmares reflect a method
> of re-experiencing the traumatic event and can be very disturbing. In avoidance, some
> residents will isolate themselves. With hypervigilance, the resident is always on heightened
> alert; they perceive danger at any time. For many Vietnam veterans the war still rages in the
> minds, and when in a nursing home, it can continue to play out there.

Soreff gives the example of a 65-year-old man, a combat veteran of Southeast Asia, who repeatedly experienced flashbacks and nightmares. In one flashback triggered by a flash of lightning, he suddenly threw three other residents out of the way as he ran for cover.

It is important to recognize that PTSD among elders is underreported and undertreated. Some elders are reluctant to discuss their traumatic experiences. For example, many veterans underreport combat-related symptoms.[97] As explained by Macleod,[98] "These veterans often had a masking of symptoms in midlife and had been reluctant to come forth and discuss their traumatic wartime experiences." Reasons may include reluctance to acknowledge psychological distress, somatic manifestations of stress, and use of alcohol and drugs to mask symptoms.[97] An additional reason for the underreporting has to do with the fact that PTSD has only been included as a separate diagnostic category since 1980, when the *Diagnostic and Statistical Manual, Third Edition (DSM-III)* was published, whereas the United States was engaged in several wars (World War II, Korean War, and Vietnam War) that ended long before.

A comprehensive individualized assessment is essential in the evaluation of an older resident who has suffered a trauma.[97] Ongoing efforts by the IDT are needed to identify and diagnose residents with PTSD; clinicians should proactively consult with close family members when the resident is unable to report on past traumas due to advanced cognitive impairment. According to Weintraub and Ruskin,[97] the assessment should include "the resident's view of how the trauma has affected him or her, obtaining a complete history (i.e., psychiatric, medical, developmental) and physical examination, assessing social support, and performing a complete mental status exam, including a cognitive assessment." Heightened sensitivity must be practiced in order to avoid causing the person emotional distress during the assessment due to his or her recall, if not re-experiencing, of the traumatic events.

It is important to know the life history of all residents with dementia, but especially in the context of PTSD. Care partners should sensitively and empathically review with close family members the nature of traumatic events as they occurred during the person's life. Attention should be given to traumatic events during early childhood, as these have been found in research to be a vulnerability factor for PTSD and subthreshold PTSD among elders.[99]

Document these traumatic life events in the resident's clinical chart; ensure that direct care partners are informed about the traumatic events if your IDT determines that it is essential for providing care, enhancing the resident's psychological well-being, and/or understanding the origins of the resident's distressing and harmful behavioral expressions. At the same time, develop ways to protect the confidentiality of the deeply personal and sensitive information (such as sexual abuse early in life). Seek written permission—from cognitively capable residents and from close family members/legally authorized representatives of residents in advanced stages of dementia—to use this information to improve the person's care, emotional support, and daily efforts to prevent DHRRIs.

Direct care partners should pay special attention, be sensitive, and remain vigilant to avoid events that may remind the resident and/or reactivate the traumatic experiences. Previous research among war veterans found that reminders of war-related traumatic experiences caused these individuals to become upset.[90] As explained by Mittal and colleagues,[95] "The intense emotions at the time of trauma initiate a long-term conditioned response to the reminder of events."

Exposure to symbolic representations of old traumas, such as wartime trauma, and situations that induce a sense of lack of control, such as deteriorating health or death of a loved one, may cause an onset or worsen manifestations of PTSD in residents.[97] Direct care partners should decrease residents' exposure to events that may remind them of traumatic experiences from their past. Examples of documented reactivating events include entry of a male resident into the bedroom of a female resident who was sexually abused as a child (an intrusion of private space that frequently caused her to feel threatened and fearful), images from a recent war shown on television that reminded Holocaust survivors of World War II, showerheads reminding Holocaust survivors of gas chambers, and a fatal car accident shown on television reminding a resident of a tragic car accident in her or his family.

A scary episode in the present may trigger fear in a resident who was a victim or witness of violence at some point during her or his life. Physical restraint procedures used on residents with dementia may reactivate victimization and/or past trauma.[100] Moreover, "flashbulb" memories, which are vivid and detailed memories of the moment when an individual first learned the news about an important, shocking public event (such as the German invasion of Denmark in 1940 or Japan's attack on Pearl Harbor in 1941), could trigger a posttraumatic stress reaction in elders.[101] Finally, the varied losses, physical and functional changes, and social isolation associated with very old age may reactivate symptoms of PTSD.[97]

When a resident with dementia and PTSD has already been exposed to reactivating events and is re-experiencing the traumatic event, a trained and skilled direct care partner should empathically validate his or her emotions and subjective experiences. An important goal is to "tune into" the emotional reality of the resident (for example, using the Validation Method's techniques) and avoid insisting the person come back to objective reality when the resident has already lost the cognitive ability to do so. Remember that the person is reliving these awful memories *as if they are real.* Many residents in mid-to-late stages of dementia become even more frustrated, upset, fearful, and angry—increasing the likelihood that they will engage in DHRRIs—when care partners try to contradict or convince them that what they are experiencing is not real or is not occurring in the present. For example, telling the 86-year-old woman in the example given earlier, "Stop it. You are not having a baby," will likely make things worse and escalate the situation.[63] As explained by Feil, "Painful feelings that are expressed, acknowledged, and validated by a trusted listener will diminish. Painful feelings that are ignored or suppressed will gain strength and become 'toxic.'" Direct care partners should use the Validation Method's principles and communication techniques[63] when working with older residents with Alzheimer's disease in general and during situations of reactivation of old traumas. Formal training in this communication method is essential to handling these distressing situations effectively (for information on training, visit the website of the Validation Training Institute).

Addiction

A subgroup of residents experiencing addictions (past and current) to alcohol and drugs may be prone to involvement in DHRRIs as exhibitors. Residents who are addicted to nicotine represent a common challenge in LTC homes in general (such as fire hazards) and in the context of DHRRIs. With regard to the effect of substance abuse on DHRRIs, the primary focus here is on past and current alcohol addiction and abuse. The important role of drug addiction as a risk factor for DHRRIs is only minimally addressed here, given the highly specialized knowledge and expertise required to address it.

◆ Past Addiction to Alcohol or Drugs

A study by Messner[102] examined history of alcohol use and levels of "aggression" in community-dwelling people with dementia by using a survey of 100 family care partners. Although the methods used in the study do not allow us to infer causality, the study found that an increase in levels of alcohol consumption (from 1 to 5, where 1 represents an occasional drinker, 2 is a moderate drinker, 3 is a frequent/heavy drinker, 4 is a problem drinker, and 5 is an alcoholic) was associated with verbal and physical harm to others. In accordance, Soreff[78] states that past substance abuse can result in DHRRIs. For example, a long history of heavy alcohol use may result in cognitive impairment or dementia such as Korsakoff's syndrome. Cognitive impairments (for example, an inability to recall recent events such as having already eaten breakfast) may lead to verbal expressions (such as repetitive questions) that could frustrate other residents and thus contribute to DHRRIs.

To mitigate the potential risk of DHRRIs related to a history of heavy alcohol use or drug abuse in your care setting, the following preventive measures should be considered.

1. First, conduct a preadmission behavioral assessment (including a thorough assessment of alcohol and drug use history) to determine potential risks and whether your direct care partners have the resources, staffing levels, specialized training and skill set, and ability to care for and treat the individual safely. If the IDT determines that the person's condition and accompanying care challenges are beyond your direct care partners' ability to meet his or her care needs and keep him or her and other residents safe, the individual should not be admitted to your care setting.

2. If your care setting has the ability to meet the person's care needs and keep him or her and those nearby safe, ensure that an initial care plan is completed before admission; the care plan must be updated within the timelines specified in the regulations governing your care home. The care plan should include specific measures required for this person such as general supervision, monitoring of roommate assignment (if private bedroom was not assigned) and sharing of bathrooms, personally meaningful engagement, and ways of meeting the person's unique care and safety needs.

3. Carefully monitor residents who are at risk of resuming heavy alcohol drinking, even after significant periods of abstinence. Resuming heavy alcohol drinking is likely to increase the resident's risk of involvement in DHRRIs and harmful behavioral expressions toward direct care partners. An evaluation during admission and periodically thereafter—in consultation with the resident and his or her family—should assist the IDT in making specific instructions in the resident's care plan with regard to access to alcohol, including the amount of drinking permitted each day and week, if any.

It is important to note that not every resident with a history of heavy alcohol drinking or drug use engages in harmful verbal or physical expressions toward others in the present. Sometimes, a person's heavy alcohol drinking decreased substantially or was discontinued years ago and its negative effects may have reduced substantially or been eliminated altogether. Whether or not the person discontinued heavy alcohol drinking years ago or recently, we should avoid labeling the person as an "alcoholic," as this label carries with it a profound stigma that is likely to reduce rather than enhance empathy and adequate care and treatment to the individual. If the person feels labeled and excluded, in turn, that may increase the likelihood that he or she will be involved in DHRRIs.

◊ Current Addiction and Use of Alcohol or Drugs

A substantial portion of nursing home residents experience alcohol-related problems and alcohol use disorders.[103] In one study, half of elders in veterans' nursing homes were found to have lifetime alcohol abuse or dependence, and nearly one-fifth of residents continued abusing alcohol.[104] Furthermore, a study in eight nursing homes in France found a high prevalence of chronic alcohol consumption among residents with MMSE scores greater than 15 (almost 20% were heavy drinkers, which was defined as three or more glasses of wine or equivalent per day).[105] Another study, in assisted living residences in the United States, found that alcohol misuse and abuse may be a problem in this fast-growing LTC setting. Based on nursing assistants' reports, the researchers found that more than two-thirds (69%) of the residents drank alcohol; one-third of these residents were drinking alcohol daily.[106] According to Nicholas Castle[36]

> Misusing and abusing alcohol can have a profound negative impact on health, safety, and quality of life. Nursing home residents with alcohol abuse problems are more likely to suffer from depression and anxiety and behavioral problems such as wandering, leading to falls and fractures.

Substance abuse, such as excessive or heavy alcohol drinking, is a major risk factor for residents' engagement in behavioral expressions labeled as aggressive toward others. The aging of the baby boom generation in the United States, in combination with high rates of substance abuse in this population, suggests an urgent need to identify and treat it in elders. Drug abuse has been known for decades to be a risk factor for aggressive behaviors and violence in the general population,[107] and there is no reason to think that it does not continue to be a contributing factor for DHRRIs in care homes. Readers interested in learning more about the increasing problem of drug abuse among elders, including risk factors, consequences, assessment, and interventions, are advised to read the excellent article by Kuerbis and colleagues.[108]

There are several general actions to consider when addressing the challenging and complex issue of excessive alcohol use and abuse in LTC homes. First, as mentioned above, avoid making the mistake of admitting a resident with a current alcohol or drug addiction when your care setting does not have the specialized capabilities and skills for treating and caring for the person and those around him or her safely.

Second, if the person is already a resident at your care setting when an addiction is discovered, work closely with alcohol and drug addiction centers and specialists on developing a care and treatment plan for the individual; regularly re-evaluate and update the care plan as care needs and safety issues change. Beyond meeting the person's care needs, the care plan should detail specific measures for preventing the resident from consuming excessive amounts of alcohol or drugs. For example, develop instructions for careful monitoring of use of alcohol by at-risk residents in public spaces and inside their bedrooms, or during cocktail hour in care homes where such a social activity is offered.[103] Third, closely supervise and monitor the resident for alcohol consumption but also for distressing behavioral expressions. Residents with addiction may experience a lack of impulse control, which may contribute to quick escalation of negative emotional states (such as anger) during interactions with other residents, resulting in harmful incidents. If you find that your efforts to prevent the person from consuming excessive amounts of alcohol fail, carefully consider the possibility of discharging the person to a more suitable care setting that specializes in caring for and treating elders with such addictions.

Fourth, routine individualized assessment and treatments for depression, anxiety, and distressing and harmful behavioral expressions associated with excessive alcohol drinking should be a standard practice in your care home. Fifth, address residents' drinking histories and their potential negative effects in your policies and procedures about alcohol consumption.[109] For example, policies may include those that instruct direct care partners to retain possession of a resident's alcohol (when considered by the IDT and the resident's close family members to ensure the health and safety of the person or those around him or her), monitor and document alcohol use, and require a physician's permission for at-risk residents (i.e., residents with a known history of excessive alcohol use with harmful effects) to consume alcohol.[103]

Policies and procedures should aim to strike a good balance between the dangers of adopting and implementing a paternalistic approach toward the resident with excessive alcohol consumption and the need to keep all residents and direct care partners safe. While respecting all residents' choices regarding their lives is an important value, the rights and safety of other residents and direct care partners should not be violated as a result of such alcohol consumption.

Train all direct and non-direct care partners in detection and management of alcohol abuse. The following signs of potential alcohol misuse and abuse should be included in the training:[106] falls, forgetfulness (significant change from baseline), ulcers, stomach or pancreas inflammation, liver disease, high blood pressure, mood swings, speech problems, tiredness, isolation, and changes in mood and behavioral expressions. Auto accidents could be a sign among residents in early stages of dementia who are still driving (such as those living in assisted living residences). Training non-direct care partners such as housekeeping staff is important because they regularly enter residents' bedrooms to complete housekeeping tasks, so they are in a good position to detect signs of alcohol abuse (such as the smell of alcohol or empty beer cans in the bedroom or trash can).

Importantly, direct care partners, nurses, and physicians need to stay alert to the negative effects of mixing prescription and certain over-the-counter medications with alcohol and drugs.[106]

Finally, consider allowing low-risk residents to enjoy moderate amounts of alcohol occasionally, if such consumption clearly does not have negative effects on their and other residents' health and safety. If this approach is taken, it is important to practice ongoing monitoring of the resident's access to alcoholic drinks and regular and careful individualized assessment of the effects of such drinking on the person and others; open, respectful, and clear communication with the resident and, when appropriate, her or his close family members; and good communication and timely information transfer across all direct and non-direct care partners and other IDT members (including detailed documentation).

◊ Cigarette Addiction

Beyond its various negative health effects, the physiological dependency on nicotine is a problem for a significant number of older adults[110] and for the majority of the population with severe chronic mental illness.[111] As Kathryn B. McGrew states, "This issue represents extraordinary challenges in nursing home daily life. This problem is a product of the combination of addiction, restrictive smoking policies, and limited financial resources for the purchase of cigarettes."[112] Cigarette addiction may exacerbate mental illness symptoms and become a source of conflicts between staff and residents and DHRRIs.

Smoking in nursing homes and assisted living residences is a complex and serious issue with potentially far-reaching safety implications. It is complex and challenging partially because it is a quality-of-life issue and a matter of choice in a care setting where vulnerable and frail residents with diverse medical, functional, and cognitive abilities reside.

One approach to addressing this unique and complex challenge is to institute a smoking schedule in which smoking times and clearly defined spaces are designated, so that smoking is integrated into the routine of the LTC home.[112] One reason for using this approach with residents with serious mental illness, as explained by a direct care partner, is that some residents may "have no control or judgment about cigarettes." A person may forget when she or he had a cigarette and then, as mentioned above, repeatedly demand it from direct care partners or other residents. For some people with dementia, it may be helpful to use a smoking diary in which direct care partners log each time a resident smokes a cigarette. The diary can then be used to remind the resident with short-term memory deficit when she or he had a cigarette last time and when, according to the smoking schedule, she or he will receive the next cigarette. However, it is important to refrain from arguing with residents with dementia about the facts when they insist that they did not receive a cigarette, even when the last log of their smoking is shown to them. Such arguments are likely to cause the resident to experience an increased level of frustration and anger and therefore to escalate the situation. When using a smoking schedule and diaries, it is important to inform all direct care and non-direct care partners as well as float staff, external agency staff, and the resident's family about their use.

Balancing residents' autonomy and right to choice with the need for supervision is a constant challenge in general, but especially when the care home is understaffed. "That's my one thing, please don't take that away from me. That's the one thing I can enjoy," said an 83-year-old nursing home resident who was partially paralyzed from a stroke, when she was asked by her family to give up smoking. The family had been informed of burn holes in the resident's clothing and on her wheelchair. Three months later, the resident, who was left unattended on the patio before dinner, suffered very deep (third-degree) burns while smoking a cigarette. She died two days later. "Our goal is to raise awareness to this . . . ," said her daughter-in-law. "No one who can't get up and walk away should be allowed to smoke unsupervised."[113]

Cigarette Addiction and DHRRIs

Repeated requests for cigarettes from other residents, or for the money to purchase them, can trigger conflicts between residents. These repeated requests are not uncommon, and they trigger DHRRIs either because of their verbally intrusive and persistent nature or because they are perceived as disruptive to other residents who may respond negatively toward the individual. Alternatively, one can easily see how taking cigarettes or money without permission (for example, from another resident's bedroom) could lead to DHRRIs.

Fire Prevention

Pay special attention to potential fire hazards and proactively prevent them. Residents with dementia, who have short-term memory impairment and decreased awareness to personal safety, can put themselves and others at risk when they smoke. They may forget and leave a burning cigarette that will cause a fire. A resident with dementia could, for example, leave a burning cigarette by the bed, go to use the bathroom, forget she or he had left a cigarette burning, and leave the bedroom without going back to the bed to put it out. In addition, many residents with advanced Alzheimer's disease may not be able to recognize a fire hazard or know what to do when fire erupts, or they may not be able to call for assistance during an emergency.

Consider having at-risk residents use a smoking apron (a silicone-coated fiberglass fabric that covers a person from the shoulders to below the knees) designed to protect wheelchair users from accidental cigarette burns. Train all direct and non-direct care partners in helping residents use these aprons safely. Using it can help prevent serious burns and deaths.

Be sure that multiple fire extinguishers and burn blankets are placed in key locations in the care home in case of a fire. Train all direct and non-direct care partners in quickly and skillfully using fire extinguishers and burn blankets during life-threatening emergencies. Finally, make sure that installation of smoke detectors and fire sprinklers meet fire codes as well as state and federal regulations applicable to your care home.

Mitigation of Second-Hand Smoke

To protect the interests of nonsmokers and help prevent conflicts between smokers and nonsmokers, consider implementing a strict policy in which residents with dementia are allowed to smoke only with care partners' direct supervision, within their individual smoking schedule, and only in a secured garden or backyard next to the care home, when such space exists. If space allows, your care home might consider setting up a small area within the garden or backyard for residents to smoke in order to respect the wishes of others who want to enjoy the outdoors without inhaling smoke. Although this approach may not resolve the problem completely—residents may still be found smoking in bedrooms, bathrooms, and other parts of the care home outside of their smoking schedules—when implemented consistently by all direct and non-direct care partners and visiting family members, a strict policy will likely reduce the risks involved in unsupervised smoking. It will also help keep the care home free of smoke and a smell that is offensive to many people.

In general, any policy, procedure, or approach chosen should be based on whether the resident addicted to cigarettes has dementia (including the unique manifestations of the person's cognitive impairments and the ways in which these are assessed by the IDT to affect the person's ability to smoke safely), and/or serious mental illness, such as schizophrenia or personality disorder.

In any care home where smoking is permitted and cigarettes are available, staffing levels are critical at all times, as direct care partners must provide constant supervision to residents with dementia and those with significant physical limitations during smoking periods. All care employees need to remain vigilant and proactively seek to identify and immediately but gently and respectfully redirect residents who try to smoke cigarettes beyond the individual resident smoking schedules or in smoking-restricted locations.

Past Behavioral Expressions and Convictions

Knowing the past history of distressing and harmful behavioral expressions exhibited by elders with dementia as they have manifested before admission to the care home often proves invaluable in the IDT's preparations for the person's arrival and timely development of preventive measures for potential similar expressions while in the care setting. Knowledge of elders' past convictions for violent acts is equally important.

Both types of information are critical for decision making, first of all regarding whether the person should or should not be admitted to the LTC home. Thorough collection and careful examination of such information in sufficient time prior to admission should, in most situations, make it clear to the administrator and IDT whether the care home has the resources, safe staffing levels at all times, specialized training, risk assessment, and personalized strategies necessary to meet the person's needs and keep him or her and other residents and care employees safe.

Although access to reliable and complete information prior to admission is not always realistic, the standard practice should be that the IDT makes all possible efforts to collect this information in as complete a way as possible and review it in a timely manner. Failure to do this has led to a significant number of severe injuries and deaths as a result of incidents involving residents who should have never been admitted to certain care homes.

Finally, attention and effort should be dedicated to discerning what information is reliable, so as to avoid labeling elders as aggressive, violent, and abusive when such stigmatizing labels are not warranted. As mentioned earlier, the majority of elders with dementia are not inherently aggressive or violent but rather they do their best to cope with very distressing and frightening situations while living with a serious brain disease. Previous well-meaning but undertrained and under-resourced care partners (family or paid), care professionals, and care settings unable to meet their varied care needs can be too quick to label these individuals using these terms. This labeling can leave a lasting record that follows the person into the new care home, limiting direct care partners' ability to collaborate with the new resident to help meet his or her emotional and physical needs and to keep the resident and others safe.

◆ Behavioral Expressions Reported as Aggressive Before Admission

Behavioral expressions reported as aggressive prior to admission among people with moderate to high levels of cognitive impairment can often predict whether they will engage similarly while living in the care setting.[77] After a resident with a long history of these behavioral expressions severely injured another resident, a manager at his care home in England stated,

"We weren't aware of that information. If we'd have known that, we wouldn't have accepted that gentleman into this home." The injured resident died 3 weeks later.[114] Some people with dementia have had lifelong tendencies to engage in arguments, altercations, and aggressive or even violent behaviors toward others. Ryden[115] reports that 40% of community-dwelling people with dementia who exhibited these types of behavioral expressions had been reported to engage in them before the onset of the disease. That said, many others do so only after the onset of dementia.[116]

The dangerous but fairly common practice of admitting residents to a care home without adequate preadmission behavioral assessment must be avoided. The following tragic incident illustrates how risky this practice can be.[117] A 74-year-old man with cognitive impairment who had engaged in physically aggressive behaviors toward his wife and son at home was admitted on an emergency basis to a LTC home in Toronto. Within 8 hours of his arrival, two of his roommates were found dead; he had injured them using a wheelchair footrest. He managed to cross the hallway and go into another bedroom, where he started to attack another resident, but a housekeeping staff member was able to defuse that incident.

In short, it is essential to conduct a behavioral assessment and review of any past violence-related actions before a candidate is admitted. If the assessment and review show that direct care partners may be unable to meet the person's care and safety needs and prevent future behavioral expressions that may harm other residents, the individual himself or herself, and/or direct care partners, the candidate should not be admitted. For more detailed considerations and suggestions, see "Admission Criteria and Residents with Behavioral Expressions Reported as Aggressive" in Chapter 7.

However, it is important to recognize that a subgroup of elders with dementia living at home are mistakenly labeled as aggressive and violent by their caring but burned-out family care partners who may not have received adequate education in dementia-specific approaches, communication techniques, and prevention and de-escalation strategies. These individuals are not truly aggressive or violent; instead, unskilled approaches by their well-meaning family members and their own unmet needs have often triggered their behavioral expressions. It is not uncommon to see reductions in these behavioral expressions after admission to a high-quality care home with adequate staffing levels of well-trained direct care partners.

In certain situations, the history of aggressive or violent behaviors may be discovered only after the resident with dementia has been admitted to the care home. This often occurs when the resident does not have involved family or when the family is involved in his or her care but does not share this key background information—sometimes, out of fear that the application will be rejected by the LTC home. It is also not uncommon for residents with dementia to be transferred from an acute care hospital to an LTC home without complete information about previous behavioral expressions.

When such information is discovered after admission, a careful and ongoing IDT assessment of potential safety risks must be promptly conducted; the evaluation should be repeated within a reasonable time interval determined by the administrator as appropriate to the resident. If the team determines that the risks—those uncovered from the resident's past *and* those related to his or her current behavioral expressions—are beyond the care home's ability to address effectively, a thorough discharge planning process may need to be considered. The IDT must work to identify a suitable specialized care setting to increase the likelihood that the transfer will result in safe outcomes for the person and for all involved.

Moving a resident with dementia to a new care home can be traumatic to certain individuals, and specialized care homes for elders with cognitive impairment and behavioral expressions considered aggressive are lacking in many communities across the country. Therefore, the decision to discharge these individuals should not be made lightly or in a rushed manner, unless an imminent danger exists to the resident or others in the care home; in such extreme situations, a temporary psychiatric hospitalization might be needed. Working closely and in a supportive manner with the resident's family during these stressful times is a high priority. In addition, key information about the resident's behavioral expressions and potential safety risks should be fully and clearly communicated with the managers of the new care setting. A responsible transfer process will assist the new care setting in its preadmission screening process and determination as to whether that setting could realistically meet the care needs of the resident in a safe way.

Finally, it is important that owners, administrators, and managers of care homes be fully aware of and adhere to current state and federal regulations pertaining to wrongful and involuntary discharges. Inappropriate evictions, also called involuntary wrongful discharges, are among the most prevalent complaints lodged by consumers—usually families but also residents—against U.S. nursing homes and assisted living residences.

◆ Past Convictions for Violent Acts

A subgroup of people who have been convicted for violent behaviors at some point in their lives may develop dementia and exhibit similar or worse behaviors while living in a care home. The U.S. Government Accountability Office[118] (GAO) found that in 2005 about 3% of all nursing homes that received Medicare and Medicaid funds housed at least one person who was a convicted sex offender (these estimates are understated because of data limitations). The GAO report showed that 204 LTC residents were paroled non–sex offenders, and 700 were registered sex offenders in the eight states reviewed in the study. Some of these residents may exhibit physically violent or sexually aggressive behaviors that put other residents and direct care partners at risk. Care advocate Wes Bledsoe identified more than 50 crimes allegedly committed by 44 sex offenders and other convicted criminals in LTC homes between 2002 and 2006.[119] However, contrary to widely held beliefs, a substantial portion of people who are registered sex offenders are not dangerous sexual predators. Rather, it is only a subgroup of registered sex offenders who may pose a risk of harm to other residents.

In a recently reported horrific case in a nursing home in New York,[120] a registered sex offender—a convicted "known sexual predator"—sexually abused a woman with advanced dementia on three different days over a 5-month period. The investigation report stated that the abuse resulted in "actual harm" to the woman. State investigators found that the man sexually abused two other residents and cited the nursing home for failing to protect residents from abuse, not reporting the incidents to police and the state health department, and not properly investigating the incidents. According to the investigation report, the director of nursing and the nursing home's doctor said that they were unaware the perpetrator was a convicted sexual predator. Clinical psychologist John Brose reflected on this disturbing case (Brose, e-mail communication, June 9, 2021):

> The perpetrator was on the sexual predator registry, which should have given staff a heads up to be hypervigilant. . . . [m]ost people who abuse people sexually never end up on the registry. Therefore, staff and managers need to be hypervigilant 24/7 to protect the people that pay their salary. Our residents pay their salary to keep them safe.

As importantly, Brose reminds us,

> If you remove the fact that he was a sexual predator, the issues are exactly the same. The staff did not adequately protect the residents. They did not create a behavior plan or environmental plan to keep all parties safe. Even someone who is not a sexual predator but because of deficits in brain chemistry starts acting out sexually, the staff have a responsibility to provide safety for all involved. In this case, the staff fell short by a football field. They did not get a behavioral health specialist involved. They did not refer for a sexual assault examination at the hospital. They did not produce evidence that they had multiple

team meetings to make sure all staff are trained in the possibility of future problems from a sexual point of view.

Consider the following factors when addressing risks posed by people who have prior convictions for violent behaviors. First, your care home should not admit a candidate resident if a thorough review by the IDT of past violence-related convictions suggests that the home does not have the resources, staffing levels at all times, or specialized training and skill sets among direct care partners to effectively address and prevent the person's aggressive or violent behaviors in ways that keep other residents and themselves safe. When considering the risk of a person's reoffending, use a risk assessment with well-researched and validated methods. The factors should include the following:

- The nature of past offenses and convictions, including the seriousness of the offenses;

- The time period since they occurred;

- Evidence of rehabilitation, including length of time as a law-abiding citizen;

- Successful completion of and responsiveness to required treatment and counseling;

- Written opinions of qualified professionals who have worked closely with the person over the past several years, such as a written statement that he or she is unlikely to reoffend;

- Recommendations from courts, parole or probation officers, and former landlords;

- Absence of substance abuse;

- Stable employment and housing, to the extent that the known status of "sex offender" does not prevent the person from securing housing;

- Any reports of other violent criminal activity;

- Prior psychiatric hospitalizations;

- Medical, functional, physical, cognitive, or mental health conditions that may minimize the risk of reoffending; and

- The availability and use of family and community supports.[121]

If your state is one of the few that has laws specifying LTC homes as entities to be notified for at least some registered sex offenders who entered them, use this information to proactively and immediately implement strong measures to keep other residents and direct care partners safe.

Keep in mind that many people with dementia who are not registered sex offenders may express themselves sexually toward other residents in ways that are perceived as threatening by those other residents, or they may engage in actual sexually aggressive behaviors toward other residents; these may include a subgroup of people with dementia, traumatic brain injury, frontal lobe injury, or serious mental illness. Therefore, the admission team should conduct a preadmission behavioral risk assessment (verbal, physical, and sexual) for *every* candidate resident. As thorough an assessment as possible prior to admission would increase the likelihood of an appropriate and safe placement and decrease the inappropriate admissions. Such an assessment can also serve to gather key information to inform proactive implementation of measures aimed at prevention of risk during a person's residency at the care home. For more information about preadmission behavioral assessment, see "Conduct Thorough Preadmission Behavioral Evaluations" in Chapter 7.

4

Situational Causes and Triggers

Rarely is behavior a random act;
all behavior has a cause or a triggering event.

Paul Raia[122]

This chapter describes more than three dozen factors reported in the care practice and research literature as leading to distressing and harmful incidents among residents with dementia in long-term care (LTC) homes. The contributing factors (see Table 4.1) are classified as modifiable (◇), partially modifiable (◈), and nonmodifiable (◆).

A close look at distressing and harmful resident-to-resident interactions (DHRRIs) reveals that they are usually the result of residents' unmet emotional, psychological, social, and physical or medical needs, as well as situational frustrations, intersected with their cognitive disabilities. Careful attention to a resident's needs and proactive anticipatory and timely fulfillment of them will reduce the likelihood that they will result in these incidents. Geriatrician G. Allen Power[65] invites us to reflect on the situation that a person with dementia may face:

> Imagine that tonight you are at home having dinner with your family. There is a knock on the door, and two men come into your house or apartment, carrying a mattress and bedspring. The men set the bed up in your bedroom across from your bed, hang a thin curtain between the two beds, and then escort a stranger into the home who will share your bedroom for the rest of your life. How many of you are ready and willing to take on this type of living arrangement?

Routine daily efforts to identify and systematically document the causes and triggers using the Behavioral Expressions Log (available for download at healthpropress.com; see p. viii for access instructions) can enable direct care partners to detect critical patterns that should serve as the basis for development and implementation of individualized prevention and de-escalation strategies.

Feelings as Triggers

This section identifies a series of negative emotional states experienced by residents with dementia that, when left unaddressed, can lead to DHRRIs. Although cognitively intact people can experience all of these negative emotional states, a large number of elder residents with middle- to late-stage dementia have difficulty regulating these states, especially when they are facing distressing daily situations. It is very important for direct care partners to understand this critical but often under-recognized disparity between the residents' preserved ability to *experience* the full range of emotional states and their diminished ability to *regulate* their negative emotional states. When residents with a serious brain disease such as Alzheimer's disease are left on their own with no adequate, timely, and skilled attempts from care partners to assist them in meeting their needs and to help defuse the negative emotional buildup, interpersonal frustrations can develop and escalate to the point of psychological and/or physical harm—the

Table 4.1   Factors That Can Be Situational Causes and Triggers

Factors	◇ Modifiable	◈ Partially modifiable	◆ Non-modifiable
Feelings as triggers			
Feelings of the person with dementia			
Functional frustration	X		
Sadness		X	
Loneliness and feelings of abandonment	X		
Difficulty waiting		X	
Feelings about other residents			
Jealousy		X	
Conflicts between roommates		X	
Impatience toward residents with greater cognitive impairment		X	
Perceiving another resident's behavioral expression as inappropriate		X	
Angry disputes about a topic		X	
Triggers related to institutionalization			
Institutional life			
Institutionalization and lack of autonomy	X		
Lack of interest in an activity	X		
Competition for limited resources		X	
Competition for direct care partners' attention		X	
Perception of unfair treatment at mealtime	X		
Institution-specific triggers			
Lack of consistent daily routine	X		
Boredom and insufficient meaningful engagement	X		
Evenings and weekends as risk factors			X
Repeated but unmet requests for assistance	X		
Problematic seating arrangements	X		
Clearing a way through a crowded area		X	
Unwanted entry of animals into the care home	X		
Triggers related to other residents			
Violations of personal space			
Invasion of personal space		X	
Unwanted touch		X	
Repeatedly following another resident		X	
Unwanted entry into the bedroom or bathroom of another resident		X	
Triggers related to personal objects			
Eating or drinking from another resident's plate or cup		X	
Sitting in another resident's seat	X		
Perceived theft of personal belongings		X	

Table 4.1 Factors That Can Be Situational Causes and Triggers *(continued)*

Factors	◇ Modifiable	◈ Partially modifiable	◆ Non-modifiable
Interference between residents			
Interfering with a resident's activity		X	
Trying to protect a resident from another		X	
Trying to assist another resident (unwanted help)		X	
Angry attempts at social control		X	
Other triggers			
Vocal expressions experienced as irritating		X	
Angry verbal and/or physical reaction after reaching a "breaking point"		X	
Language mismatch			X
Racist comments and ethnic stereotyping		X	
Intolerance based on sexual orientation and gender identification		X	

"breaking point" described elsewhere in this text. As Mary Marshall and Margaret-Anne Tibbs state,[123] "Having dementia can feel as if it is all about failure in every aspect of life and leads to loss of confidence, low morale, and great anxiety. We have to do everything we can to reduce the sense of failure."

Care partners can prevent or at least mitigate these incidents by adopting a strength-based approach that focuses on the skills and abilities the person has not yet lost, ensuring that all residents have meaningful, person-directed activities, and by developing trusting and supportive relationships with residents who may become sad and lonely. It can be very helpful to find out each resident's lifelong and current sources of pleasure, meaning, purpose, and hope and continuously work to promote and nurture these feelings. Additionally, an organization may consider providing regular one-on-one psychotherapy sessions to sad or depressed residents with early-stage dementia.[124] An evaluation of six 10-week psychotherapy groups for 19 people with early-stage dementia showed reductions in levels of depression at the end of the group (the effects were maintained at 10 weeks' follow-up).[90] Providing these essential support services on a regular basis can have tremendous value in improving the psychological well-being of these individuals.[89] For an overview of psychotherapy with people with dementia (including components and techniques), see the article by Junaid and Hegde.[124]

Feelings of the Person with Dementia

◇ *Functional Frustration*

Because of worsening impairments in physical, cognitive, and executive functions, many people with dementia find completing certain self-care tasks independently very difficult or even impossible. Examples of these functions are bathing, toileting, dressing, eating, and walking; communicating effectively (understanding others or expressing themselves clearly and coherently); initiating personally meaningful engagement in joyful and enriching activities; reaching their desired destinations (such as bedroom, bathroom, or dining table); and remembering recent events.

Complicating these disabilities is the frequent fear of failure, uncertainty, and doubt, combined with limited awareness of cognitive deficits, especially as the disease progresses. The

Table 4.2   Relatively Preserved Abilities in Elders with Dementia

- Long-term/remote memory, such as memories from childhood and young adulthood
- Procedural memory/"hardwired" lifelong, overlearned, habitual skills, such as swinging a golf club or playing the piano (with cueing in later stages)
- Musical abilities such as the ability to enjoy listening to personally preferred old music, singing, humming, whistling, or drumming
- Primary sensory functions, such as touch, massage, personally preferred soothing aromas or essential oils, such as lavender
- Primary motor functions, such as walking, exercising, movement, dancing
- Ability to perform repetitive tasks such as raking leaves, mowing the lawn (with a hand mower), shelling peas, dusting
- Sociability and social skills, such as enjoying the company of others, ability to be polite; however, in many individuals with Alzheimer's disease, awareness of social graces may become compromised at some point
- The ability to reach out to someone in need
- The ability to read, which remains in many elders well into Alzheimer's disease, when vision abilities are good. The DEEP guide entitled *Writing Dementia-Friendly Information*, which is co-produced with people with dementia, recommends choosing "an uncluttered font without serifs or 'curly bits.' Use Arial rather than Times New Roman." (dementiavoices.org.uk)
- Aesthetic experience and appreciation, such as the ability to enjoy artwork or beauty in nature, such as a garden, forest, lake, or river
- Sense of humor and the ability to smile and laugh; one resident with early-stage Alzheimer's disease said, "Humor is the only prescription that never fails"
- The ability to be present ("in the moment"), not 10 minutes ago, or 5 minutes from now, but in this very second
- Ability to be genuine, as lifelong social masks fall away

Adapted with significant modifications from Bowlby[127] and Zgola.[59] DEEP, Dementia Engagement and Empowerment Project.

inability to do things that they once took for granted can cause tremendous daily frustration for these individuals. Decreased frustration tolerance may contribute to irritability, restlessness, and anxiety, emotional states that can make these individuals more susceptible to engaging in distressing and harmful interactions with other residents. One director of nursing in an assisted living residence for people with dementia said, "They need changing. That's a biggy. Some of them become agitated and hit others because they need to be toileted."[34] Having soiled underwear or incontinence briefs has been reported to cause a person living with Alzheimer's disease to engage in behavioral expressions (of unmet needs) that were mistakenly labeled as aggressive.[125]

It is important to assess and identify the source of functional frustration and proactively compensate for the resident's functional deficit while preserving the resident's self-esteem and sense of independence. For example, care partners should carefully document each resident's toileting needs and typical schedule and anticipate the person's needs by providing proactive assistance in reaching the bathroom in time and using the toilet. The primary focus should be on focusing and gently supporting the resident's remaining abilities (persisting cognitive assets) and identification of ways to compensate for lost functional abilities. As Power[49] states, "We need strength-based care, not deficit-based care."

Take care not to create "excess disability"—disability not due to disease alone—by helping the resident with tasks or portions of tasks that she or he is able to complete independently.[126] Tables 4.2 and 4.3 present examples of relatively preserved abilities in elders living with dementia.

Table 4.3 Relatively Preserved Emotional Capacities

- Experiencing and expressing the full range of emotions and feelings of any human being

- Perception of emotional states of others, such as facial expressions, tone of voice, gestures, and posture (although this ability can be limited in some people)

- Responding to others' emotions, as in "mirroring"; increased sensitivity to emotional states of others, although in certain dementias such as frontotemporal dementia this ability can be impaired early in the disease

- Learning and remembering, sometimes with cueing, emotionally significant events and experiences—especially early, well-established, personally emotional memories

- Sensing who has real concern for the person, who is honest, and who can be trusted; this can often be seen when observing the person's verbal and nonverbal reactions during interactions with the care partner

Partially adapted from Raia.[128] Keeping in mind these relatively preserved emotional capacities, Raia reminds us that it is important to remember that people with dementia "may be less able to control their emotions, like frustration and anger, when they are upset."[129]

◆ Sadness

A study by McShane and colleagues[130] followed 86 community-dwelling people with dementia for at least 4 years or until death. Family members were interviewed during this period to assess their relative's cognitive function, mood, and behavioral expressions considered aggressive. Sadness (appearing particularly sad, miserable, or depressed) was found to predict onset of "physical aggression" (such as hitting, kicking, scratching, or pushing) over 1 and 2 years. One reason residents with dementia experiencing these emotional states may be at risk of engaging in DHRRIs is that they can have a lower level of tolerance of others around them than that of residents who are more content and happy.

As explained elsewhere, it is helpful to develop a close, trusting relationship with the resident and emotionally support her or him. Whenever possible, provide compassionate and warm companionship and care, especially when the resident appears to be sad. If there is an identifiable root cause, try to address it. For example, provide regular emotional support for a resident who recently lost his or her spouse.

◇ Loneliness and Feelings of Abandonment

A focus group study by Rosen and colleagues[14] found that direct care partners perceived loneliness and feelings of abandonment as triggers of DHRRIs among nursing home residents. Residents experiencing these feelings may try to stay away from others and therefore be less likely to become involved in DHRRIs, but others who are frequently in close proximity to other residents (either by choice or not) may engage in distressing interactions with them, partially due to sadness, frustration, restlessness, anxiety, and irritability.

Besides the general advice to provide ongoing emotional support, reassurance, and companionship, it is especially important to help residents experiencing loneliness to engage in personally meaningful activities that promote socialization and friendships with others, as well as feelings of meaning and purpose in their lives. Visiting with other residents or with toddlers and trained pets can be very effective in bringing joy and alleviating loneliness for some residents with dementia. Another way to help lessen loneliness and feelings of abandonment is to recruit and train volunteers to visit regularly; these people can serve as companions who can engage the resident in personally meaningful conversations and one-on-one activities, such as sharing a poem, a hand massage, or a walk in the garden.

Depending on the resident's relationships with family members and longtime friends, a care employee might encourage and facilitate relationships with them, perhaps teaching them evidence-based techniques for having meaningful communication, engagement, or other joyful experiences during visits. Another approach is to show the person that she or he is a valued, loved, and cherished member of the care community by, for example, seeking their input and advice into various matters affecting life at the home and engaging the resident in activities that contribute to the larger community, such as preparing packages and encouragement letters for hospitalized children or soldiers serving overseas.

◈ Difficulty Waiting

Many residents with dementia experience difficulty waiting for a group activity or special event, a meal, a visit to a secured garden, or medical or nursing care. In these situations, residents may become restless and anxious, which may irritate and annoy other residents around them. While waiting for a musical performance to start, a resident with dementia might become anxious and say repeatedly, "How long will this be going?" "I don't feel like staying that long," and "I don't think I can wait here forever . . . *please*."[34] Others around the resident, becoming annoyed and angry, may react verbally or physically in an effort to stop her repeated verbal expressions.

To avoid escalation resulting from difficulty in waiting, care partners should plan ahead and try to have only a limited number of residents with dementia in each waiting area—for example, waiting in the hallway to be weighed—and start structured group activities on time as noted on the daily activity schedule. Residents with Alzheimer's disease have short-term memory deficits (such as difficulty or inability to recall events or statements made minutes ago), so it is important to provide these residents with frequent reminders of the expected waiting time. These reminders need to be communicated gently, quietly, and respectfully, in a way that helps to preserve the person's self-esteem and to help him or her "save face." When a resident is having difficulty waiting for an activity to start, a care partner can invite her or him to take a walk together, returning to the activity room shortly before the activity starts; if you do this, remember to ensure that the resident's preferred chair is reserved.

Feelings About Other Residents

Some DHRRIs arise from conflicts between individuals. Jealousy, disagreements between roommates, and even differences in cognitive function levels can contribute to conflicts. Knowing and understanding the resident's unique history and care needs can help care partners make decisions on room placement, dining schedule, and other factors for maximum compatibility among residents. Understanding a person's history can also help to shape direct care partners' strategy for mitigating a DHRRI.

◈ Jealousy

Jealousy among residents with dementia can be the result of various factors. A resident who rarely receives visits from family members may become jealous that her or his roommate receives frequent visits. A resident who is not socially accepted by other residents or is treated as an outcast may become resentful and jealous of other residents who enjoy high social status and respect from others at the care home. Or, for instance, resident A, who wants to feel close to resident B, may become jealous of resident C, who develops an intimate relationship with resident B. In one incident, a woman with dementia threw a glass of water on another woman; then the two tried to hit each other. Direct care partners intervened in time and prevented the hitting, while the first resident called the second "a whore." During a conversation with the nurse, the first resident said that the other was gossiping about her with others. Later, the nurse explained that the first resident often felt jealous and threatened by the second resident when she would spend time with a particular man who lived in the care home.

In other care homes, such episodes have been reported to lead to serious injury and even death. A 79-year-old male resident with dementia in a nursing home near Toronto developed a close relationship with a female resident (also with dementia), believing she was his wife. The two were seen walking around the care home together as a couple. One day, he yelled and screamed at a 69-year-old male resident with dementia that the woman was his wife and demanded that he leave them alone: "Get your own wife." A couple of minutes later, the younger resident walked fast toward him and kicked him in the stomach. He fell backward and struck his head on the tile floor. The head injury led to deterioration in his health, and he died about 3 weeks later.

Feelings of jealousy may stem from a lack of intimacy, defined as "the feeling of being in a close personal relationship."[131] Being intimate is "marked by a warm friendship developing through long association" or by "a very close association, contact, or familiarity."[132] Care partners should assist where possible by creating regular opportunities to fulfill a resident's needs for intimacy, such as with close family members, supportive friends, toddlers or children, or trained dogs.

If a resident is cognitively able and feels comfortable sharing, the care partner can gently explore how she or he feels about the need for intimacy (it is important, however, to do it in a private space to protect the person's privacy; also, sensitive issues may arise during the conversation). A social worker or psychologist could discuss it discreetly with residents who have early-stage dementia. As mentioned elsewhere, it is a good idea to consider the life history of the resident, particularly how his or her needs for intimacy were met in the past, and as much as possible to explore the current hopes and expectations for intimacy. Ask what the resident sees as good qualities in an intimate partner. Reminisce with him or her about positive experiences and cherished memories from past intimate relationships that were sources of joy and happiness. While respecting current family relationships, consider whether helping the resident find a new intimate partner would be appropriate. Consult with the IDT about the best course of action and, when appropriate, inform and consult with the resident's close family members.

◆ Conflicts Between Roommates

It should not be surprising that nursing home roommates with positive emotional bonds are happier and more content with their living situation than those with conflictive relationships.[133] The negative impact of conflictive relationships on residents' quality of life is demonstrated by studies showing frequent, distressing, and harmful verbal and physical interactions between roommates in LTC homes.[24] My close examination of 77 deaths resulting from resident-to-resident incidents showed that 33 (43%) of these fatal incidents took place between roommates.[29]

As explained by Marsha Frankel,[79] "Most seniors had not had a lot of experience living communally. Unless they were in the military, they were unlikely to have lived in a dorm at college . . . or to have gone to a sleepaway summer camp . . . so they are not used to sharing space with other people." Following are examples of issues that can escalate to conflicts between roommates:

- One roommate being perceived as too loud or noisy by the other
- Preferences for television shows or volume of the radio or TV
- Opening versus closing windows and shades
- Whether to have the door open or closed
- Use of closet space

- Lighting-related issues (e.g., turning the lights on at night)

- Preferred bedroom temperatures (e.g., too cold or hot)

- Preferences around using the shared bathroom (e.g., preferred and conflicting times of usage, leaving a door open while using the toilet, and cleanliness)

In addition, disputes over placement of the beds have contributed to DHRRIs between roommates.[134] In one case, resentment over a 100-year-old roommate's window-side bed reportedly contributed to conflict and, subsequently, the strangling death of the roommate.[35] It is common for residents with cognitive impairment to enter a shared bathroom when their roommate is using it. Additionally, as noted elsewhere, conflicts between roommates are often triggered by things a roommate with dementia may verbally express or do, such as urinating in a trash can or drawers inside a shared bedroom.

Previous research suggests that elders without cognitive impairment generally prefer not to share a bedroom with individuals living with dementia.[135] Rooming assignments between individuals with and without cognitive impairment can result in a worsening of the mental and emotional status of the latter. In one study,[136] 2 weeks after this kind of placement, 17 of the 20 nursing home residents without impairment expressed feelings of depression and loneliness, 12 of the 20 expressed feelings of anxiety and insecurity over having a roommate who had cognitive impairment, and five became less friendly and more irritable. By contrast, two residents became *more* friendly and considerate, with an increased concern for the roommate who had cognitive impairment. Although it is important to encourage and nurture supportive relationships between residents without cognitive impairment and those with dementia, situations causing emotional distress to one or both residents must be closely monitored and addressed—including the timely consideration of a bedroom reassignment when the distress is ongoing and/or poses a safety risk.

Prevention of roommate conflicts begins with a thoughtful room assignment. It is important for assigning staff to carefully assess the resident's life background, such as lifelong sleeping habits; current functional and cognitive limitations; and preferences related to personal living space. Once roommates are assigned, care partners should consider the need to facilitate their getting to know each other and to promote a sense of fairness, compassion, and compromise around use of limited resources in the shared room. Most elders have at least one piece of precious life background information a roommate will appreciate knowing; using it thoughtfully while respecting the person's right for confidentiality could be helpful in building a close supportive relationship between the two individuals. In fact, discovering the life history of fellow residents can sometimes lead to meaningful surprises, such as when two families discovered that their parents, who were living with dementia in a VA nursing home, had served in the same unit during the Korean War.[137]

It is important to take into account the wishes and preferences of residents regarding their experience of living with roommates, no matter their level of cognitive impairment or verbal ability (carefully observe the nonverbal reactions of residents with advanced dementia to various daily situations involving their roommates). As explained by Miles and Sachs, "The concept that decision-making capacity is *task-specific* reminds us that persons who are unable to reflect on or manage health care decisions or personal finances may still retain strong preferences about rooms, roommates, or personal space."[138]

Regular monitoring and documentation are also important in helping to prevent conflicts among roommates with dementia, as cognitive impairment levels and behavioral expressions can change, and, even when they do not, people in any stage of cognitive decline can simply reach a breaking point. In certain situations, what appears to be a successful roommate assignment may eventually turn out to be less than desirable, if not harmful. Consider the case of Albert F., who was matched with Riley C. As described by the administrator,[134]

They're both Alzheimer's patients and Albert had had a private room and Riley, I guess, virtually had a private room. His roommate had passed away, and we had not filled that bed. There was some concern when we moved them together. And they got along really well. Everybody was really pleased and it was a nice move. And then, after they were together for a while, I guess it started to get hard. Started, you know getting into each other's way, and they started spatting, and then they started hitting, and then they started pushing, and we were actually afraid somebody was going to be hurt.' One night during the 11:00 to 7:00 shift the two men came to blows and a decision was made by a concerned and exasperated night staff to move Albert into another room.

To assess the quality of the relationship between the roommates, direct care partners might consider using the Emotional Bondedness Scale (EBS),[139,140] which includes 12 statements aimed at evaluating the amount of personal support, positive affect, and sense of mutuality derived from the dyadic relationship. Examples of items from the EBS are "R makes me angry or upset," "R is sensitive to my feelings and moods," "R sometimes hurts my feelings," and "We have trouble getting along." If a resident is unable to report on the relationship with her or his roommate, the items can be modified for use with a close direct care partner and/or family members. Another approach may be environmental modifications to the shared bedroom. These are discussed in more detail in Chapter 5.

Most importantly, it is critical to remember that for all long-stay residents, the LTC home is their home, and their bedroom is their last frontier of privacy. The standard of care should be private bedrooms, with a relatively small number of bedrooms designed for two people (two unrelated residents or a couple) at most. Some elders with dementia, such as those who tend to develop restlessness, anxiety, and fear when left alone for significant periods, may benefit from having a caring and supportive roommate. The socialization and friendship could assist in reducing feelings of social isolation, and some roommates may also be able to alert care employees when a resident is in need of assistance but is unable to do so on her or his own such as due to cognitive disability.

It is no longer acceptable to have three or more people sharing a bedroom in a nursing home or assisted living residence. Many care advocates consider this practice a gross violation of the rights of residents (such as the right for privacy). At least one province in Canada—British Columbia—requires newly licensed LTC homes that are publicly funded to have 95% of the bedrooms as private spaces (under the Community Care and Assisted Living Act).[141] Some innovative care models in the United States, such as the Green Houses of the Eden Alternative, are already providing private bedrooms to all residents.

◆ Impatience Toward Residents with Greater Cognitive Impairment

Whether they are roommates or not, some residents who are cognitively intact or have mild cognitive impairment or early-stage dementia may lose patience or become restless or angry with residents who have more advanced dementia. They may perceive the verbal or behavioral expressions of the other persons frustrating and annoying, and they may respond with potentially harmful comments or actions of their own—for instance, angrily shouting at another resident to stop yelling, demanding that she or he stop invading one's personal space, or even making physical contact with the other person in an attempt to discontinue whatever it is that they perceive as frustrating.

In one reported instance, a female resident in a care home for people with dementia entered the lounge. "Am I in the right place?" she asked. Another female resident answered, crossly, "Come in and sit down," then commented, "She is a right clown." The resident who had just entered asked, "Is that right, sitting here?" The other responded sternly, "Sit, sit," and raised her eyes to the ceiling with a look of disapproval. The resident who had entered asked more questions, such as "Can I come down there?" and "Can I get something from here?" These additional questions provoked the other resident to shout, "Shut your mouth."[142]

As explained by Michael Ellenbogen, who lives with dementia in his home in the community, "I am not sure I could handle dealing with people who progressed to the next stage. That scares me very much because I have some idea about how they may act. That is a reflection of what I might be one day. I just don't want to see it."[143] A study by Teresi and colleagues[55] showed that residents who were cognitively intact and lived with or adjacent to, or shared a bathroom with, cognitively impaired roommates exhibiting behavioral expressions reported experiencing substantial distress. "Half of these cognitively intact residents reported being disturbed by arguments, suspiciousness, and moods of roommate or unit mates, and . . . two-fifths found direct exposure to a roommate with dementia upsetting and distressing." Among problems reported were lack of privacy, loss of dignity, being disturbed by noise in the bedroom, lack of privacy in using the toilet, and negative effects on personal habits, sleep, and health. "Facilities placing cognitively impaired persons with nonimpaired persons may be placing the nonimpaired at risk in terms of their quality of life."[144]

Although these scenarios are fairly common, it is important to recognize that a significant number of elders without cognitive impairment get along well with residents who have substantial cognitive disability, and they do not feel that their quality of life is reduced by living in close quarters with them. In fact, some of these individuals find it meaningful and rewarding to be able to support and assist these residents as they struggle to cope with the effects of their serious brain disease and various stressful daily situations. Hubbard and colleagues found that not all residents were unsympathetic to residents with cognitive impairment, and some were willing to protect them from other residents. For example, one female resident, referring to another with a perceived cognitive impairment, was heard saying to a male resident, "They should be in another place, folk that are confused," to which he replied, "That's not very Christian-like."[142]

Power[65] cautions against stage-specific grouping of residents. "No two people are alike, even if they display similar degrees of cognitive ability." He suggests that care partners should take into consideration the fact that as residents' abilities change and they no longer "fit the program" or the care unit and they are moved to another unit, important relationships for these residents are disrupted (which can be especially challenging for residents with dementia, who have difficulty initiating and forming new relationships with others). He reports[65] on a potential benefit of having residents with different cognitive function levels living in close proximity:

> While friendships undoubtedly occur between people living with dementia, the incorporation of people with normal cognition provides a different level of stimulation that can help keep people connected in a more durable way, which in turn can promote growth and maintenance of abilities.

Indeed, as I mentioned earlier, some of the most compassionate acts occur between residents with higher cognitive function toward those with lower cognitive function levels. It is nevertheless a persistent challenge in many care homes trying to reduce widespread fears, stigma, and misconceptions held by residents who are cognitively intact or have early-stage dementia about those whose disease is more advanced, especially regarding what they perceive as frustrating verbal and behavioral expressions.

It is important for all care employees to promote a sense of community, interdependence, and empathy among residents by encouraging, nurturing, and rewarding compassionate and helpful acts between them and to send a clear and consistent message that psychological and physical retaliation toward residents with more severe cognitive impairments is unacceptable. For residents with short-term memory loss, you will need to provide frequent reminders. As in the discussion above regarding roommate assignments, direct care partners and IDTs need to do their best to be intentional in their assignment of residents to activities or areas of the care community. Resident clustering—matching residents of similar abilities together, not only in their bedroom assignments but at other times, such as dining and activities—is one approach.[144,145]

Individualized and group-level resident assessments are essential to weigh the disadvantages of shared living across cognitive function levels and the potential advantages of such living arrangements.[65] The estimated impacts (positive and negative) of moving a resident with advanced dementia to another care home for both the resident and the group of residents in the former care home should be carefully taken into consideration when making these decisions, and these decisions need to be made in close consultation with their family members.

All direct and non-direct care employees must remain vigilant and immediately defuse or meet unmet needs underlying a person's behavioral expressions perceived by others as annoying (such as repetitive questions, screaming, mishandling food or utensils, or undressing in public) by redirecting or providing gentle guiding cues. When intervening, it is important to preserve the dignity of the resident engaged in the behavioral expression and enable him or her to save face. As mentioned previously, residents with higher cognitive function have been found to engage in acts of hostility toward residents with lower cognitive function, including labeling their behavioral expressions. Beyond the potential for psychological and physical harm, a concern identified by Hubbard and colleagues is that, "Once 'labeled,' their behavior was repeatedly interpreted in this way."[142] Care employees must actively seek to anticipate and identify any potentially hurtful comments and ask residents with higher cognitive functioning to refrain from making them and, as always, provide gentle but clear reminders to those with short-term memory loss.

◆ *Perceiving Another Resident's Behavioral Expression as Inappropriate*

In my early study,[34] each of the following behavioral expressions was found to trigger angry and potentially harmful reactions by residents who observed them, including the following:

- Walking in repetitive circles in the middle of an activity room

- Reading a large newspaper during a music group activity

- Continuously looking at one's food but not eating it (for example, staring at a slice of bread)

- Eating in a way that was perceived as inappropriate, such as trying to pour ketchup into a glass and drink it or insisting on eating sweet and sour sauce, or mishandling utensils (for example, trying to eat an unpeeled banana or eating a dinner roll with a fork)

- Picking at one's nose during a meal with other residents

- Continuously cracking one's knuckles at the dining table

Other examples of behavioral expressions that may trigger DHRRIs between residents include taking out a dental plate and putting it on the table during a meal, chewing a napkin, spilling food, putting bread in the milk glass, emptying a water glass over a dinner plate, eating jam with fingers, eating out of a jam dish, or drinking from a milk jug. Reactions and insults heard from other residents, include "Tweets like him should stay at home" and "Look at him! He eats like a pig!"[146] It is important to emphasize that beyond the risk for DHRRIs, these situations also put the dignity of the resident who engages in the behavioral expressions at risk. As Grethe Berg explains, "The experience of doing something shameful is powerful and painful, even for a person who suffers from a dementia illness."[146]

It is important to keep in mind that no matter how irrational or annoying a behavioral expression may appear, there are unmet human needs underlying nearly all of these human expressions. Direct care partners should proactively create and maintain the conditions for the resident with dementia to succeed (not fail) in everything she or he does, and where possible to help the resident save face after engaging in behavioral expressions perceived as annoying or inappropriate by others. The key is to observe the resident carefully to proactively detect the earliest signs of his or her distress, anxiety, and behavioral expressions and to promptly and skillfully intervene before other residents become frustrated and their angry reactions are triggered. For example, one resident who had middle-stage Alzheimer's disease was sitting in the dining room having her lunch. At some point she opened her purse and took out of it dry feces wrapped in a toilet paper. The resident, who was known to misidentify objects, was looking at it while being seated close to her tablemates. A direct care partner noticed, approached her quietly, and asked her to come with her. She guided the resident to the bathroom in her apartment and assisted her in throwing the feces into a trash can and washing her hands. By immediately but gently and quietly redirecting the resident away from her dining room table, the care employee enabled the resident to save face. One can only imagine the reaction of her tablemates if they had noticed it before the care partner did.

It is important to use an anticipatory care approach, not a reactive one, and try to proactively address residents' unmet needs before behavioral expressions develop, or at their earliest observable signs, in order to avoid any triggering of negative reactions from other residents. Once a behavioral expression has been noticed, calmly and quietly acknowledge any frustration or annoyance experienced by other residents and, if needed, explain that the behavioral expressions are caused by cognitive disabilities and are not done intentionally to upset them. Seek residents' help by nurturing their feelings of empathy and tolerance toward other residents, especially those with more advanced dementia.

❖ Angry Disputes About a Topic

Tense interactions and conflicts between residents with dementia often develop from arguments about various topics. When direct care partners are not present or do not promptly and skillfully intervene, these arguments may intensify and escalate into DHRRIs.[24] For example, two tablemates were engaged in a lengthy and distressing verbal interaction during lunch. The episode intensified when the residents disagreed on the extent to which a third tablemate needed assistance with eating. One resident told the other, "You are outrageous. She is a poor helpless girl that can't help herself." In response, the second resident told her angrily, "Yes, how do you know? You don't even know yourself . . . so keep your mouth shut."[34]

With these types of conflicts, as with others, direct care partners should calmly intervene at the earliest signs of residents' restlessness, distress, and anxiety; quietly and calmly acknowledge and validate the feelings and frustrations of both residents; and, where possible, divert the residents' attention to something else (e.g., during a meal, reminisce about a favorite childhood food, or share a personally interesting story from the daily newspaper). However, be aware that this may be only a temporary solution; care partners must still try to identify and address the underlying needs behind the interpersonal tensions. Examples of these may be two residents with strong personalities who are used to managing others and must have it their way; competition over who identifies more correct answers in a crossword puzzle; different worldviews, value systems, or cultural backgrounds; and situational misunderstandings due to cognitive impairment.[34] Whatever the underlying issues, encourage residents to compromise and help them find ways to remain respectful of each other and sensitive to each other's needs, abilities, disabilities, and preferences; if the arguments recur, consider changing seating arrangements in the dining room or activity room, or otherwise keeping them separate from each other. Of course, without an organizational commitment to safe people-to-people ratios (staffing levels) at all times, the ability of direct care partners to implement these recommendations may remain limited.

Triggers Related to Institutionalization

This section identifies a series of situational causes and triggers that stem from life in a LTC home. Most residents with dementia did not choose to move to the residence, and most probably would have preferred to live in their homes. Not being able to enjoy many of the things we often take for granted in our own homes, residents with dementia must cope with their cognitive disabilities while, for all practical purposes, being forced to be in the presence of a significant number of strangers many hours of each day, evening, and even at night when they have a roommate or when another resident enters their bedroom. Examples of some of those things we all enjoy in our homes in the community include having a sense of freedom, privacy and safety, being in a quiet and calm environment, doing nearly anything we wish to do such as having a meal or grabbing a snack whenever we want to, going to sleep when we are ready (without interruptions), taking a shower when we want to, and engaging in personally meaningful and enriching activities in our free time. In short, in the words of John Zeisel,[147] "Home means who I am ('me'), home means family, and home means safety."

By contrast, residents' ability to control the many factors affecting their life, care, and rights—such as which television channel and program to watch in the lounge and what types of food or meaningful engagement program will be offered each day—is often limited in many care homes, which can lead to tremendous frustration. Chronically low staffing levels and high staff turnover combined with the fact that the resident's lifelong history may be insufficiently known to many direct care partners impacts the ability to build and maintain close, trusting relationships with the residents—the single most important asset direct care partners can have when caring for them. Making things worse is the lack of adequate specialized dementia care training for direct care partners in many care homes (including knowledge about approaches for meeting residents' psychological needs, emotion-based communication techniques such as the Validation Method, and personalized psychosocial strategies for prevention of various forms of distressing and harmful behavioral expressions, including DHRRIs).

Taken together, residents' dignity, personhood, identity, trust, sense of control, and emotional and physical security are often threatened in many LTC homes, which in turn may contribute directly to the development of DHRRIs. Increasing direct care partners' awareness of these factors can go a long way toward enhancing their sensitivity to the potential negative effects of these factors and the need to proactively minimize their impact on residents with dementia.

Institutional Life

Between 43% and 46% of people turning 65 years old are estimated to have a lifetime risk of entering a nursing home at some point in their life (more than half of women and one-third of men).[148,149] This means that there is a good likelihood that *you* will also live in a nursing home at some point in your life. To the best of your ability, make the residents feel as much at home as possible, as you would expect if you were to become a resident in a care home. Full commitment by owners and administrators of care homes through appropriate resource allocation and support of direct care partners is a necessary first step in making this important vision a reality.

◇ *Institutionalization and Lack of Autonomy*

Moving into a care home causes many people with dementia to experience a loss of independence and control over their lives and care.[150] It can be frightening to many individuals, and for a subgroup of these people it can be a traumatic and devastating experience. This major life event and the need to adjust to it while living with a substantial cognitive disability often contributes to residents expressing their sadness and frustrations through the only means available to them, behavioral expressions. A focus group study with direct care partners that examined DHRRIs in a large nursing home in New York City[14] and a report by Susan Snellgrove and colleagues[151] found that residents' adjustment from a lifetime of independence to institution-alization and communal living was a contributing factor of DHRRIs.

Feeling loss of control is considered a major component of behavioral expressions labeled as aggression among people with dementia.[49] One resident explained "aggressive" behavior be-tween residents this way: "Some of them are angry because they are brought in here by [their] family."[152] The majority of elders prefer not to live in a care home, and the decision is usually made by a family member or recommended by a nurse, physician, or social worker.[153] Many people with dementia have little involvement in decisions about the move.[150] Instead, their inability to live independently and safely in their home because of their cognitive and other functional limitations leads to the decision by family members to move them to a long-term care setting. Many receive limited opportunities to participate in decision-making processes about their care arrangements and feel that they are not listened to sufficiently in these major life transitions.[154] Some residents with dementia do not understand why they need to stay in a care home.[155,34] "Why am I here? I haven't done anything wrong," one resident asked her daughter. Another, who had vascular dementia and experienced repeated anxiety, said, "I am stuck here. I am afraid of this place. I want to go back to my work."[34] Another woman with early-stage dementia reported, "They took me by force and put me here by force. I am incar-cerated here. Because I don't have anybody to be with, I am here . . . for the rest of my life."[34] These heartbreaking statements reflect deep frustration and trauma among individuals with dementia who are struggling with making sense of their current living situation. According to Desai and McFadden,[156]

> Most persons with dementia are often abruptly admitted to a LTC residence, often being given the news just a few days before the move and sometimes even after the move. A small but not insignificant number of persons with dementia have an even more harrowing expe-rience of going into a psychiatric unit for "stabilization of their agitation" and, from there, are admitted directly to a long-term care residence. Such a radical and sudden change in one's living situation frequently triggers "aggressive behaviors," as these represent the only way for many persons with dementia to express how deeply and persistently their needs and rights have been ignored.

Jayne Clairmont, owner and CEO of English Rose Suites in Minnesota, warns, however, that some people with dementia may lose the cognitive ability to process information conveyed to them during the decision process related to their move to a care home. She adds that involving these people in the decision process may not work and may cause them avoidable distress (oral communication, September 28, 2015). Every person is different, and therefore individualized assessment is essential for determining the extent to which the person has the cognitive ability to understand and meaningfully participate in the process without causing her or him signifi-cant distress. In the middle stages of Alzheimer's disease, such an assessment can often be quite challenging because of a significant "gray area" and variability across individuals with regard to their ability to understand the implications of a move and to meaningfully participate in the decision-making process.

In short, initial and ongoing grief over admission to a LTC home (especially unwanted ad-mission) is widely recognized as a cause of distressed behavioral expressions in people with de-mentia.[157] It is easy to forget this fact when a resident with dementia expresses frustrations due to the constraints imposed daily on her or him by the care setting's rigid policies, operations, procedures, and care practices. This represents a major concern because many low-performing nursing homes and assisted living residences still base their policies and operations on institu-tion-centered rather than person-directed care practices.

With the participation of the person with dementia (when adequately assessed to be cog-nitively capable) and, if appropriate, his or her family, a qualified care employee such as a nurse or social worker should plan for the placement over weeks or a few months when possible, providing emotional support, education, and guidance to both the person and the family in the decision-making process related to the move and preparations for it. In some cases, encouraging and supporting the person's participation at a local adult day health care program specializing in caring for people with dementia for a year or two prior to the move to a LTC home could assist in the individual's adjustment to life in it during the weeks and months after admission.[156]

Following are suggestions for residents already living in the LTC home, to prevent or address a distressing loss of autonomy.

- *Promote the resident's sense of control.* To the extent possible, enable the resident to participate in small and large decisions affecting her or his life, care, and meaningful engagement. Ask the resident with early-stage dementia (and if not possible, her or his close family members) what she or he finds as most helpful in enabling her or him to feel a sense of control over her or his life and care. Use this information to develop and implement the person's care plan.

- *Provide flexible, individualized care schedules* (for example, mealtimes, bedtime, awake time, and personal care tasks such as bathing and grooming) based on the resident's lifelong habits and current preferences, abilities, and disabilities.

- *Promote choice* with clothes, food and drinks, meaningful engagement, music preferences, and bedroom decoration. As the resident's cognitive function declines, provide only a small number of choices (two or three) within each of these domains to avoid overwhelming the person and causing frustration.

- *Always protect the privacy of residents* in public spaces and inside their bedroom and bathroom. For example, use warm, large towels to cover the resident well before and immediately after assistance with bathing. Preserving a sense of dignity during provision of personal care will strengthen the person's sense of control.

- *Enable the resident to be outside and decompress in a secured area* (such as an outdoor garden) when she or he wants to, when it is safe and weather permits, and always with adequate supervision. It is easy to forget, as many of us take the ability to go outside for granted. The need to be outdoors on a daily basis and to enjoy the health and psychological benefits of doing so does not change in most individuals after developing dementia and moving into a care home.

- *Regularly offer meaningful and enriching outings* to residents in the community (for example, visits to a museum; an orchard for apple or peach picking; or an arboretum, lake, or restaurant), but only with an adequate number of direct care partners and trained volunteers to ensure meaningful engagement and adequate supervision. Outings should be based on residents' preferences; if they cannot verbally express them, seek input from close family members. Review the person's life story for ideas.

- *Look for and develop programs customized* to the needs of people with dementia, such as "Meet Me at the Movies,"[158] a film-based program developed by *ARTZ* (Artists for Alzheimer's™). As explained by the developers of the program,

  The films are selected based on focus group interviews with potential participants to determine which films would most resonate with the audience. The chosen clips are famous or iconic. Many people remember these famous scenes, which are embedded in their long-term memories, so they naturally become engaged in the process. To accommodate for shorter attention span, ten 4-minute film clips are projected during the performance instead of the entire movie. To increase focus of attention and participation, two "guides" onstage gently coax memories, opinions, and feelings from the audience.

- *Eliminate institutional features from the physical environment*, such as nurse stations, medication carts, multiple-occupancy bedrooms, bright fluorescent lights, and overhead paging). Incorporate features that encourage familiarity and provide a sense of being at home (for instance, allow people to bring in and use personally meaningful belongings from their home, or allow the smell of muffins baking to spread throughout the kitchen and dining room).[159] A person's sense of control decreases in a care setting that looks and feels like a hospital and increases in one that looks and feels as close as possible to a home.

- *Make the residents feel at home*, to the best of your ability. Zeisel states that a sense of home is created by the scale of rooms and bedrooms (as in a large family house), easy wayfinding (clear destinations), personal furniture and décor (not like in a hotel), and people who smile and hold your hand. Zeisel explains,[148,149]

    > The more a person feels at home, the more she is relaxed, in control, and the more she will treat others there as family and friends. The more a person (staff or family) is treated as family and friend, the more they relate to the other person as a whole person, which leads to person and relationship centered care.

◇ Lack of Interest in an Activity

A resident who is not interested in participating in a group activity can become frustrated and/ or can contribute to frustration among those who are participating. In one instance, two residents with dementia were sitting at the same dining room table during "activity stations" and were building a Lego structure. Resident A clearly was not interested in participating. Over the course of 20 minutes she asked eight times to discontinue her participation in the game ("Can we put this away?" and "Are we finished?"). Direct care partners were present in the area and heard these requests but did not respond to them. The repeated requests from resident A eventually caused resident B to become frustrated. At one point, resident B angrily pounded on the Lego structure with her hand and then picked it up and slammed it on the table. It crashed on the table and floor and broke into many small pieces.[34] Needless to say, no one at the table was able to enjoy the activity after that.

Intervention is crucial at the first signs of a resident's disinterest and willingness to discontinue participation in an activity. Do not wait until the resident's frustration builds up and triggers angry reactions from other residents. The care partner should help the resident to disengage from any activity she or he is clearly no longer interested in, and may want to offer an opportunity to participate in a different, personally meaningful activity or help the resident leave the activity area if desired.

Direct care partners need to pay close attention to the nonverbal signs and body language of residents that may indicate frustration or lack of interest in the activity, such as repeatedly looking outside the activity room, facial expressions indicating boredom, and so forth. Some residents do not want to continue to participate in an activity, but because of cognitive impairment, lack of ability to verbally articulate their need, and/or physical immobility, they are unable to leave the area on their own. Others may express their needs verbally only after being prompted by care partners. For example, one resident repeatedly said, "I need to go," and after she was asked about it, she added, "Pee." This resident often had difficulty locating the public bathroom and her bedroom.

◆ Competition for Limited Resources

Many DHRRIs develop during arguments over who is entitled to use which resource and when, often exacerbated by misperceptions driven by memory loss and other cognitive disabilities caused by dementia. Examples of such resources include a preferred chair in the main activity or dining room, a table in the dining room, and television channel or remote. The nature of living in close quarters with many other residents with dementia often contributes to disagreements and conflicts over these and other limited available resources. This problem is typically more common in larger care homes that have 30 or more residents on a unit than in small-scale ones with 10 or so residents, although it also depends on the unique features of the care home's physical environment (such as layout), easy access to various shared resources, and other factors.

To avoid the development of these kinds of conflicts, all direct and non-direct care employees need to regularly work on instilling an atmosphere of sharing, fairness, and compromise; it is important to nurture, acknowledge, and reward acts of kindness, empathy, compassion, and generosity between residents. When faced with conflicts over a particular item or resource, care employees should avoid arguing with a resident who has a substantial cognitive disability about the facts (such as to whom a chair belongs) because in most situations this is likely to escalate the situation. Instead, encourage a compromise while taking into consideration the cognitive functions and disabilities of the residents involved.

Strive to understand the functional, psychological, or social meaning of the resident's preferred resource (such as a chair or table). For example, one resident repeatedly insisted on sitting in a chair located near the entrance to the main activity room over a several-month period, which often irritated and frustrated several other residents. Although she was unable to express it verbally due to cognitive deficits caused by her Alzheimer's disease, one possibility suggested by direct care partners was that she often needed to use the bathroom and wanted to avoid interrupting residents during group activities—something she was not articulating in words. This might have been an example of behavioral expressions driven by her attempt to meet her physical needs.

Identify and document patterns of recurring circumstances of competition for limited resources that trigger DHRRIs. It is not uncommon for these episodes to repeatedly take place among the same pairs of residents with dementia. Identifying these pairs should guide your care team's decisions regarding care partners' work assignments, residents' supervision, and targeted individualized preventive strategies with the two individuals. Typically, each resident in a pair involved in repeated DHRRIs has a unique role in the development of these episodes. For example, one tends to be the exhibitor while the other is more often harmed, although at times roles within certain dyads may reverse.

Ensure effective information transfer between direct care partners, including insights gleaned from direct observational assessments, to increase the likelihood of fair distribution of the limited available resources at the LTC home. As importantly, make sure that float staff, weekend staff, and external agency staff are all informed about triggers of DHRRIs that tend to occur in relation to competition between particular people for limited available resources at your residence.

◆ Competition for Direct Care Partners' Attention

Although the number of direct care partners is often insufficient in LTC homes,[160] it is important to make every possible effort to attend to residents' requests for attention. Competing for a direct care partner's attention has been reported as a trigger of DHRRIs.[14,6] One direct care partner reported the following: "When he sees me attending to another resident, he says, 'Come. Come. Come. Come.'"[14] Berg reports on a resident with dementia who swore and slammed the door when she did not get the full attention of direct care partners.[146]

A better, more accurate way to describe most of these requests is to view them as expressions of the basic need for recognition, affirmation, reassurance, and emotional support. The institution-centered term "request for attention" (or worse, the label "attention seeker") can easily lead to a lack of interest in proactively detecting residents' unmet needs. It is, of course, common for residents with dementia to make these repeated requests due to short-term memory loss, such as when a resident forgets that she or he already received, for instance, food or medication not long ago. The use of gentle and frequent reminders is obviously important, but there is an equally important need to identify the emotional or other needs underlying these requests. For example, a resident with dementia continuously deprived of human touch may tend to feel anxious when left alone for significant periods and thus may repeatedly seek comforting touch.

Knowing the resident and her or his physical, emotional, psychological, and social needs and addressing them proactively and promptly is key. If requests are ignored, the unmet needs underlying them tend to grow, which is likely to result in distressing and harmful behavioral expressions. Until adequate staffing levels are required, funded, and implemented, this problem is likely to continue and present a daily challenge for residents and direct care partners. It is, however, first and foremost an area to be addressed during care employees' training programs.

On a regular basis, the direct care partner should carefully assess the resident's underlying physical and psychological needs and the causes behind repeated requests for attention. Direct observation and timely physical and medical examination—such as noting facial expressions or body language that may indicate pain or skin irritation—are essential to identifying the causes of some of these requests. Psychological causes may include loneliness and the need for companionship or human touch, as noted earlier.

My own qualitative study[161] has shown that a subgroup of residents with dementia experience restlessness and anxiety when left on their own for significant periods. The study concluded that direct care partners need to do whatever they possibly can to provide these residents with timely reassurance and emotional support to alleviate their emotional distress and optimize their psychological well-being.[161] Direct care partners can serve as a lifeline for these residents with dementia during these times.

Often, a resident's requests are situational and relate to factors in the physical or social environment. For example, a resident may become irritated by glare coming from outside or cold temperature in the room. Timely identification of these factors can often bring about discontinuation of these requests when the source of irritation is eliminated.

Remember to always look for the underlying human need before labeling the resident as "attention seeker"; do not automatically assume that a resident's repeated requests are solely for attention. Once a resident has been labeled, direct care partners are much less likely to seek to identify and fulfill her or his underlying needs.

In the context of low staffing levels, it can help to train volunteers in dementia-specific supportive approaches and communication techniques. One of the best examples of a successful volunteer program is the Volunteer Services Department of Baycrest Centre for Geriatric Care (Toronto, Ontario, Canada). Among other essential roles, these trained volunteers serve as eating assistants, companions to residents with advanced dementia who have difficulty eating independently. The attentive presence of these carefully selected and well-trained volunteers often helps prevent, detect, and resolve many problems caused by direct care partners' limited ability to attend to every request for assistance from residents with dementia. For information about the Eating Assistance Program, including the training material, see Robertson and colleagues[162] as well as Szpiech.[163]

◇ *Perception of Unfair Treatment at Mealtime*

Distressing and harmful episodes between residents can often result from their perceptions of unfair treatment during mealtime. In one case, a resident with dementia became anxious and angrily yelled at direct care partners and other residents when he thought his meal portions were smaller than those received by other residents. In another episode in the dining room, a resident asked a care partner, "Why are you serving her before me?"[35] Mead[164] describes how a similar situation was resolved: "After staff learned that, as the head of his family, he had always been served first, they began giving him his meals before other residents, and the outbursts stopped."

It is important to learn about former dietary habits and mealtime routines. Review a resident's lifelong and current eating habits to help assess whether the meal portions are meeting her or his dietary needs. Consult with the resident's close family members and dietitian to identify ways to provide personally desirable meal portions within the resident's nutritional needs and restrictions.

Serving every resident in the order he or she desires in care environments with a large number of residents and insufficient direct care partners is often not realistic. In these situations, it is helpful to (1) try to understand why the resident wants to be served first (unmet need, need to use the bathroom, difficulty waiting, or fear that the food will run out and the resident will remain hungry); (2) determine whether this is an isolated or repeated request; and (3) use your best judgment while balancing between providing equal treatment to all residents and preventing contagious frustration, anxiety, and anger leading to conflicts in the dining room.

As mentioned elsewhere, avoid arguing with the resident about the facts. You can apologize sincerely if for some reason it is not possible to meet a resident's request. For example, you could say, "I am sorry, Mr. Smith, but we ran out of sandwiches. I will make sure to save you one tomorrow. Would you like me to make you toast with cheese instead?"

Institution-Specific Triggers

Beyond the many restrictions on one's life that often result from living in any congregate care setting, and the triggers that arise from them, some triggers can result from the rules and practices used in a particular care home. These are factors that, once discovered, can be addressed by owners, administration, or direct care partners.

◇ Lack of Consistent Daily Routine

Many people with dementia struggle to cope with changes in daily routine and structure in various domains of their lives (examples include self-care, personally meaningful engagement, nighttime sleep, and transitions into an unfamiliar environment). Lack of structure or change in routine often cause may residents with dementia to feel distressed and anxious, which can contribute to the development of distressing behavioral expressions, including engagement in DHRRIs. Joyce Simard states, "It is generally accepted that structure and routine help residents who have Alzheimer's disease feel less anxious and will increase their active participation in activities."[165]

Remember, small changes taken for granted by people who are cognitively intact may be extremely difficult for people with dementia to cope with, and they can be a major source of distress for these individuals. Ellenbogen,[143] who lives with dementia, shares, "If my routine is different on a particular day, it throws me off very quickly."

It is important for the LTC home and care employees to provide a consistent, fairly repetitive daily routine. However, this does not mean that the exact same type of activities should be provided to the residents every day. Occasionally introducing reasonable changes in the daily routine may work well as long as the changes are based on residents' or close family members' input and as long as direct care partners provide frequent reminders to the residents about the planned changes. Changes in the daily activity schedule should be communicated in a timely manner to residents verbally *and* in writing (using elder- and dementia-friendly font and contrast) to accommodate for short-term memory deficits. Certain residents with dementia tend to become irritable and anxious when they wait too long for an activity to start or when an activity is canceled and they were not adequately notified about the change or offered an alternative activity to engage in. This in turn can lead to their expression of repetitive questions (e.g., "Why am I sitting here when nothing is going on?"), which can frustrate other residents and trigger DHRRIs.

As much as possible, bring medical, dental, podiatric, and other diagnostic and treatment services to the LTC home to limit disruption in the person's daily routine caused by the need to go out to appointments in the community.

Although offering a consistent daily routine is very important to residents with dementia, there are times when common sense warrants flexibility. Being flexible and ready to change the daily routine is helpful when the advantages of doing so clearly outweigh the disadvantages. For example, in one assisted living residence for people with dementia, residents and direct care partners started dancing spontaneously to the music being played in the activity room during downtime. It started when a care employee invited a couple of residents to dance with her. As the dancing continued, other residents joined the unplanned activity, which clearly brought joy to the residents. After about 5 minutes of dancing, a recreation assistant walked into the activity room and said that she had to turn off the music, saying, "Our schedule says trivia, and then we will do short stories." The positive momentum of the enjoyable dance abruptly came to a halt. In this case, adhering too strictly to the activity schedule represented a missed opportunity to improve these residents' emotional states.[34] As explained by Simard,[165]

> Although there is a schedule of when programs begin and end, it can be very loose. Although most days follow a predictable routine, the routine may change because a program residents enjoyed the day before does not work on this day or a group of children are visiting and all eyes are on them. "Go with the flow" is the motto of most activity professionals.

Cindy Kincaid adds,[166]

> It's okay if the activity doesn't work. How many times have we started an activity and after 10 minutes we see that nobody is paying attention except us? It's okay to stop it. Do something else. Be willing to switch gears on a drop of a dime.

Care homes that provide high-quality care to people with dementia typically offer a structured, consistent, and repetitive daily routine including a rich, diverse, meaningful, enriching, appropriate, and dementia stage–specific activity program. These programs, however, also pay careful attention to incorporating adequate rest periods between activities that are ideally tailored to individual residents' needs and preferences. It is important to provide these programs not just during the day, but also in the evening and, as needed, during the night (for those experiencing repeated and extensive nighttime wakefulness).

When such programs are successful in engaging residents with dementia meaningfully over the course of the day and evening, the residents tend to experience lower levels of anxiety and distressing behavioral expressions.[167] According to Ashok Bharucha, "It is precisely during unstructured time spent in shared spaces free of care-related activities that residents are likely to receive the least staff supervision, and episodes of resident-to-resident physical aggression are likely to go unnoticed."[168]

Simard proposes a "lifestyle approach" to establish a daily routine for residents that is familiar and fills their days with meaningful activities,[165] and leading experts from the Alzheimer's Association (Massachusetts Chapter) recommended that structured activities should be offered 7 days per week for at least 8 hours per day in LTC homes.[169]

◇ Boredom and Insufficient Meaningful Engagement

Boredom, understimulation, and insufficient meaningful engagement are factors that commonly contribute to distressing behavioral expressions among people with dementia.[170] Research studies show that nursing home residents are not engaged in activities during the majority of their time[171,172] and, thus, many manifest a greater number of distressing behavioral expressions when not occupied in structured or social activities.[171] One direct observation study in 36 LTC homes examined the activity patterns, behavioral expressions, and affect of

406 residents (average age 84 years), the majority of whom (77%) had dementia. When residents were left to self-initiate activity during unstructured time, they were found to be more disengaged, spent most of their time doing nothing, and were more anxious, sad, or "agitated" than when they were engaged in organized activities.[173]

In addition, preliminary findings from my early study on DHRRIs[13] in two dementia care homes found lower levels of these episodes during residents' participation in structured activities than in times when the same residents did not participate in activities. As observed by a direct care partner, "Maybe they're sitting around with nothing to do, and that's when they get on each other's nerves."[14] When a nursing home resident was asked, "What is the worst thing about living here?" he answered quickly, "Having nothing to do. Sitting in the chair like a goddamn idiot."[63] Crump adds that "failure to provide opportunities for activities is tantamount to abuse of persons with dementia."[174]

Regarding the meaningfulness of activities, Power cautions that "failure-free" activities are usually devoid of meaning. Instead of offering failure-free activities, he suggests asking, "How can we facilitate an activity where people can succeed, but where they can also (safely) fail from time to time?"[65] For example, one resident with dementia was asked by a recreation therapist to write her own name on a whiteboard in front of a large group of other residents with dementia. She was unable to do so, which not surprisingly caused her tremendous frustration and embarrassment in front of her peers. Had the therapist known the resident's current cognitive and writing ability, this heartbreaking situation could have been avoided. Instead, if this resident had been interested in trying and if she could tolerate it without causing her significant frustration, a one-on-one activity with her in a private room may have enabled her to practice writing her name with a trained facilitator. Having someone be fully present with her, providing reassurance and encouragement as well as gentle cueing, could have enabled her to gradually improve her ability to write her name (if her cognitive deficits required for this task were not already permanently damaged). "Failing safely" with a trusted facilitator during this more dignified process would probably not have caused this woman the level of frustration and humiliation she experienced during the group activity.

Many residents with middle- to late-stage dementia have difficulty initiating engagement in personally meaningful activities and need encouragement, assistance, guidance, reminders, or cueing to start such engagement. These and other residents with dementia may also experience difficulty sustaining their engagement in activities and similarly need guidance, cueing, and encouragement to continue and to benefit from it without becoming frustrated or irritable. Every person is different, and brain disease affects each individual in unique ways. Therefore, meaningful engagement should always be individually tailored to the person's current preferences, abilities, and disabilities.

◆ Evenings and Weekends as Risk Factors

Evenings and weekends are time periods of increased vulnerability for residents with dementia. One study in Connecticut nursing homes found that half of DHRRIs requiring police involvement occurred between 4 and 10 p.m.[6] My study found that 44% of fatal resident-to-resident incidents occurred during the evening hours, 14% took place during the night, and 38% took place during the weekend.[29]

The cumulative effect of several factors may contribute to these findings. These include, among others, lower staffing levels, less active presence of managers, lower levels of meaningful engagement in activities, and increased tiredness and irritability among residents with dementia during the evening hours. These factors, along with higher numbers of float and external agency staff, make weekends vulnerability days.

To avoid DHRRIs during these periods, it is important to educate owners, administrators, and all direct and non-direct care employees that evenings and weekends represent serious vulnerability time periods requiring care community–wide attention. In planning evening care and when allocating resources for this time period, they should take into consideration the fact that tiredness among residents with dementia during these hours is very common and that it often contributes to increased irritability, restlessness, and anxiety, and thus risk of involvement in DHRRIs. Coping with a serious brain disease every single minute of the day means that, without adequate rest periods, many individuals are physically and emotionally exhausted in the late afternoon hours and evening.

As has been noted previously, it is essential to provide adequate staffing levels of well-trained direct care partners, including the active presence of experienced and skilled managers (to provide guidance, experiential learning, support, and supervision to direct care partners). In one LTC home, half of DHRRIs were reported to have occurred between 5:00 and 8:00 p.m. A study in the home evaluated the protective role of staffing levels on DHRRIs during evening hours and found that a higher number of direct care partners during the evenings was associated with reduced DHRRIs.[175]

In addition to safe staffing levels, it is important to provide meaningful engagement to residents during the evening hours and on weekends. Enjoyable evening activities that are calming, quiet, low intensity, and cognitively less demanding than daytime activities should be developed and implemented thoughtfully, with the aim of avoiding overstimulation of already tired residents. Striking a good balance between periods of rest and organized meaningful engagement is key. Some of the best care homes offer meaningful engagement to residents with dementia until 8:00 p.m. The owners and administrators of these care homes know that meaningful engagement is one of the best ways to prevent DHRRIs and other problems. They know that the benefits and healthcare savings gained through investment in recreation staff time during evening hours and weekends outweighs the short-term costs.

In one care home dedicated to caring for elders with dementia, frequent distressing resident-to-resident incidents took place during the evening hours. An intervention was developed to prevent these incidents. Immediately after dinner, trained volunteers led a 30-minute walking group for three consecutive days; these were compared with four days of the week in which walking groups were not offered. The outcome was a 30% reduction in incidents classified as aggressive (resident-to-resident and resident-to-staff) during the 24 hours after the walking groups.[176]

In general, the use of float and external agency staff during the weekends should be eliminated, or if not possible, reduced to a minimum. These individuals are typically less familiar with the residents with dementia, their life histories and unique care needs, abilities, cognitive disabilities, preferences, behavioral expressions, and their risk of involvement in DHRRIs. As mentioned elsewhere, building and maintaining close trusting relationships with residents is critical for prevention of DHRRIs.

◇ *Repeated but Unmet Requests for Assistance*

Deficits in short-term memory may contribute to DHRRIs. Certain residents with dementia who have already received their medications but do not recall this can start swearing when denied by care partners; this kind of expression can trigger harmful interactions with other residents. When a resident with dementia walked around the care home repeatedly asking in a concerned voice, "When is my daughter coming?" and "Is my daughter coming today?," another resident who was waiting for his breakfast gradually became irritated by her questions and said angrily and loudly, "Stupid lady."[34]

It is important for the direct care partner to immediately address any request for information or assistance, no matter how repetitive, made by a resident with dementia. If you are busy, approach the resident and reassure her or him that once you finish the task you are currently engaged in, you will assist her or him. Make sure you tell the resident how long you anticipate it will take you to return. If your task takes you longer than expected to complete, provide frequent reminders and reassurance to the resident or ask another direct care partner to provide updates on when you'll return, or ask that co-worker to assist the resident.

It is helpful to conduct assessments to identify and document the time periods during which a resident tends to seek assistance from direct care partners, so that this assistance can be proactively provided *before* the requests get to a point in which they annoy other residents. Document these times in the person's care plan so all direct and indirect care partners as well as float staff, weekend staff, and external agency staff are aware of them.

◇ Problematic Seating Arrangements

Problems in seating arrangements, such as in dining rooms and activity rooms, are a frequent trigger of incidents between residents with dementia; one study showed that seating arrangement was the primary trigger in 30% of DHRRIs.[13] In one reported case, two residents with a long history of DHRRIs were seated next to one another during an organized activity. One resident grew frustrated with the other, who she said spoke "endlessly," put her hand on the resident's mouth in an intrusive way during a group activity, and said, "Would you shut up?" In response, the resident whose personal space was invaded threatened to stab her, grabbed her shirt, and pushed her.[13]

Grethe Berg, author of the book *The Importance of Food and Mealtimes in Dementia Care: The Table Is Set*,[146] describes the problematic nature of mealtimes in a care home with unstable staffing patterns and breakfast routines that changed from day to day: "Mealtimes were characterized more by accidental circumstances than being a safe and secure element of daily life in the unit. There was lack of routines and continuity both for staff and for residents." Specifically, lack of intentionality and thoughtfulness in planning the seating arrangement during meals contributed to tensions between residents as well as avoidable situations that threatened their dignity and personhood.

Many DHRRIs can be prevented or at least mitigated by implementing a consistent seating arrangement policy, such as predesignated seating in the dining room with name tags placed on the tables that can be easily read by older adults and those with dementia. The predictability created by this consistency can be tremendously helpful for residents with dementia, especially those experiencing visuospatial disorientation and wayfinding difficulties. However, care partners need to regularly assess the need for changes in seating arrangements, as residents' dementia may progress and their new cognitive disabilities may contribute to misunderstandings and misperceptions between tablemates who previously got along well.

Consider changing the seating arrangement when residents who sit together repeatedly irritate and upset each other or engage in DHRRIs. Avoid allowing too much time to pass before making a change. Carefully monitor tense arguments between tablemates with dementia and consider making a prompt change when you are concerned about psychological and/or physical harm to one or more residents involved. When implementing a change in the seating arrangement, offer the resident an equally good chair whenever possible. Going forward, make sure the residents who do not get along or have a history of DHRRIs do not sit close to each other.[177] Of course, constraints dictated by the physical environment (such as lack of alternative spaces for mealtime) may make the implementation of this recommendation complex and challenging. Do your best to brainstorm creative solutions with your co-workers.

Research has found that the same pairs of residents with dementia tend to engage in recurring DHRRIs.[13] Being proactive in identifying, documenting, and carefully supervising pairs of residents can increase the likelihood that repeated episodes are identified early and that changes in seating can be implemented before such episodes escalate and result in harm to one or more residents. In one extreme case, two tablemates engaged in repeated tense and upsetting verbal interactions over a period of 3 months and 10 days before a new direct care partner noticed it and advocated for a change in the seating arrangement shortly after she started working at the care home. The change of seating took minutes to implement, and no incidents were observed between the two residents after the change was made.[34] The distressing arguments between the two residents with dementia had been *normalized*; it took the arrival of a new care employee to notice them and advocate for a solution.

Finally, to the extent possible, it is usually a good idea to have residents with similar cognitive function levels sit next to each other, while direct care partners regularly observe and monitor how they get along. At times, though, as mentioned previously, residents at different stages of dementia may get along very well, enjoying companionship and peer support during mealtime.

◆ Clearing a Way Through a Crowded Area

A common situation that has been found to contribute to DHRRIs in a nursing home is hindrance of a resident's easy movement throughout certain areas in the home.[24] A resident's movement may be impeded by the presence of other residents, such as when an area is too crowded to move through easily or when the resident in a narrow hallway is walking behind a frail resident who uses a walker or walks more slowly.

Cluttered space and crowding of equipment—for instance, medication carts, cleaning carts, walkers, and wheelchairs positioned in ways that limit or block walking paths in public spaces—may cause residents to experience frustration as they try to navigate their way around them or move them, which can contribute to verbal and physical conflicts between residents, whether or not they have dementia.[177,178] We can imagine the frustration of a resident with dementia who needs to use the public bathroom but is stuck behind a line of residents trying to reposition a medication cart that blocks the path in the hallway. It is important to remember that tasks that are simple for cognitively intact and physically able people, such as moving a wheelchair that is blocking one's way, can be very challenging and complex for a frail resident with middle- to-late-stage dementia who uses a walker.

All care employees (direct care partners and non-direct care staff such as housekeeping, dietary aides, maintenance, front desk, and office staff) need to regularly observe physical spaces and make sure hallways and other common walking paths are not overcrowded with residents or cluttered with equipment that could restrict free and safe passage by residents. All care employees should be trained, and reminded, to anticipate and proactively address this issue.

In addition to minimizing clutter and other hindrances, care employees should plan ahead to minimize crowded situations, such as the transition period between the end of a group activity and the arrival of a group of residents for a meal in the dining room. Timely assistance to the group leader by a direct care partner prior to the end of the group activity and immediately after its conclusion is critical for a smooth, stress-free, and safe transition of the group of residents to their destination.

Pay special attention to frail residents, whether or not they have dementia, who tend to walk slowly. Proactively and gently redirect them aside when you notice a resident behind them and becoming impatient and frustrated. Also, if you know that a certain resident tends to become impatient with the walking pace of other residents, plan ahead of time and when possible encourage him or her to walk before the residents who walk slowly or take another route, when the physical layout of your care home allows it.

It is important to try to understand what makes a particular resident walk fast in overcrowded places. Some residents may walk faster than usual when they are concerned that their seat in the dining room or television lounge will be taken by another resident. In these situations, it can be helpful to reassure the resident that her or his seat will be saved (to the extent that it is possible to do so).

◇ Unwanted Entry of Animals into the Care Home

When planned carefully, facilitated professionally, and supervised attentively, interaction with trained pets (also called animal-assisted therapy) can bring tremendous joy to many residents with dementia, and this meaningful engagement can have calming effects on them.[127,60,179] Although many elders love dogs and cats, others prefer not to spend time with them; this wish must be fully respected.

It is important to conduct a survey with residents and close family members to identify residents who prefer not to participate in activities with pets or for whom the presence of certain animals may be a source of distress. Include in the evaluation information about fears, allergies, and other possible sensitivities residents may experience in the presence of certain animals. Document the results of your survey in the residents' care plans and make the information accessible to all direct care and recreation therapists. Then, make every effort to avoid exposing these residents to animals. As importantly, observation of residents' verbal and nonverbal signs during pet therapy activities should provide helpful insights into the ways in which certain individuals react to particular pets. Lifelong preferences tend to continue in many elders with dementia, but they may also change at some point into the disease.

Make sure that each trained animal (whether visiting or living permanently at the care home) goes through timely health examinations and receives vaccinations as required by state and federal regulations governing your care home. This will assist you in avoiding exposing vulnerable and frail residents to unhealthy or unvaccinated pets.

Unwanted visits from animals at the care home, however, may distress certain residents with dementia and, in some cases, may be perceived to or actually compromise their personal hygiene. One morning, for instance, a cat entered a secured dementia care home from the backyard. A tense argument about the cat developed between two residents. Resident A, who did not like cats and was concerned that it would bring diseases into the care home, tried to make it go back outside by chasing it, shouting at it, and attempting to hit it with her shoe. Resident B, who had had several cats in the past, could not stand the potential harm to the cat and tried to protect it. The argument intensified, and the two residents cursed each other. Later on the same day, a physical altercation developed between the two residents after another cat entered the care home from the backyard. Resident B pushed resident A when she tried to direct the cat out of the care home with her shoe. The push caused resident A to fall to the floor, where she started cursing resident B, who responded, "I'll kill you." The care employees intervened too slowly—only after resident A had fallen.

After these recurring episodes, a simple and brief observation in the backyard of the care home revealed that a large dumpster had been placed very close to the external fence of the backyard. Cats were regularly attracted to the food remnants and other garbage in the dumpster. From there, the smell of the food served to residents attracted them into the care home. My colleague Nurit Shtruzman and I drove to the Health and Sanitary Department of the local municipality and asked that the dumpster be moved to another location. Once it was removed, the cats stopped entering the care home, which eliminated the trigger for these distressing and potentially harmful episodes.

Triggers Related to Other Residents

This section addresses factors largely triggered by the actions of other residents that threaten or are perceived as threatening the sense of privacy and personal safety of a resident, who in response reacts in a defensive way to protect his or her own rights and safety. Many of these factors have to do with violations or perceived violations of personal space and private space (such as a bedroom), as well as those factors related to actual or perceived right to possession of personal belongings and objects. Other factors and triggers are verbal and physical disruption of one's activity or enhanced frustration caused by distressing vocal expressions by other residents and other verbal, physical, or behavioral expressions that bring a resident to a "breaking point."

Finally, the section also addresses the important but largely overlooked issues of racist remarks as well as harassment of residents who are lesbian, gay, bisexual, or transgender in care homes. Awareness and sensitivity to these factors should motivate owners and administrators of care homes to ensure that adequate staffing levels of well-trained direct care partners are provided at all times so that all employees will be able to remain vigilant and well positioned to detect and promptly respond to early signs of distress, anxiety, and fear underlying these triggers. Most importantly, they will be able to proactively identify and meet the residents' unmet human needs that often contribute or directly cause these episodes.

Whatever occurs in reaction to other residents, though, it is up to the care partner and team to investigate and, where possible, anticipate the needs of the residents in their care. As advocate Kate Swaffer,[180] who lives with young-onset dementia, says, "Of course we will display 'challenging behaviors' if no one bothers to understand our frustrations, or our needs."

A review of 85 resident-to-resident incidents in two secured care homes for people with dementia found that in the majority of them, an observable situational frustration contributed to the development of the episode.[13] Another study examining the circumstances surrounding the deaths of 105 elders as a result of resident-to-resident incidents identified situational frustrations (for instance, invasion of one's personal space, unwanted entry into one's bedroom, and distressing episodes between roommates) as frequent triggers of these traumatic and tragic deaths.[29]

Violations of Personal Space

A common trigger of DHRRIs revolves around the various ways in which a resident's personal space is invaded by another resident with dementia. These incidents include invasion of the immediate area around the resident, unwanted touch, a resident following and/or staying close to another resident, and unwanted entries of a resident into another resident's bedroom. According to Phair and Good,[181] entering the "intimate zone" of 6–18 inches from a person with dementia without an invitation or explanation may result in an "aggressive" reaction. More accurately, these reactions by residents with dementia whose space is invaded should be considered defensive and protective in nature, not truly aggressive, even if the consequences of such reactions (such as pushing away the invading resident) could result in serious physical injuries.

◆ Invasion of Personal Space

Invasion of other residents' personal space, especially by residents with middle- to late-stage dementia who are able to walk or move independently (including with the aid of a cane, walker, or wheelchair), is a very common trigger of DHRRIs. Personal space is defined as "the invisible boundary that each person maintains between [him- or herself] and others, which serves as a buffer from real or perceived threats."[182] It is important to emphasize that many residents who are unable to walk independently are still able to invade other residents' personal space, such as by using their wheelchair in a way that gets too close to or makes physical contact with another resident, whether intentionally or not. Worse, there are several reports in the research literature of residents either with or without dementia who used their wheelchairs in ways that physically harmed other residents (for example, bumping or ramming the wheelchair into another resident). In my early study,[13] one resident's foot was observed to frequently touch other residents' legs during mealtimes, causing angry verbal and physical responses toward her. It is possible that the touch was uncontrolled (i.e., due to nervous leg movement), although it may have been done deliberately, as was suggested by certain direct care partners.

It is interesting to note that residents who were physically injured during resident-to-resident incidents have been found in previous research to be more physically independent than residents with no injury; in other words, needing extensive assistance and being severely dependent in activities of daily living was associated with reductions in being injured by other residents.[26] This finding might be explained by the fact that cognitively impaired residents who tend to be more ambulatory are more likely to engage in or find themselves in situations that instigate DHRRIs (such as invading other residents' personal space or bedrooms). The association between residents' "wandering" (the biomedical term used in the cited study; traditionally describing "unpredictable pacing without a goal" or "aimless, meaningless movement"[183]) and being physically injured during these incidents may provide indirect support for this possibility.

A word about words is warranted here. The term "wandering" should no longer be used in the context of continual movement by residents with dementia within the various physical spaces of their care home. A more suitable person-directed care term may be "searching"[184]; in other words, the resident with dementia *searches* for something meaningful to do, people she or he feels close to, or even a bathroom.

These movements in this population are nearly always purposeful, even when it is not immediately clear to us what that purpose is and the person is unable to convey it in words. One study in a care home for people with dementia reported that direct care partners rarely used the term *wandering* during months of the researcher's observations and interviews. Instead, the care partners used terms such as "getting busy," "moving," "moving on," "pacing," or "walking" to describe residents' continual movement in a meaningful way. These words connote or connect with purpose. They represent the important but often overlooked difference between a biomedical "language of limits" (which restricts language to the realm of medical concerns and excludes the experiential and interpersonal context of the resident) and a "language of openings" (which "focuses on the self and the lifeworld of the person, thereby honoring context").[183]

It is crucial for all direct care partners to observe residents vigilantly and to promptly and gently redirect those who tend to invade other residents' personal space. Avoid waiting until the invasion results in a verbally or physically harmful reaction by a resident who feels that his or her space has been violated. Remember that a substantial portion (44%–63%) of deadly incidents between residents were classified as "push–fall" incidents; many of these harmful physical contacts occurred as a result of invasion of personal space (as Chapter 1 demonstrated).

All employees (not only direct care partners but also food service, housekeeping, maintenance, and clerical staff, as well as clergy) should be trained in early recognition and timely redirection techniques and should be expected to redirect residents away from other residents' personal space when they notice such impending intrusions. In one incident, a resident with more advanced dementia stood very close to another resident who was sitting quietly at the dining room table, waiting for her breakfast. All direct care partners were in residents' bedrooms providing personal care. The resident whose personal space was being invaded gradually became frustrated and angry and eventually pushed the other resident away from her. A housekeeping staff member who was vacuuming the hallway noticed the episode. She quietly turned off the vacuum cleaner, approached the "invading" resident, and redirected her away from the area. No additional episodes were observed between the two residents for the rest of the morning.[13]

It is important to proactively engage residents with tendencies to invade other residents' personal space in personally meaningful activities to decrease the likelihood that they will become intrusive during downtimes. However, continue to pay attention to these residents during group activities, as invasion of other residents' personal space is not uncommon during participation in group activities. Having a second care employee next to or inside the activity room, to assist the group leader in meeting residents' varied needs (including the need to keep one's personal space free of invasions), is a good practice. I have seen this help prevent many DHRRIs.

Care employees should be reminded to avoid normalization of invasion of residents' personal space. Although such invasions are common in LTC homes where residents with dementia are cared for, each person has a right to privacy and protection of their personal space. Normalizing invasions can violate this right and put these and other residents at risk of harm. Direct care partners need to remain vigilant and proactively engage in efforts to extend and protect the personal space of all residents with dementia but especially those who tend to respond to these intrusions with defensive and protective behavioral expressions that could result in harm to other residents or themselves.[185]

◈ *Unwanted Touch*

Unwanted physical contact can represent a form of invasion of personal space and is a frequent trigger of DHRRIs. A study[185] among 24 nursing home residents with severe cognitive impairment experiencing high levels of distressing behavioral expressions examined the relationship between interpersonal distance, including touching, and behavioral expressions classified as aggressive. The study found that "the amount of 'aggressive' behaviors manifested when residents were touched was greater than when they were displayed at any other interpersonal distance" (i.e., less than 1 foot, between 1 and 3 feet, more than 3 feet, and being alone). The findings suggest that residents with dementia may interpret unwanted touching as a violation of their personal space.

A common occurrence is when a resident with advanced dementia touches the hand of a tablemate during mealtime. For example, resident A often reached out to touch people in a friendly way. Resident B did not like to be touched. In the lounge one evening, resident A reached out to touch B, who in response struck her in the head, causing a 2-inch laceration above her left eye.[6] Another resident, with vascular dementia, often reached out with her hand toward direct care partners and other residents in an attempt to grab their arms as they walked by her dining room table. Close observation over several days suggested that she tended to do it when she was worried and anxious.[34] Merrie Kaas[186] explains this need for physical contact: "If I am feeling fearful, I want to touch someone and maybe bring them in to make me feel less fearful." The need to identify the unmet human needs underlying these physical expressions (otherwise potentially perceived as annoying) is clear.

It is incumbent on care employees to remain as alert as possible to these attempts and promptly but gently redirect the resident's hand from the other resident. Each resident's comprehension level should guide your approach from nonverbal to verbal and/or gentle physical redirection. If the attempts persist despite your efforts, consider repositioning the resident's seat out of touching range. Provide frequent emotional support and reassurance to residents for whom anxiety may underlie these physical contacts. Try to find out whether the resident is seeking assistance but is unable to express it in words.

As in all cases of behavioral expressions, try to identify the root cause (unmet need) that leads to the physical contact (such as feelings of loneliness or anxiety and need for emotional support or companionship, or a need for assistance with a task). It is not uncommon for the nature of the physical touch itself to be useful in identifying its underlying human need. Looking closely and continuously at the person, her or his nonverbal expressions, and the actual physical touch can sometimes reveal it.

Provide frequent but gentle reminders (quietly) to the resident with dementia who is able to understand and sufficiently retain this information to respect the personal space of other residents. Remember that if the resident were cognitively intact, she or he would probably be embarrassed by her or his intrusive physical contact. Respond and intervene in ways that helps the resident save face and preserve dignity.

If the unwanted touching continues despite all your efforts to detect and fulfill the unmet need underlying it, consider assigning more tolerant residents to sit next to the person.

Encourage and instill a sense of empathy and compassion between residents who are more cognitively intact and those with more advanced dementia.

◆ Repeatedly Following Another Resident

Occasionally you may see a resident with advanced dementia following another resident. This individual may do so frequently and/or for prolonged periods of time in ways that are perceived as annoying or intrusive by the other resident. At times, it can result in a defensive verbal or physical reaction that can result in harm. There are several reasons why a resident might tend to stay close to another resident in this way. Below are some examples:

- Anxiety or fear of being left alone

- Not knowing what to do next

- Not knowing where one is

- Difficulty reaching desired destinations in the care home

- Wanting to initiate engagement in a personally meaningful activity but being unable to

- Perceiving another resident as providing a sense of security

- Misidentifying the resident as a relative or old friend

A spouse of a resident with dementia said, "I found out that when they are alone, they are frightened. That's why they follow you." Sometimes, the behavioral expression may be psychologically beneficial for the resident and is received well or at least tolerated by the other resident. However, in other situations it can be annoying and frustrating to the other resident, who may experience it as a violation of privacy, an intrusion of personal space, or an interruption of solitary activities. These situations can lead to a buildup of increased frustration or negative emotion, resulting in the resident reaching a breaking point and pushing away or hitting the resident in an attempt to create some space and privacy.

Remember to avoid labeling a resident with dementia with stigmatizing terms or comments such as "the stalker" or "She is like Velcro" (I heard these unhelpful terms used in an assisted living residence dedicated to caring for elders with dementia). Instead, observe the resident closely to identify the underlying needs behind this tendency and to find out the extent to which it is emotionally, psychologically, socially, or physically beneficial to the resident. Address the underlying needs, such as by providing frequent reassurance, companionship, reminders of upcoming events, and engagement in personally meaningful activities. In certain situations a trained volunteer or private companion can assist in meeting the resident's needs for companionship and reassurance in an environment the resident may perceive as becoming less familiar and more distressing or frightening.

Determine the extent to which the tendency to follow another resident annoys and frustrates the resident on the receiving end or whether it is tolerated or even encouraged by her or him (in some dyads, it may take place in the context of friendship between the two residents). In my early study of this phenomenon, one resident with dementia was compassionate and helpful to another resident who also had dementia (the two shared a bedroom), but she also yelled at her and occasionally even hit her when she became frustrated by the things she said or did.

It is important to develop and consistently implement an individualized strategy that respects the emotional and psychological needs and wishes of both residents. Document the intervention and its outcomes and modify it when it does not bring about the desired outcomes. To the extent possible, consult with residents (who have the cognitive ability to do so) and their families to learn about their wishes, needs, insights, and suggestions for more effective approaches and strategies.

Remain vigilant and redirect a resident to another location when her or his following another resident annoys and frustrates the latter. Try to engage the resident in a personally meaningful activity to keep her or him away from the other resident. Remember, however, that simply redirecting the resident to another part of the care home may bring about temporary relief to the other resident, but the resident may still return to that resident. When this happens, try to figure out the unmet need driving it and then proactively meet it.

There can be situations where the attempts to walk after another resident are frequent and clearly annoy the other resident. When all efforts to identify the resident's underlying unmet need do not succeed and when ongoing redirection efforts do not work, consider having one of the residents participate in a local day program specializing in caring for people with dementia for several hours during the day (when such a program is available in a nearby location). The structured separation of the two residents can reduce the negative effects of the intrusions on the resident during those hours. However, direct care partners at the adult day center should be advised to monitor the resident's emotional state in case she or he becomes distressed by being separated from the other resident. When the resident taken to the day center is the one following the other, care partners should observe her or him to determine whether she or he initiates walking repeatedly after one of that center's participants.

In situations of serious concern for the safety of one or both residents involved in these episodes, the IDT, in close consultation with the resident's family, may need to consider moving one of the residents to another suitable care unit within the care home (when one exists), or to a different care home, to prevent potential physical harm during these interactions. That said, the emotional reactions and psychological states of both residents should be carefully assessed after the separation to determine the effects of the intervention, because in certain situations one of the residents may experience a loss of a meaningful relationship or friendship due to the move.

◆ Unwanted Entry into the Bedroom or Bathroom of Another Resident

Unwanted entry into another resident's bedroom is a very common situation in LTC homes in general and in those specializing in caring for people with dementia. It is also a common trigger of DHRRIs. My own study[29] showed that among the 50 fatal resident-to-resident incidents that took place inside bedrooms, 19 (38%) occurred in the fatally injured resident's bedroom and seven (14%) occurred inside the exhibitor resident's bedroom; the remainder occurred between roommates in a shared bedroom (38%) or other location such as an area between two bedrooms. Another study[30] in U.S. nursing homes found that of 69 fatal resident-to-resident incidents, 34 (49%) took place inside a bedroom; of these, 12 incidents occurred in the exhibitor's bedroom, 11 in the deceased resident's bedroom, and 11 inside a shared bedroom.

For example, a resident with dementia may believe that another resident is her or his spouse and enter his or her bedroom to seek company or even intimacy. There are many reasons for these unwanted entries. Whatever the reason, they may be perceived by other residents as intrusive and threatening and cause these residents to become frustrated and upset, and they often lead to DHRRIs (such as when the resident whose bedroom has been invaded attempts to push the invading resident out).

Some residents are so disturbed by other residents entering their bedrooms that they place gates or other devices on their doors for prevention. A resident who tended to walk up and down the corridors and enter the bedrooms of other residents in a care home for people with dementia said about a resident whose bedroom was invaded, "He's crying when you go to the room with the gate. . . . He forces us away."[142] In another LTC home, resident A was trying to block resident B from entering his bedroom. In response, resident B started hitting him, the two men struggled, and then resident B pushed resident A to the floor, causing a hip fracture; resident A died 4 days later.[187]

Sometimes the intruder is a source of fear for the resident. In one case, a resident found another resident, who was reported to frequently engage in harmful behavioral expressions toward others, in his bed. The resident said,[152]

> When I told him to get out as this was my room, he would argue with me that this was his room, and one time he pushed me and actually punched me in the shoulder. I was angry and fearful . . . he was bigger than me. As quickly as I could, I got to the alarm to call someone and they finally came to get him out of there.

Other residents with dementia may not be able to call for help, a situation that can lead to physical injury and death. In one tragic incident, a resident with dementia was hit repeatedly over the face and head with an activity board by another resident with dementia who had entered his bedroom. His wife said: "My husband couldn't defend himself or yell for help."[188,189] His physical condition deteriorated after the episode, and he died 3 months later.

It is helpful to remember that repeatedly walking around the care home (such as in the hallways) and entering another's bedroom may appear aimless, but it is often purposeful and can serve as a form of communication when the resident is unable to convey it in words. It may be an expression of a basic human need that needs to be proactively addressed. Examples include the need to do something useful; a need for companionship or sense of security; or a need to respond to environmental irritants such as too much noise or poor lighting, physical discomforts like pain or constipation, emotional or psychological distress, or tiredness (being unable to locate one's bedroom and entering another resident's bedroom instead).

In your efforts to understand and resolve unwanted entries into other residents' bedrooms, consider the lifelong history of the resident. In one case, an 83-year-old man repeatedly entered the bedrooms of other residents, removing magazines and papers from their nightstands and tray tables (a common trigger of DHRRIs). After consulting with his family, the care team learned that this man had been a letter carrier for the postal service for more than 40 years; it was suggested that he be given a canvas shoulder bag. Direct care partners asked families to bring in old magazines and empty envelopes, and they strategically placed them around the nurses' station and common areas where he would see them. He quickly became preoccupied with collecting the materials they had placed for him, and the intervention reduced the frequency of unwanted entries into other residents' bedrooms.[190] His unwanted entries were reframed as an effort to feel useful again and engage in a meaningful activity.

Make sure that residents with dementia are able to move about freely and are monitored carefully so that they remain safe and do not leave the premises. According to Tilly and Reed,[190]

> Many people interpret the term "wandering" to suggest that the activity should be stopped when, in fact, it is often better to support a resident's movement. Beneficial effects of moving about and exploring include: Stimulation and social contact, maintaining mobility, strength preservation, prevention of constipation, and enhancement of mood.

Brawley[191] suggests engaging residents in a sufficient number of personally meaningful activities throughout the day and evening because "without anything meaningful on which to focus and to alleviate boredom, many residents with dementia explore inappropriate places such as co-resident rooms." Lucero and colleagues,[192] who used video to record the movements of residents labeled with the unhelpful and stigmatizing term "wanderers" found that "unstructured and unguided freedom can have harmful consequences," including DHRRIs.

One meaningful activity that could be offered on a daily basis to residents with dementia who tend to walk around the care home and enter other residents' bedrooms is a structured (individual or group) walking activity—preferably outdoors, if weather permits. Led and supervised by direct care partners or volunteers, residents could walk on a well-designated circular path in a secured garden. Although engagement in this or other activities throughout the day and evening is critical for prevention of unwanted entries into other residents' bedrooms, it is important to provide rest times or breaks; these might be accompanied by calming music or nature sounds.[190]

Camp[193] reports on a resident with dementia who routinely entered other residents' bedrooms and cleaned them up. On one occasion, the invasion caused a distressing interaction (shouting) with a resident whose bedroom was invaded. Camp asked the resident who entered, "Do you ever go into other people's rooms?" Resident: "No. Why should I do that? That would be crazy!" Camp: "What do you like to do in your own room?" The resident said that she liked to keep it nice and tidy but that many times people had come into her bedroom and messed it up while she was out, so she had to fix it up. Camp: "Where is your room?" Resident: "I have no idea."

It turned out that the woman entered other residents' similar-looking bedrooms thinking they were her own. Using the remaining abilities of the woman in reading and learning, Camp developed an inexpensive intervention in which he basically practiced with the woman locating her bedroom by reading her first name, which was printed in black ink on a page of blue pastel-colored paper and placed at eye level next to her bedroom door (while distinguishing it from other residents' bedrooms by printing their names with a pink background and placing them next to their bedrooms). From this approach, the resident learned to locate her bedroom and avoid entering other residents' bedrooms, and requests from the nurses to give her medications for "agitation" discontinued.

If appropriate, the walls of different hallways and rooms could be painted a different color. These visual cues may help certain residents with dementia navigate more easily to their own bedrooms and bathrooms. Another practical strategy to promote residents' identification of their own bedroom is to place a "shadowbox" filled with personal and family pictures and other personally meaningful and recognizable items next to each resident's bedroom door.[84]

For residents who do not recognize current pictures of themselves or their family and friends, consider replacing them with photos the resident recognizes and likes.[194] Prominent displays of personal memorabilia and cues of long-term significance have been shown to increase resident orientation to the bedroom by 50% compared with non-personalized cues.[195]

A LTC home may want to consider installing assistive technologies such as the Vigil® Dementia System[196] to alert direct care partners in real time to residents' unwelcome bedroom entries. For a description of this technology and other strategies, see the "Use Assistive Technology" section in Chapter 8.

General vigilance and proactive redirection are key to avoiding unwanted entries. It is important to redirect the resident as soon as you notice her or him moving toward another resident's bedroom. Remember: The resident's bedroom is her or his home and last frontier of privacy. Think about how you would feel and react if someone entered your home without your invitation.

Triggers Related to Personal Objects

Issues surrounding use of personal objects or objects perceived as personal, as with personal spaces, frequently operate as triggers of distressing and harmful interactions between residents. Living in close quarters with other residents who have dementia often poses a daily challenge in terms of timely detection of these situational triggers that could potentially take place in any part of the care home.

◆ *Eating or Drinking from Another Resident's Plate or Cup*

Taking food or drinks from other residents in the dining room is a common trigger. One resident with dementia in my early study repeatedly tried to take food from other residents' plates during mealtimes. During one episode, the resident from whom she tried to take the food threatened her angrily, saying, "I'll hit you. I'll break your neck." In a separate episode, another resident hit her on her hand when she took food from his plate and told her, "You're a thief."[34] Similarly, a videotaped study by Lucero and colleagues showed residents with advanced dementia walking around the care home after completion of morning care and, "when they become aware that food has arrived, if they are not served immediately, they walk among tables and take food from trays of those served. The residents currently eating often were observed to yell at the residents and slap their hands away."[192] Residents in that study were also observed drinking from other residents' cups or containers left on the nursing station counter, which could also instigate DHRRIs.

It is important to observe residents vigilantly and to redirect, promptly but gently, any attempts to take food or drinks from other residents at the first sign of these attempts. As in all cases, try to identify and address the underlying needs and conditions behind a resident's attempt to take food or drinks from other residents. Some possibilities to consider include feeling hungry or thirsty, difficulty waiting for one's meal or drink, not knowing or recalling where one's food or drink is located, loss of impulse control, or not recalling having eaten shortly before. When a resident's attempts are repeated and cannot be prevented by direct care partners, consider changing the seating arrangement in the dining room to decrease the likelihood of angry and potentially harmful verbal or physical reactions by residents whose food or drinks are being taken.

Ensure that residents who tend to take food from other residents while walking by dining tables are served their meals first, in an attempt to decrease these expressions.[192] For residents who prefer not to eat sitting down, consider offering finger foods (bite-sized foods that are easy to pick up, such as chicken nuggets and orange segments) to enable them to meet their nutritional needs "on the go" and hopefully minimize their need to take food or drinks from other residents.

Be informed about residents' dietary restrictions (such as those due to diabetes, food allergies, irritable bowel syndrome, and diverticulitis) and increase the level of direct care partners' supervision accordingly. Make sure that the lists of dietary restrictions are updated in a timely manner (for instance, immediately after a new dietary assessment), and see that all care employees including float staff, external agency staff, and weekend staff are aware of these restrictions. Not adhering to dietary restrictions could lead to medical complications and harm to certain residents. There are many reported instances of residents under strict dietary restrictions reaching out and taking food they are not supposed to eat. In one case, a cognitively impaired person on a pureed diet due to risk of aspiration had frequently tried to take food from other residents. A tray with sandwiches was left in reach, unsupervised, for more than an hour; the resident picked up a sandwich, ate it, choked, and then died.

Recruit and train volunteers to strengthen supervision of residents with substantial cognitive disability. As noted earlier, one innovative program to consider implementing is the volunteer Eating Assistance Program developed at Baycrest Geriatric Centre, Toronto, Canada.[162,163]

◇ *Sitting in Another Resident's Seat*

Disputes over seating are often reported in the literature as a trigger of resident-to-resident incidents, particularly in the context of dementia. Factors such as memory loss, visuospatial disorientation (e.g., difficulty remembering or locating one's table or seat), deficits in executive functions, as well as inconsistent seating arrangements often contribute to these tense and harmful episodes. In my early study on DHRRIs, resident A, who had early-stage Alzheimer's disease, discovered resident B, whose disease was in the middle stage, sitting in the chair where resident A would usually sit during snack time. Resident A said to a direct care partner, "That woman is a fruit loop." Then she told resident B, "You are nuts" and added, "She is more nuts than a fruit cake." Then she approached resident B and told her angrily, "You are a fruit loop" and "Next time you sit in my seat your food will be poisoned."[13]

In a case such as the one described above, it is important for the direct care partner to assess the resident's visuospatial deficits and wayfinding difficulties and in the future, proactively assist the resident to her or his seat. Although deficits in short-term memory are often a contributing factor, it is also important to evaluate the role of the resident's executive functions, such as the ability to plan, initiate, sequence, monitor, and discontinue a complex task, in the development of these episodes. Identification of specific deficits in executive functions should guide the development of individualized strategies to proactively assist the resident with dementia to locate her or his table and seat.

As has been emphasized before, try to remain vigilant and proactively but gently and skillfully redirect a resident with dementia who is about to sit in another resident's seat. Avoid arguing with a resident with dementia who insists that a chair is hers or his or refuses to move from it. As suggested by Zgola,[59]

> Instead of trying to convince the resident of her error, say, "Mrs. K., I know you really prefer this chair. However, could you do me a favor just this time, and sit in this chair over here? I would really appreciate it."

You can also say, while pointing to her table, "Your soup is getting cold right here" or "Your friends are waiting for you" (but say it only if it is true). If this does not work, quietly ask the resident who *usually* sits on that chair to help you out this time around by allowing the other resident to sit there. Then, thank and praise the resident for this concession and offer her the best available alternative seat.

◆ Perceived Theft of Personal Belongings

Perceptions and accusations of theft of personal belongings by residents with dementia are a common challenge in many care homes. Bethel Powers states,[197]

> Persons with dementia often lose or misplace their belongings, or forget that they have given them away, thrown them away, or hidden them. Alternatively, things may have been taken by other residents who cannot discriminate between the belongings of others and their own or have been deliberately stolen by employees.

These situations can pose a serious risk to the safety of residents involved. In fact, several residents have died as a result of physical conflicts with another resident over personal items such as a quilt, blanket, sweater, or housecoat.

It is important to try to understand the deep symbolic meaning of personal belongings to residents with dementia. A particular object can serve as an identity marker for the person, provide familiar comfort or a sense of security, bring back cherished memories, bind the person to other people, nurture pride, entertain, or provide pleasure in the nearness of an item that signifies a compelling interest. Examples include a gift passed down through generations, offering a sense of continuity and personal connection, or a necklace given by a husband for a golden wedding anniversary.[197] Some items may have aesthetic meaning, such as clothes or cosmetics.

There is also a need to recognize the important functional meanings that some items have for residents, such as eyeglasses, hearing aids, and dentures. The loss or misplacement of these devices is common in care homes, and can cause significant distress to residents, as they can result in substantial limitations on their ability to function independently and safely. Qualified specialists should evaluate residents' visual, hearing, and dental status regularly and as needed, document specific needs, and make recommendations for addressing them. Residents with dementia may remove or reject glasses, dentures, and hearing aids for several reasons. These appliances should be checked regularly for proper fit, function, and cleanliness. Hearing aid batteries should be tested and replaced as needed, and residents' ears should be checked for impaction with cerumen. Residents with dementia who need to use these appliances need to be routinely assisted in doing so.[197] Proactively addressing these issues will reduce the likelihood that they will put away or misplace these devices, or that they will mistakenly accuse other residents of taking them.

Avoid arguing with a resident with dementia who claims that her or his belongings have been stolen, even if you know that they have not. Do not make a big scene. Remember that short-term memory loss experienced by elders with Alzheimer's disease may cause them to believe that the item was stolen. Show that you care about any resident's complaint about missing items and take it seriously.

Validation and Real or Perceived Theft

Naomi Feil, developer of the Validation Method, reports[63] on an 83-year-old resident, Frances, who blamed another resident for stealing clothes from her. At some point Frances said, "Last night she stole my pure silk lace panties. Raw silk!" Feil noted, "there was not one shred of truth in her accusations . . . I showed Frances her raw silk lace panties, with her name sewed in them, hidden under a napkin in her bottom drawer. The more I tried to convince her that no one was stealing her underwear, the angrier she became. Reality orientation made her abusive." Feil then validated Frances's accusations. Reflecting on her approach later, she suggested that the loss of Frances's husband and feelings of jealousy underlay her distressing behavioral expressions:

> I learned not to contradict, patronize, argue, or try to use logic or give insight. When she told me about her stolen panties, I should have rephrased her words by asking 'Your best silk panties? When did she steal them, Mrs. Blake?' Feeling my concern, Frances Blake would have begun to trust me. 'Who gave them to you?' I should have asked, to encourage her to reminisce. Mrs. Blake might have expressed her real grief—the loss of her husband and the loneliness of living alone. By validating her grief and anger, I would have helped alleviate some of her stress. With someone to listen to her, her blaming would probably have diminished and she would have been accepted by her friends and neighbors

Consistent with Feil's approach, Teepa Snow[198] provides the following example:

> Resident: "My things are missing. They are taking my things." Snow: "They are stealing your things. Oh, so they are not where you left them. You put it somewhere and they are not there." Resident: "Yes." Snow (genuinely and respectfully): "Woo, you hate that." Resident: "I do." Snow: "I don't blame you. That shouldn't be happening." Resident: "No." Snow: "No, that's wrong. Let me see if I can figure out what is going on here." Resident: "People are coming into my room." Snow: "Yeah, people are coming in and you don't want them here. I understand that. They shouldn't be coming in. That's not okay. Let me see if I can figure out what I can do about it. I am sorry that's happening."

When Items Are Taken

Often, personal items are being taken by residents with advanced dementia without permission from other residents.[197] Those residents may mistakenly believe that these items belong to them, or they may simply find comfort in using them.

When it is not possible to engage these residents meaningfully, you may need to temporarily distract or redirect them to another part of the care home. However, remember that the unmet human needs underlying these attempts to take other people's items will probably not be met by this kind of temporary solution.

When a person with dementia is blamed for stealing, it is crucial to help the accused person save face and retain his or her dignity in this potentially hurtful situation. Offer to help find the missing item. Promptly and discreetly conduct a floor-wide search in all bedrooms (starting with those of residents who you know tend to take other residents' personal belongings) and public spaces of the care home.

The direct care partner should connect with the person blamed for taking the personal items and with what they are feeling. Raia and colleagues[129] give the example of a resident who is found rummaging through her roommate's closet. They suggest: "Don't say, 'Stop that Mrs. Suarez! You are making a mess and those aren't your clothes!' Instead, you could say, 'Hello Mrs. Suarez, I'm Martha. I was just looking for you. You seem upset. Have you lost something?'"

Some additional practical suggestions include the following:

- Name label *all* of a resident's clothes and personal belongings before admission to the care home (using elder-friendly and dementia-friendly font type, size, and contrast). Mark assistive devices such as glasses, engrave dentures, and tag prosthetic devices.

- Take inventory of all of the resident's personal belongings, and be sure to update these lists throughout her or his residency.[199] Provide a copy of the inventory to the resident or her or his family (including at each time the list is updated).

- Ask the resident's family to take pictures of valuables such as jewelry and other cherished and expensive items (and keep a copy of these photographs in a locked safe). Encourage them to keep copies of receipts from any items brought into the care home. Such documentation can assist during internal and external investigations of missing items and those allegedly stolen.

- Use locks for drawers and cabinets where only the resident or her or his family and a small number of designated care employees and managers have a key.

- Be alert and routinely look for residents' personal items that could end up in the wrong place (for instance, wastebasket, laundry hamper, food trays, or toilet bowl).

- Promptly report missing items in writing and verbally to all co-workers and managers. Make sure to inform the resident's close family members about the lost item as soon as possible—preferably, immediately after the search for the missing item does not result in locating it.

- Continuously evaluate bedroom placements when roommates take each other's items or when items are taken repeatedly during unwanted entries into another's bedroom, causing distress and potential harm.

- Ensure respectful, thorough, and timely investigation of all residents and families' complaints regarding missing items. Document the circumstances surrounding these incidents, their investigation and outcomes, and make suggestions for prevention of similar incidents in the future.

Employee Theft of Resident Items

Although the vast majority of direct and non-direct care partners will never steal from residents, some care employees take advantage of the asymmetry of power they have with vulnerable and frail residents who are dependent on them for, and trust them with, their basic care and safety. The first national study on thefts in nursing homes examined this concerning phenomenon in 47 nursing homes in ten states.[200] The study found that a substantial proportion of employees reported seeing or suspecting their co-workers of stealing from residents. Almost one-fifth of family members suspected that their relatives' possessions had been stolen by nursing home employees. A small minority of employees self-reported that they had stolen from residents, and most had done this more than once.

Thefts by care employees also take place in assisted living residences. In one study,[201] I examined 63 Minnesota Department of Health investigation reports substantiated as "financial exploitation" in assisted living residences between March 21, 2013, and July 12, 2018. A total of $116,917 worth of personal belongings (i.e., money and jewelry) had been stolen from 103 residents (on average, $1,135 was stolen from each resident). Personal items stolen included cash, credit cards, gift cards, jewelry (such as wedding rings and necklaces), and a radio.

As a first step to avoiding this problem, it is essential that the care home establish a zero-tolerance policy for theft of residents' personal belongings by employees.[197] This means that the right of residents to be free from all forms of financial exploitation must be clearly described (in writing and verbally in person) prior to employment (such as in the employee orientation handbook), in the care home's policies and procedures, and during training programs. In addition, ensure that all employees know that thefts of residents' belongings (money, jewelry, or all other items) will result in disciplinary action, termination, a report to the state survey agency, registration in applicable (discipline-based) state maltreatment registries (such as a nurse aide registry), and notification of law enforcement. In many cases, immediately after a strong suspicion arises about a care employee, temporary suspension of the individual will be required until internal and external investigations are completed. This initial step is often needed to ensure that similar crimes will not be committed by the care employee against the victim or other residents during the duration of the investigations.

Interference Between Residents

There are various ways in which a resident's interference of another resident's activity operates as a trigger of DHRRIs. Examples of these scenarios are described here.

◈ Interfering with a Resident's Activity

Many residents with dementia that is in a middle or more advanced stage may say or do things that other residents find intrusive, which often triggers an angry verbal and/or physical response. A resident might repeatedly trying to speak with another person who is reading a newspaper, for example. In one case, a resident stood blocking the television from the view of a resident who was trying to watch a show. The resident who was trying to watch TV shouted at her, "Get out of there!" When the resident did not move, he called her "idiot" and "stupid." As she left the area, she told him, "Shut your mouth."

The direct care partner should proactively anticipate the interference and then quietly and gently redirect a resident away from the area where the intrusion occurs—in the above case, away from the television set to ensure other residents a clear view of the screen. Remaining vigilant and working to detect early warning signs of interference with another resident's activity is key for prevention. However, do not assume that this will necessarily resolve the problem; sometime after you leave the area to attend to other residents' needs, the resident may return and do the exact same thing again because he or she has a need that is not being met.

When interference occurs, quietly apologize to residents whose activities were interrupted and thank them for their patience, understanding, tolerance, empathy toward other residents, and helpfulness. Try to understand what the interfering resident is trying to communicate, without words, through his or her verbal expressions and actions. Identify the unmet needs and develop an individualized plan to proactively meet them. Recognize that residents with advanced dementia may unknowingly interfere with other residents' activities. Therefore, it is important to respond quietly, gently, and respectfully to help residents save face and preserve their dignity when trying to resolve these situations.

Know that episodes of interference like this often follow a pattern (for example, related to time of day, location, residents involved, or objects). Systematic documentation of the circumstances and sequence of events leading to these acts often reveals these patterns, which should serve as the basis for development of individualized preventive strategies.

◆ Trying to Protect a Resident from Another

Some residents with dementia may become involved in episodes while trying to protect one resident from another.[13] Resident A may try to stop annoying, frustrating, threatening, or potentially harmful verbal and/or behavioral expressions exhibited by resident B toward resident C. The attempt to discontinue the behavioral expressions may trigger a verbal and/or physical incident between residents A and B.

As always, it is important to observe the residents carefully, assess the potential for harm, and intervene at the earliest signs of distress or anger, such as by redirecting one of the residents to another area in the care home where she or he can engage meaningfully in a different activity. Identify the reason behind a resident's effort to protect another resident. For instance, a resident without cognitive impairment or with early-stage Alzheimer's disease may notice that someone with advanced dementia is fearful after being threatened or bullied by another resident because of his or her engagement in verbal expressions perceived as irritating or annoying. In the case of the veteran described in the next section, you might want to hold an IDT consultation with the resident (if cognitively able) and his family to develop a care plan that will enable him to fulfill this need. The plan will need to be adapted to his current cognitive and physical abilities, disabilities, and preferences. For example, serving on a New Resident Welcome Committee might be suitable to residents with early-stage Alzheimer's disease, and preparing basic Healing Wish cards for children in the hospital might be suitable and beneficial to certain residents with middle-stage disease.

While trying to keep the resident safe, be sure to acknowledge the good intentions behind the resident's effort to protect others. Rewarding residents' compassionate acts on a daily basis is critical in every care community. It will also go a long way toward instilling the expectation that every resident's safety matters and that all people working and living in the care home have something to contribute to realizing this important goal.

◆ Trying to Assist Another Resident (Unwanted Help)

Certain residents with dementia may try to give unwelcome support, assistance, and advocacy to other residents (often, residents with earlier-stage dementia assist those with more advanced disease). A few examples of unwanted help that have been documented are giving instructions to a resident in an attempt to take the role of the care partner; feeding a resident or even forcing the resident to eat against his or her will; and pushing a resident's wheelchair when he or she does not want help. A 63-year-old Vietnam veteran who had PTSD, traumatic brain injury, and traumatic amputation was placed in a care home due to his dementia. His previous occupation was as a counselor for disabled veterans; his inclination to assist disabled veterans and invade their personal space contributed to his being the target of harmful verbal and behavioral expressions from other residents.[202]

There are also examples of especially unsafe efforts, such as trying to help a roommate (thinking she is not being well cared for) by pulling out an intravenous tube. These incidents, besides being potentially risky and dangerous to the resident on the receiving end, can lead to DHRRIs between both residents. In one episode, a resident with Alzheimer's disease attempted to hit another resident who was trying to calm her when she became anxious, upset, and angry while demanding to leave the secured dementia care home unattended.

It is important to monitor any resident's efforts to assist another, and try to identify which actions are welcomed by the other resident, are actually helpful, and are done safely, and which ones are done against the other resident's will, compromise her or his remaining self-care abilities (in other words, contribute to excess disability), or violate her or his rights, preferences, autonomy, and safety. Document in detail any unwanted and unsafe "helping" acts and make sure all direct and non-direct care partners are aware of those individuals who tend to engage in them. Remain vigilant, intervene at the earliest sign of distress, and proactively redirect residents who tend to assist other residents in unwelcome and/or unsafe ways. Think about creative things residents with strong inclinations to assist others can do so in helpful and safe ways for other residents. Find out what kinds of nonprofessional assistance certain residents may need and appreciate receiving. Use this information as the basis for harnessing the good will of residents who are cognitively and physically capable of providing such assistance.

For example, develop creative and respectful ways to create a meaningful role in the care community for a former social worker who now lives with early-stage dementia and wants to continue her lifelong work by assisting and advocating for other residents with dementia (such as appointing her as the head of a welcoming community for newly admitted residents or by encouraging her to become a companion and emotionally support residents who may feel lonely or depressed).

As with other factors described in this chapter, it is worth remembering that a resident's unhelpful and unsafe attempts to assist others may occur in patterns (such as between the same pairs of residents, locations, and times), and they may recur if you do not proactively identify and fulfill the human need underlying them in an intentional and structured way. Always acknowledge residents' attempts to assist other residents while explaining that certain attempts are unnecessary or even potentially harmful (your approach will need to be adjusted to the resident's cognitive function and comprehension level). In consultation with your IDT, think about other constructive and safe ways in which they could assist fellow residents and direct care partners. Consulting with the resident himself or herself (when cognitively able) and close family about ideas based on their intimate knowledge of the person's lifelong history can prove invaluable in resolving these situations.

Remember that the universal need to assist others remains well into the late stages of dementia. The goal should be to nurture and support the continued expression and fulfillment of this need, while working hard to find creative and safe ways to do it.

◈ *Angry Attempts at Social Control*

It is fairly common to see some residents trying to dictate to other residents what they should or should not do, as part of an attempt to control their actions and behavioral expressions. These demands have been reported to trigger verbal and physical conflicts between residents.[201] Because of their losses (aging and dementia related) and declining sense of control over their lives, some residents may try to regain control over frustrating daily situations by attempting to control other residents' actions. Examples include imperative statements and commands in attempts to change or discontinue another resident's verbal and behavioral expressions (for instance, the repetitive questions of an elder living with a short-term memory loss) or prevent a resident from engaging in an action that is perceived as annoying and disruptive, such as an unintentional invasion of one's space. Depending on the nature, frequency, and severity of these attempts, they might be seen by other residents as aggressive, and they can trigger angry verbal and physical responses from other residents.

Some residents may have lifelong tendencies to control others in their family or at work, and these tendencies may continue or worsen after they develop dementia and move to a care home. It is easy to imagine that a former high-ranking military officer, police officer, or high-powered lawyer, accustomed to telling others what they should do, would try to maintain this lifelong role in an overcrowded, overstimulating, and noisy care environment where other residents may not be receptive to and tolerant of this communication style.

Direct care partners observing this type of behavioral expression should acknowledge the concerns of a resident who is trying to discontinue another resident's actions and expressions, while preserving the dignity and personhood of the resident engaged in them. As always, try to identify and meet the underlying human need behind the behavioral expressions that cause the other resident to become frustrated and angry. If it is not possible to readily identify and address the underlying unmet need, quietly and gently redirect the resident away from the area, invite her or him to join you for a walk or coffee, or try to engage the resident in an activity she or he enjoys.

Other Triggers

Other common triggers of DHRRIs not addressed earlier in the chapter are discussed here.

◈ *Vocal Expressions Experienced as Irritating*

Various forms of verbal expressions by residents with dementia often frustrate and annoy other residents and direct care partners, and they frequently trigger DHRRIs. Examples include repetitive speech, questions, and requests for assistance; calling out or making noise; screaming; and moaning. Care employees who ignore these situations—sometimes mistakenly considering them as "normal"—"are demonstrating an act of neglect," according to Teresi and colleagues.[203] In general, the term "disruptive vocalizations" should be avoided when describing residents with advanced dementia because most of these vocal expressions in this population have a cause, meaning, and purpose *to the individual*, even if she or he is unable to verbalize what it is and/or when direct care partners are unable to identify the cause. In the vast majority of situations an unmet human need underlies these expressions, such as frustration, boredom, fear, or physical pain. The term "disruptive vocalizations" is a stigmatizing biomedical term reflecting the old culture of institution-centered care. The term *disruptive* can suggest that these expressions are done intentionally by the resident in advanced dementia. In the words of Cohen-Mansfield and Martin,[204] "Sometimes the main purpose of treatment is change in subjective perception of disruptiveness of behavior rather than change in the behavior itself."

That said, these behavioral expressions can be very frustrating and annoying to other residents. For example, when a resident angrily walked around yelling, "Horse! Horse!," direct care partners labeled him as "agitated" and usually avoided him because his yelling was annoying. By consulting his family, though, they learned that, in his 20s, he had taken care of horses. The care partners brought in a saddle, reins, cleaning supplies, and pictures of horses. They filled his room with these items that were familiar to him. His yelling diminished, and he would clean the saddle and reins for long periods of time.[205]

Direct care partners often face significant daily challenges when attempting to address residents' distressing verbal expressions. Inadequate staffing levels can limit care partners' ability to proactively identify and fulfill a resident's underlying emotional and physical needs and to skillfully respond to these expressions when they cannot be prevented. In one example,[206] resident A was sitting in a wheelchair in a common area, yelling out. Resident B went over and said, "Be quiet, stop yelling." Resident A was seen hitting resident B on the hand. The nursing aide separated them, and then she saw another resident needing assistance and had to leave the area. When she did, resident B began kicking resident A, and the cycle continued.

One of the most common types of vocal expressions that can be irritating—screaming[207]—is addressed below. A literature review by von Gunten and colleagues[208] provides useful information about other types of vocal expressions.

Screaming

Research has found that nursing home residents who tended to scream were depressed, were more prone to falling than other residents, were more often physically restrained, slept less well, felt more pain, had reduced cognitive functioning and autonomy, and had a poor social network.[171,209] The finding related to sleep is consistent with a study by Cariaga and colleagues,[207] which showed that residents with verbal expressions classified as "disruptive vocalizations" (as mentioned above, a biomedical term that should not be used in the context of elders with dementia) experienced more sleeping problems than their counterparts without such verbal expressions. This is an important target for intervention because the occurrence of these vocal expressions at night is a common trigger of conflicts between roommates, beyond the emotional and/or physical suffering potentially experienced by the resident who is screaming. The studies by Cohen-Mansfield and colleagues[171,209] showed that screaming occurred mostly in the evening and most often when the residents were alone, in the bathroom, and receiving care. Another study found that residents who screamed had less time dedicated to their care, were more dependent on assistance in activities of daily living (ADLs), were more disoriented in space, manifested more anxiety, maintained better speaking abilities, and experienced more hallucinations than the control group who did not scream.[210,211]

Some researchers insist on the importance of considering screaming as meaningful. For example, Norberg acknowledges that screaming may have neurological rather than social/emotional causes but emphasizes that it is important not to neglect the experience of these elders.[212] A study by Bourbonnais and Ducharme examined the meanings of screams among residents, the majority with moderate to severe dementia.[155] The study found that screams can have many different meanings and may express mental states or physical needs. Among the mental states that screams may express are dissatisfaction, satisfaction, vulnerability, existential distress, suffering, inability to understand one's situation, yearning for a parent or other loved one, or emotions such as fear, anxiety, frustration, or loneliness. Screams can also alert care partners to physical concerns, such as pain, hunger or thirst, fatigue, uncomfortable room temperature, the need to eliminate (or wetness from having done so), a needed change in position or place, the desire to modify the environment, or some other form of assistance. Other related explanations of screaming include understimulation,[210,211] attempts to communicate unmet needs,[207,213] fear of being abandoned or dying, feeling insecure or humiliated, and difficulty recognizing oneself.[214]

Bourbonnais and Ducharme state that the meaning of screams by an individual resident may change within the same day and over time[155]; new types of screams may emerge while others discontinue. Also, the screaming of a resident can have two meanings. For example, the baseline characteristics of continuous screaming due to feelings of vulnerability and dependency may worsen by thirst or pain and return to baseline after the physical need has been met or pain alleviated. It is also helpful to know that some residents with dementia may be unaware of their screaming or, if they are aware, unable to stop it.[155] Taken together, the underlying message is that screaming expressed by residents in advanced dementia has varied manifestations and causes within and across individuals in general and over time.

When a resident screams repeatedly, care partners should conduct a thorough interdisciplinary assessment that includes close observation and careful description of the expressions and the effort to understand the underlying messages they convey.[208] Triggers that bring on or worsen these expressions must be sought through careful observation, possibly over several days. During the individual resident assessments, use the Behavioral Expressions Log and the Interdisciplinary Screening Form (available in the downloadable files accompanying this text at healthpropress.com; see p. viii for access information), which could further assist you in detecting situational causes and triggers of screaming among residents with dementia. A medical and physical examination with targeted laboratory testing can help detect medical, physiological, and functional causes and triggers of a resident's screams (such as an old fracture causing pain or a skin rash causing discomfort and irritation).

If not already done, assess the resident's premorbid history, both medical and personal. This assessment could point to potential measures for addressing the cause of the distressing verbal expressions. In a case reported by Naomi Feil, an older man with dementia regularly screamed at the director of the adult day health center not to lock him in the attic; however, the director never did so, nor did he threaten to do so, and no attic existed at the center. Care employees learned that during his childhood, his father would punish him by locking him in the attic, which left lifelong emotional trauma. This resident needed validation, empathy, emotional support, and reassurance from a trusted care partner to be able to alleviate the fear caused by this early life trauma.

Direct care partners could also conduct a more formalized assessment, such as those aimed at determining the type of a distressed verbal expression. One such typology takes into account the quality, purpose, and response to the environment as well as the quantity of the expressions; this is known as the Typology of Vocalizations and Screaming Behavior Mapping Instrument.[215,216] von Gunten and colleagues assert,[208]

> Verbally disruptive behaviors must be analyzed according to a considerable number of potential etiopathogenic or causative factors before deciding on the course of treatment. The assessment will form the basis for a reasonable treatment plan that usually comprises a combination of various components.

It is important to develop and implement individualized interventions, and consider providing multiple interventions concurrently, in light of the complexity involved in understanding screaming and difficulty in achieving improvements, to increase efficacy and meet individual residents' underlying needs.[208,213] For instance, a 93-year-old woman with dementia who screamed was found to be experiencing a lack of social and sensory stimulation and to have difficulty communicating her needs and pain. The intervention consisted of positive reinforcement by talking to her when she was not screaming, informing her in advance of planned care, providing affective contact, including her in activities, and reducing her discomfort before she started screaming. Following the implementation of this intervention, the woman's screaming decreased from 46% of the observation time before the intervention to 8% after.[217] In their review of the literature,[155] Bourbonnais and Ducharme describe other strategies for addressing residents' screaming.

Social isolation may be one important trigger of screaming among residents with dementia. When touch is appropriate, accepted, and tolerated well by the individual, it is helpful to provide frequent human contact, reassurance, and gentle touch. One study by Cohen-Mansfield and Werner[218] found that when direct care partners offered sensory stimulation and presented video recordings of family members, screaming decreased by 56% and 46%, respectively, during the interventions.

Assess, proactively identify, and address unmet needs and physiological problems the person with advanced dementia may experience but be unable to express verbally (for instance, sleeping problems, pain, infection, fever, thirst, or hunger) or distressing factors in the social or physical environment, such as boredom, crowdedness, excessive noise, uncomfortable room temperature, or glare. In one case, a resident was constantly shouting, "Ow, ow, ow." This caused other residents to become upset and angry at her. A physical examination revealed that she had an open wound on her back. The resident's shouting was an expression of a clearly unmet physical need.

According to Bourbonnais and Ducharme,[155] residents' screams may constitute a unique language that can be learned. Identification of the meaning of screams should precede and guide the choice of individualized interventions.[213] They argue that "when the intervention matches the meaning, screaming often stops." To decode the meaning and causes of screams, direct care partners need to closely observe the nonverbal communication (facial expressions and body language) of residents with advanced dementia when they scream. Voice characteristics such as tone, intensity, and speed and the look in the resident's eyes are important elements indicating the meaning of screams.[155]

Raia[122] stresses the importance of distinguishing between different subtypes of screaming by residents with dementia. He describes the following three subtypes of screaming.

- *Rhythmic sound* (such as "Help me, help me"), often caused by insufficient brain stimulation. One way to approach it is to provide the person with a replacement for her or his auto-stimulation. For example, for Catholic residents, he suggests praying the rosary, which creates a kind of rhythmic mantra. A rocking chair or glider may be helpful to some individuals.

- *Low-pitched, constant sound,* often caused by pain. An assessment of pain would be needed, and if pain is detected, a treatment should be initiated.

- *Loud, shrill, continuous sound* that often stops when one approaches the person. This form is often a sign of panic and sometimes a sign of boredom. Making the person feel safe and secure, providing her or him with a higher level of one-on-one care, backrubs, and enhanced level of personally meaningful engagement may alleviate the person's fears or give her or him a sense of purpose and joy and thus reduce the screams.

Get to know and identify remote triggers in the resident's early life history, either from the resident or (in the later stages of dementia) from close family members and friends.[154] Feil tells of one resident with advanced dementia who repeatedly screamed the name of her beloved wooden and furry animal toy, which she received from her father as a child before he left the family; it was the only object she had left from him. No one in the nursing home made the connection, and thus she was labeled "disruptive" and sedated with antipsychotic medications. Learning about her childhood, Feil discovered that when she was a child her teacher humiliated her in front of her classmates by throwing her beloved toy in the trash. Now, with advanced dementia in her 80s, she re-experienced the early-life psychological trauma and regularly expressed it by calling out the toy's name.

Strive to provide consistent care by assigning the same direct care partners to the same resident over significant periods of time (several or more months when possible, when the assignment seems beneficial to the resident and works well for the care partner). The more contact a well-trained direct care partner has with the same resident, the more likely she or he will be able to decode the cause of the distressing verbal expressions.[155] Subtle and significant changes from baseline could more quickly and easily be detected by care partners familiar with the individual, her or his care needs, and unique sources of distress.

Work to build and nurture trust with the resident and use an affectionate and reciprocal "authentic partnership" approach during interactions with her or him. Include the resident in conversations. If the resident is unable to communicate verbally, include her or him in the conversation by using inclusive gestures and gentle touch when appropriate, tolerated, and helpful.[155]

When in contact with a resident who is screaming, try to stay calm. Use a reassuring tone of voice and a soothing, calming approach. Remember that residents with Alzheimer's disease are more likely to respond in a distressed way when you are distressed and/or anxious.[155] They will likely detect and respond to ("mirror") the core emotions that underlie the words you use more than to the words themselves.

Adjust the resident's daily care schedule to meet her or his needs, preferences, abilities, and disabilities. For example, scheduling a shower for a resident with advanced dementia at a time that is not consistent with her or his lifelong routine may cause her or him to express frustration through screaming.

Try to identify the unspoken function of the screaming; consider it an indication of liveliness and a form of empowerment.[155] As with other behavioral expressions, residents with advanced dementia scream (repeatedly) when this is their only remaining way to tell us that something is wrong and that they need assistance with something. Direct care partners should be encouraged and trained to put on a detective hat and always look for clues for underlying causes and triggers.

If the resident is sitting, assess the need to assist with repositioning in her seat to increase her or his physical comfort. If you are unable to identify the cause of the screaming, consider helping the person move to another area in the care home. One direct care partner reported, "For somebody who is yelling and screaming, especially during mealtime when residents tend to get upset if somebody is very noisy, we would take that person out of the dining room once she [had] finished eating. . . . We would remove her so that others [could] have their meal."[177] Sometimes, an unknown cause in the social or physical environment accounts for the screaming, and being outside the area eliminates its trigger. When assisting the person to another part of the care home, it is important to do so in a quiet, calm, and respectful way that helps to preserve the person's dignity. Many people with dementia can detect whether they are being treated in disrespectful and stigmatizing ways, so making every effort to help them save face is critical.

Sit and talk with the resident. If the resident cannot understand you, consider holding her or his hand, when she or he responds well to it; remember that some residents prefer not to be touched, and this wish needs to be respected in these situations. In general, be present and centered as much as possible, and show attention to the person in a way that is personally meaningful to her or him. Consider reading to the person[219] material you know she or he enjoys listening to. One person with middle-stage dementia enjoyed looking at *New Yorker* cartoons and reading their captions; this had a clear calming effect on her.

Approach the resident in a relaxed, non-harried, and nondemanding manner.[208] Remember, slower with many residents with dementia is, practically, faster because many individuals with a serious brain disease process information at a much slower pace than cognitively intact people. Doing things at a speed that is simply too fast for these individuals to process (outpacing) often creates new problems that take more time for direct care partners to address. Avoid fast and surprising movements that may startle and frighten the resident, such as approaching the person in the dining room from behind and pulling his or her chair backward without asking for permission or otherwise preparing the person.

Examples of helpful diversions and personally meaningful activities are exercise, music therapy, therapeutic gardening, a visit with toddlers, or other enjoyable sensory stimulation.[208] Holding and stroking a kitten or petting a dog, listening to favorite songs using headphones, or receiving a back and shoulder massage may reduce the frequency of screams in certain individuals with dementia. Using personally tailored music has been shown to decrease the frequency of screaming,[220] and using favorite music (10 minutes twice daily for 4 days) was shown to reduce screaming during an intervention for two out of three residents.[221] However, as has been pointed out earlier, it is important to remember that diversion often does not address the unmet need underlying the screaming, so you will still need to assess, identify, and fulfill the unmet needs if you want your approach to have lasting effects.

One individualized intervention using white noise has been shown to reduce distressing verbal vocalizations, including screaming, in residents with severe cognitive impairment (average Mini-Mental State Exam score of 1.66) with high need for assistance with ADLs. The white noise used consisted of a gentle ocean audiotape (sound of crashing waves interspersed with the more muffled sound of receding waves) and a mountain stream audiotape (a continuous sound of water rushing over rocks in a streambed).[222] This low-cost intervention should be made available in all care homes where people with middle- to late-stage dementia live. Tailoring the music to the individual's preferences could further increase its use and therapeutic benefits. When doing so, I highly recommend that you explore the phenomenal educational and training resources developed by Music & Memory®, a nonprofit organization that helps people with cognitive and physical disabilities to engage with the world, ease pain, and reclaim their humanity through the use of personalized music.

Encourage creative solutions. For example, one direct care partner reported on the following strategy she used with a resident who always screams: "I took her down to the Church. In the Church she won't scream anymore."[223] For residents with a lifelong love of horses, consider offering guided therapeutic programs with trained horses such as the Connected Horse Project (a collaboration with Stanford University Red Barn Leadership Program), in which participants and their family care partners interact and tend to horses from the ground (they do not ride the horses). For residents with advanced dementia, consider inviting an animal specialist to facilitate enriching and therapeutic interactions with trained miniature horses, as my colleague Judy Berry has done so successfully in care homes.[60]

Frequently inform and remind residents with memory loss about upcoming events and activities, as difficulty waiting, discussed earlier, can be a precursor to screaming or other distressed verbal expressions that can be perceived by other residents as irritating and frustrating.

If you are in a leadership position, consider providing education and additional support to direct care partners. For example, help care employees come to terms with their own emotional reactions to residents with distressing verbal expressions through regular guidance and supervision.[224] Direct care partners should try not to take residents' distressing verbal expressions personally, even if they seem to be directed at them.[213] It is critically important to avoid labeling, ostracizing, and overmedicating residents with advanced dementia who scream. Reflecting, acknowledging, and understanding how these distressed verbal expressions make you feel and working to alleviate these negative emotional states (such as through emotional support from peers or a social worker) are critical for any approach aimed at validating residents' emotional states, human needs, and distressed verbal expressions.

Support and educate family members who feel guilty and powerless because of their relative's screaming. In the words of one daughter, "It breaks my heart to come here and see my father screaming like that; it's like being stabbed, these screams, it's like someone was stabbing you."[155] Work with the IDT in collaboration and consultation with the resident's close family members to identify the root cause of the screams and biopsychosocial strategies that could bring physical and/or emotional comfort to the resident and reduce them.

As noted elsewhere, it is essential to provide sufficient staffing levels at all times so that direct care partners can have enough time to spend with the residents in general and those who tend to scream in particular.[155] Many direct care partners want to spend more time with residents (beyond scheduled personal care tasks) and often experience frustration when low staffing levels prevent them from doing so. The more time well-trained direct care partners can spend with residents with dementia in supportive ways, the more they can develop and nurture close trusting relationships with them. The stronger the trusting relationship, the more likely that the residents will feel secure, experience a sense of belonging and having others care about them, and feel less lonely. In general, screaming is less likely to occur under these latter conditions.

◆ Angry Verbal and/or Physical Reactions After Reaching a "Breaking Point"

The common reaction of reaching a "breaking point" was reported in a study analyzing reports by police officers called to nursing homes due to DHRRIs.[6] Selected examples of triggers include repetitive questions; continuous screaming; talking in one's sleep; repetitive coughing, sneezing, and burping; taking the personal belongings of another; repeated conflicts between roommates about preferred ways of using the shared bedroom; and inadvertently blocking the view of the television set.[13,6] One resident who repeatedly asked to go to the bathroom got on the nerves of another, who shouted, "You're not needing the toilet at all; go and give her a slap in the mouth."[142] In another episode, one resident who saw another hit direct care partners intervened by breaking his walking cane on the other resident's head.[83]

The fact that residents can easily reach a breaking point is another reason for early identification of warning signs of distress and behavioral expressions that frustrate and annoy other residents. These common warning signs need to be defused immediately. Make sure to document in a resident's care plan any recurring situational triggers for these episodes so that other direct and non-direct care partners, such as housekeeping and dietary staff, will be aware of them and proactively work to prevent and de-escalate them. Try to detect whether there are temporal and/or spatial patterns underlying these distressing interactions, as these can often guide you in meeting these needs and developing individualized preventive strategies. As always, try to identify and then anticipate and proactively meet the underlying human need behind the resident's behavioral expressions.

Recruit cognitively intact residents and those with early-stage dementia to serve as supportive companions for residents with more advanced dementia who tend to engage in these distressed verbal expressions. Often, the regular, attentive, and affectionate presence of a caring person who is a peer can decrease these expressions and help to maintain a peaceful environment for the other residents.

When screams or other verbal expressions of one resident appear to be distressing, annoying, or irritating to others, it is important to acknowledge their frustrations. Apologize sincerely and tell them how much you appreciate their patience, understanding, and help in resolving the situation. At certain times, when it is not possible to resolve the situation directly, you may need to consider offering—either to the resident exhibiting the verbal expressions or those frustrated by them—to temporarily help them move to another part of the care home (far enough where the verbal expressions cannot be heard). You know each resident and her or his reactions to such situations and offers. Use your best judgment in deciding who to offer such a change.

◆ Language Mismatch

Beyond the role of cognitive impairment in the development of DHRRIs, language mismatch can also be a contributing factor for these incidents. When two residents do not speak the same language, or when one or both residents has returned to the use of their native language (as often happens in the later stages of Alzheimer's disease), their ability to verbally communicate with each other in day-to-day situations is often compromised. Although nonverbal emotional communication often continues into the late stages of the disease, the inability to understand each other's words, and thus each other's needs and preferences, can often lead to misunderstandings, frustrations, and distressing and harmful incidents. In some cases, residents have reportedly mocked others who were speaking a different language. Pillemer and colleagues[24] report on a resident who had the habit of mocking her friend's language when she was bored or annoyed, saying, "Blah, blah, blah." The resident who was mocked reported this as being hurtful.

Recognizing language mismatch as a risk factor for incidents, managers should make sure to inform all direct and non-direct care partners about non-English languages spoken primarily by residents with dementia (this information needs to be collected during admission and updated throughout the person's residency, as changes occur). A special "Languages Spoken" sheet should be prepared containing the names of the primary languages currently spoken by these residents as well as updated pictures of them. The sheet should be placed in a central location and a protocol in place to ensure that float and external agency staff read it prior to starting their work shift.

Heightened sensitivity and proactive "anticipatory" preventive approach should be expected of all employees in direct regular contact with these residents. For example, direct care partners need to see that pairs of residents not speaking the same language and with a history of conflicts do not sit next to each other during mealtimes, organized activities, and downtimes. That said, certain pairs of residents with dementia not speaking the same language could still be supportive companions and friends (such as through nonverbal emotional interactions), so it is not necessary to automatically separate these residents when they get along well and have no history of conflict.

Consider recruiting and training a volunteer who speaks the language spoken by the resident with dementia. She or he could be asked to assist in bridging the language barrier during peak hours, such as when the residents spend significant time in close quarters with each other. Their translations, along with a calming and attentive presence, could decrease situational misunderstandings and frustrating interactions between the residents.

As noted elsewhere, direct care partners and all other IDT members need to work together to instill an atmosphere of empathy and mutual respect between residents. They need to send a clear message that making fun of another resident because he or she speaks a different language is unacceptable. A care partner could quietly and respectfully but firmly say to a resident, "We don't speak to each other like that here." Direct care partners and all other employees need to be unified and consistent in using this approach and will need to provide frequent reminders to residents who ignore these requests or simply forget them due to memory loss.

Additionally, family members should be asked to speak with their relatives and discourage them from making potentially hurtful comments toward other residents; of course, this approach would only work if the relative has sufficient cognitive function ability to comprehend and retain the information. Such an effort by family members could help reinforce the community-wide prevention effort. Family members of residents who are on the receiving end of these harmful comments should be consulted to learn from them about key words in their native language that may be helpful and calming. It is also important to ask family members for words the person will understand that can help in the prevention and de-escalation of DHRRIs.

Helpful Resources

The National Council on Interpreting in Health Care (www.ncihc.org) is a multidisciplinary organization whose mission is to promote and enhance language access in health care in the United States. The organization is composed of medical interpreters, interpreter service coordinators and trainers, clinicians, policy makers, advocates, and researchers. Readers may also want to explore evidence-based protocols[225] designed to facilitate the effective use of language interpretation services in healthcare settings for people with limited English.

◆ Racist Comments and Ethnic Stereotyping

In a focus group study by Rosen and colleagues,[14] direct care partners reported that racist comments by residents against other residents were hurtful and that they triggered and escalated DHRRIs. Many elders grew up in an era and in regions where racist practices were prevalent and accepted as the norm. Some of these people held racist views from their youth and continue to hold these beliefs throughout their lives, whether they openly express these views in public or suppress them as racism becomes increasingly unaccepted and condemned over the years. When these individuals develop dementia and move into LTC homes, some may continue to express their long-held racist views toward others, including toward other residents and direct care partners, especially under distressing day-to-day situations. As Alzheimer's disease progresses, the cognitive filters that enabled these individuals to hold these views unexpressed when they were cognitively intact throughout their lives are no longer working as they did in the past. Disinhibitions and problems with impulse control due to brain disease may exacerbate the frequency and severity of racist expressions.

Compounding the problem is the racial incongruency that often exists between residents as well as between residents and direct care partners in care homes. Specifically, the majority of nursing home residents in the United States are white, while a substantial portion of direct care partners are from minority groups, and many are immigrants. Racial slurs and ethnic stereotyping are often expressed by a subgroup of white residents with dementia toward care partners and residents from these groups. These expressions can be very emotionally and psychologically hurtful to those on the receiving end. It is not uncommon for these expressions to trigger defensive and protective verbal and physical angry responses by residents feeling hurt by these remarks. It is easy to see how these tense and hurtful interactions can escalate into DHRRIs in general and in small, crowded spaces of care homes.

The expression of racist comments by residents toward care employees, whether during routine care times or during DHRRIs, could limit some care employees' ability and/or willingness to assist them when these episodes occur. Several times during my early observational study on DHRRIs in two care homes for people with dementia in an assisted living residence, I heard care employees report, complain, and feel hurt by awful racist comments and slurs communicated by some residents toward them. One Black recreation therapist told me one day about a certain resident who frequently expressed racist comments toward some care employees. "It's pretty bad . . . it's hard to . . . care for somebody who is . . . racist."

Direct care partners should try to learn about the racial perceptions held by the resident when he or she grew up and throughout his or her life, either from the person directly when cognitively able or from close family members or friends. This may give a general sense regarding the extent to which a person has lifelong and deeply ingrained racist beliefs toward other ethnic groups. It will help in developing a realistic sense as to how much the IDT should invest in attempting to change the way the person was conditioned for decades versus directing the care team's limited time, care resources, and efforts toward modifying the response and approach toward this individual. As importantly, understanding the racial and ethnic perceptions of residents will enable care partners to proactively offer emotional support to residents and other staff members psychologically harmed during these heartbreaking situations.

In addition to learning about the resident's attitudes and beliefs toward other groups, nurses and physicians should also evaluate the extent to which disinhibition and problems with impulse control (such as due to cognitive impairment and/or frontotemporal damage) contribute to the person's expression of these racist remarks. This could help give a realistic sense regarding the extent to which brain disease and cognitive impairments limit the person's ability to control these expressions, which, in turn, could inform the approach used by care partners when interacting with this individual.

Work closely with the IDT to send a clear and consistent message to all residents (who are cognitively able to understand it) that racist comments and ethnic stereotyping are not accepted at the care home. Frequent reminders to all care employees, cognitively able residents, and family members will be necessary due to some residents' short-term memory deficits and persistent lifelong racist views.

Develop a written policy explicitly addressing the expectation of full respect for residents and direct care partners from all racial and ethnic groups. Share the policy with all cognitively able residents and their family members during admission to the care home and provide reminders during the person's residency. When possible and realistic, work with the resident's close family members on the development of an individualized psychosocial strategy that aims to reduce these racist expressions. Certain residents may be more receptive and willing to listen to a family member or friend with whom they have close trusting relationships. Family members could try to encourage and reinforce the care community's efforts to instill racially tolerant views in their relatives during their visits. This approach may work well in reducing these racial remarks with certain residents with dementia but not with others, for reasons already discussed.

Managers should ensure that all care employees in direct regular contact with residents know the residents with dementia who tend to express these hurtful remarks. The goal is not to label them as racist (even if they are) but rather to increase direct care partners' sensitivity and vigilance to the possibility that their remarks could hurt other residents, and could contribute to the development of DHRRIs. Being aware, direct care partners as well as housekeeping, dietary, and maintenance staff should be in a better position to proactively recognize and promptly prevent these situations from developing or de-escalating them before they cause psychological or physical harm to residents. It is important to pay close attention for any pairs of residents in which one person repeatedly makes racist or racially tinged remarks toward the other. Even residents who may seem somewhat indifferent or tolerant of such nasty remarks for extended periods may eventually reach a breaking point.

Publicly celebrate the life achievements of residents from minority groups experiencing these hurtful racist remarks from other residents. Their accomplishments (small or large) may be related to their roles in their family, work, volunteering, hobbies, special talents, awards, or honorable army service. This may assist in demonstrating these individuals' invaluable contributions to their families, communities, and the society. Beyond the potential for strengthening these residents' self-image, it could also improve their perceived image as it is held by other residents and care partners and thus increase the social acceptance and respect expressed toward them.

Be intentional and persistent in encouraging and nurturing an atmosphere of interracial, interethnic, and intercultural sensitivity, understanding, acceptance, and tolerance. For example, a care home can plan and hold culturally and ethnically diverse enriching events and group activities and develop creative ways to show residents the value and richness of each resident's race, culture, ethnicity, and religion. In addition, special events can be held on certain days such as on Martin Luther King Day to educate residents about the history and contributions of different groups of people. Make it clear that all minority groups have a human right to be treated with dignity and respect. Over time, a unified and persistent community-wide effort could enable you to see significant reductions in expressions of racist remarks made by residents toward other residents and care employees. This, in turn, will enable your care home to be a place where mutual respect among all people is deeply cherished as a core value. It will also assist you in minimizing the number of DHRRIs triggered by these racial remarks and keep residents safe.

◈ *Intolerance Based on Sexual Orientation and Gender Identification*

As in society at large, residents who identify as lesbian, gay, bisexual, transgendered, or queer (LGBTQ) may face harassment and discrimination in LTC homes. As discussed earlier, people with dementia may express their deep-seated, conditioned attitudes more readily than they might have before they had dementia. The culture of alertness and compassion that has been recommended throughout is quite relevant with respect to LGBTQ residents and their direct care providers.

In 2016, 70-year-old Marsha Wetzel sued[226] a senior living community in Illinois, alleging that as a lesbian she suffered slurs, threats, and taunts, including three physical attacks (such as hitting her in the back of the head and calling her a "homo") from other residents. She also claimed that the administrators did not take serious measures to protect her. After a federal court dismissed her suit, she appealed the case, and the court ruled in August 2018 that the federal Fair Housing Act holds a landlord liable when the landlord has "actual notice of tenant-to-tenant harassment based on a protected status, yet chooses not to take any responsible steps within its control to stop the harassment." On February 12, 2019, the senior housing residence and Wetzel reported that they had reached a "settlement to the mutual satisfaction of all parties." Wetzel moved from the residence and has since passed away.

Due to commonly held prejudice and stigma about their sexual orientation, a significant number of LGBTQ residents are likely targets of discrimination, hatred, intolerance, neglect, hostility, and verbal and physical threats from other residents and direct care partners. In addition, according to Doll[131] these individuals "fear not being accepted or being rejected by other residents, especially a roommate who may dislike 'different' people." One explanation has to do with the fact that, "older adults, because of their lack of education regarding sexuality in general and homosexuality specifically, may have more homophobic tendencies" (although this may be slowly changing with the aging of the baby boomers). Of particular concern are people who are transgendered, as they are much more likely to be targets of abuse and violence by others in general and in healthcare settings. Focusing on older LGBTQ residents in the context of DHRRIs in general and when they have dementia deserves special attention beyond the scope of this book.

For a good discussion of the profound challenges faced by elder LGBTQ residents in LTC homes and practical suggestions for addressing them, see the chapter "Lesbian, Gay, Bisexual, and Transgendered Residents" in Doll's book *Sexuality in Long-Term Care: Understanding and Supporting the Needs of Older Adults*. Another helpful chapter, by Coon and Burleson, outlining a framework for identifying barriers and strategies for overcoming them as well as suggested programs and services, is entitled "Working with Gay, Lesbian, Bisexual, and Transgendered Families" in the book *Ethnicity and the Dementias*. Consulting with these two resources[131,227] is a good starting point for owners and administrators of care homes who are serious about becoming LGBTQ friendly and ensuring a safe living care environment for these individuals.

It should be emphasized that federal nursing home regulations provide resident rights and stipulate requirements that are of importance to LGBTQ individuals who live in nursing homes. For example, all residents have the right to be free from abuse (by any individual—including other residents), and nursing homes must develop and implement policies, procedures, and care practices that prohibit mistreatment of residents. They must also investigate and report allegations of abuse to their state survey agencies and in certain cases to law enforcement. State regulations and various anti-discrimination laws may provide additional protections. The National Long-Term Care Ombudsman Resource Center provides additional information on this complex, challenging, and often overlooked human rights problem in a fact sheet entitled *Resident's Rights and the LGBT Community: Know Your Rights as a Nursing Home Resident* (https://www.lgbtagingcenter.org/resources/resource.cfm?r=923).

5

Factors in the
Physical Environment

Good design has to begin with the needs of the people who use it.

Thomas Fisher[228]

This chapter describes problematic features of physical environments in long-term care (LTC) homes that can contribute to development of distressing and harmful resident-to-resident interactions (DHRRIs) among people living with dementia. The majority of these factors have been found in research studies to be associated with behavioral expressions classified as "aggressive" among LTC residents (Table 5.1). The factors described here are all considered modifiable (◇), some during routine daily care and others during building planning or renovation.

It is important for direct and non-direct care partners and other interdisciplinary care team members to be aware of all potentially contributing factors in the physical environment so that they are in a position to anticipate and proactively minimize their negative effects on residents with dementia. The suggestions presented in this chapter center on the goal of proactively compensating for residents' cognitive impairments that cause them to be increasingly sensitive and vulnerable to these factors in general and as their disease progresses. One important premise underlying this goal is advanced by the Progressively Lowered Stress Threshold Model,[229] which states that people living with dementia "need environmental conditions modified as they experience progressive decline so that cues can be more easily processed and are thus less stressful." An optimal level of person–environment fit requires the commitment to providing person-directed, elder-friendly, and dementia-friendly physical environment in LTC homes. Many nursing homes built after the acute hospital model, but even many assisted living residences built after the hotel model, do not come close to meeting these basic standards.

Care homes that are successful in optimizing the person–environment fit are better equipped to enhance residents' physical function and psychological well-being and decrease their situational frustrations. In general, the greater the fit, the less likely residents with dementia will become involved in distressing and harmful interactions with other residents. A good fit often also enables direct care partners to be in a position to respond in time to protect residents in situations where these episodes have already started to manifest.

Factors That Can Be Modified During Routine Daily Care

Many factors in the physical environment can be modified during routine care by direct care partners and interdisciplinary care teams to minimize or eliminate their negative effects on residents with or without dementia.

Table 5.1   Factors Associated with Distressing or Harmful Behavioral Expressions

Point of Modification	◇ Environmental Factors
During routine daily care	• Indoor confinement or lack of regular daily access to a secured outdoor area or garden • Lack of personalization of residents' bedrooms • Inadequate separation between beds in shared bedrooms • Limited or lack of sensory comprehension of environmental input • Noisy, overstimulating, and hectic environment • Crowding • Problematic television programs and content • Lack of adequate landmarks and signage • Temperature discomfort • Glare, direct and indirect • Challenges accessing, using, and sharing elevators • Access to sharp or dangerous objects
During building planning or renovation	• Larger care homes with a high number of residents • Line-of-sight obstacles reducing the ability to supervise residents effectively • Institutional (versus homelike) qualities of the residence • Lack of private away (non-bedroom) spaces • Inadequate outdoor spaces • Lack of bedroom privacy • Shared toilets and showers • Narrow hallways • "Dead ends" in hallways • Outdoor environmental noise • Poor indoor sound quality • Inadequate lighting and daylighting

◇ Indoor Confinement or Lack of Daily Access to Outdoor Areas

Research has found lower levels of distressing and harmful interactions among residents living in LTC homes with outdoor spaces compared with residences that do not have such spaces.[230] One research group studied the effect of mandatory confinement indoors on the incidence of behavioral expressions classified as aggression and use of psychotropic medications among residents with dementia in an acute psychogeriatric unit. Changes in the frequency of these expressions and use of psychotropic medications were examined during (test) and after (posttest) a 32-day period of confinement, defined as denial of access outdoors due to construction and maintenance. Rates of verbal and physical conflicts and the use of as-needed psychotropic medication decreased in the posttest period, when residents were released from confinement and had free access to a fenced and secured garden court-yard in good weather.[231]

The lack of regular daily access to secured outdoor spaces often causes tremendous frustration to certain residents with dementia. The inability to decompress and enjoy the various health and psychological benefits of being outside represents a major missed opportunity for prevention of conflicts with care partners and other residents. Residents who are deprived of being outside regularly may experience excessive circadian rhythm disturbances (associated with cardiovascular problems, immune dysfunction, cognitive and functional deterioration, depression, and increased mortality[232]) and vitamin D synthesis deficiencies (associated with increased risk of falls).[233] By contrast, the following benefits of using secured outdoor gardens were reported by Lisa Talyaco[234] in a newsletter for a care home dedicated solely to caring for people with dementia:

> When residents have the opportunity to use an outdoor space, their quality of life improves. Outdoor space provides sensory experiences and stimulation, encourages exercise, and allows residents to make observations that they would not be able to make indoors. For people with memory loss and dementia, outdoor space can also stimulate memories of previous home life. When participants are outside, they enjoy the weather, the plants and flowers, the breeze, the sun, the space, and the quieter surroundings. The garden offers staff the opportunity for a more relaxed place to talk with folks. When people are upset, it seems like a natural place to decompress.

For Bell and Troxel, the developers of *The Best Friends Approach to Dementia Care*, the right to be outdoors on a regular basis is so important that it is included in their 12-item "Dementia Bill of Rights."[235] Direct care partners and administrators should maximize opportunities for residents to use dementia-friendly, secured outdoor spaces. Residents with dementia need the greatest possible access to a secured outdoor space where they can be apart from other residents or at least be with a smaller number of residents.

Allow residents to be outside for at least 30 minutes each day, weather permitting, with adequate supervision by direct care partners, and with appropriate safety measures. Adequate staff-to-resident ratio of well-trained direct care partners is necessary to accomplish this daily goal skillfully, efficiently, and safely. Taking residents, especially those with middle- to late-stage of dementia, out to a secured space requires constant and attentive supervision, guidance, physical assistance, and personally meaningful engagement (even if the latter means sitting and enjoying watching birds on the trees).

◇ Lack of Personalization of Residents' Bedrooms

Personalization in residents' bedrooms is defined by Zeisel and colleagues[159] as "the degree to which residents are allowed to and actually do place personal objects in their bedrooms." These researchers found that residents in special care homes for people with dementia that provided more privacy—more private bedrooms and more opportunities for personalization—had less anxiety and aggression.

Zeisel[147] states that the bedroom of a resident with dementia must be her or his sanctuary. Despite successful culture change initiatives aimed at creating LTC homes and bedrooms that look and feel like a home (such as the Green Houses of The Eden Alternative and English Rose Suites in the United States and Arcare in Helensvale, Australia), bedrooms and bathrooms in a large number of care homes still have many institutional characteristics. They often also lack personally meaningful and familiar items, such as personal or family pictures and paintings hung on the wall, decorations, plants (nontoxic), and furniture (easy chair or desk) that could increase the resident's sense of belonging, attachment, identity, personhood, self-image, and pride. A person's personal space is "an expression of who they are—as a person. If a person's bedroom—her personal space—reminds her of who she is, others will treat her more as a whole person (e.g., 'What a lovely picture of your wedding that is')."[147] Likewise, Bethel Ann

Powers[197] states, "The presence of personal effects may help staff appreciate the uniqueness of the individual and be of comfort to families."

In the earlier stages of dementia, when the resident is able to express his or her wishes, ask what personal items and furniture she or he would like to have in the bedroom; when the right dementia-friendly conditions are created for these conversations, many who have middle-stage Alzheimer's disease are also able to express their preferences. Do your best to accommodate and respect the resident's wishes and ask how she or he would like the bedroom to be furnished and decorated. Research among people relocating to nursing homes has shown that residents with cherished possessions were better adapted than those without them.[236] When the resident is no longer able to verbally express her or his wishes because of cognitive impairment, consult with close family members and friends about ways to personalize the resident's bedroom.

Where possible, encourage residents and their family members to bring furniture from the person's home (such as a bed or mattress or a favorite chair or lamp) and personally meaningful objects into the personal living space (for instance, family pictures, a personally quilted bed cover, or religious objects). Zeisel suggests that care homes should "enable walls to be hung with personal photos and paintings."[147] It is important to remember, though, that you will also need to take into consideration the potential for loss, misplacement, or theft of residents' belongings (see Chapter 4 for discussion and suggestions).

The inability to respect residents' wishes can bring about negative consequences. One resident with cognitive impairment said, "I really wanted to bring my bed, but they said 'No,' so I have a terrible time sleeping."[197] One 74-year-old resident with dementia[237] had refused to enter her bedroom since her admission to the care home. She persistently walked up and down the hallways, entered the bedrooms of other residents, or attempted to sleep in a chair in the lounge. She was labeled a wanderer, resistive, and aggressive until direct care partners learned about the lifelong sensitivity she had to the color used to paint her bedroom walls (purple and mauve). No longer able to convey it in words, she expressed it through her refusal to use her bedroom. A review of her life history revealed that she was Irish and was once a devout Roman Catholic. In her faith these are the colors of mourning. She always had a morbid dread of these colors and their distressing association with grief and death. Away from her bedroom she was psychologically comfortable. However, when confronted with her bedroom she was consumed by fear and sought sanctuary elsewhere. Once she was reassigned a different bedroom painted in different colors, she was willing to enter the bedroom without any reservation.

Finally, when possible and safe to do so, avoid using medical equipment and furniture in residents' bedrooms.[147] If medical equipment is needed in the bedroom or if it needs to remain immediately accessible to the resident and/or direct care partners, find ways to cover it so it will remain out of sight when not in use. Every decision must be based on each resident's unique care needs, abilities, and disabilities, while balancing such changes with each resident's need for timely medical care and safety. When done thoughtfully, small changes can go a long way in enabling a resident to feel more at home.

◇ Inadequate Separation Between Beds in Shared Bedrooms

Lack of adequate separation between beds in shared bedrooms reduces the perceived and actual sense of personal and private space.[159] It may also increase the likelihood that residents with dementia will invade or be perceived to invade their roommates' part of the shared bedroom. Noise, such as speaking, calling out, or loud radio or TV can travel easily across a small shared space and disrupt one's roommate. This can cause conflicts even outside the bedroom. Some residents who share a bedroom may be less social in the public areas of the care home and more "territorial" in claiming space, either in a section of the hallway or a chair in the day room.[238,239]

When it is not possible to build private (single-occupancy) bedrooms, make sure that the common space and the personal space are well delineated in the bedroom for each roommate and that a clear, residential-quality boundary exists between the two spaces, such as a wall or well-secured, attractive bookshelf when possible, *not* a ceiling-suspended curtain. In one reported instance,[240] in a nursing home in Queens, NY, a 71-year-old resident wanted the curtain divider open, whereas his 66-year-old roommate wanted it drawn for privacy. Their disagreement escalated into a physical attack one morning around 1:20 a.m., when the younger resident, who apparently had had no history of violence or outbursts, used a piece of wheelchair to severely beat his roommate, who died soon afterward at the hospital.

At the very least, it is important to adhere to the federal nursing home regulations pertaining to "full visual privacy" for each resident in bedrooms (effective November 28, 2017). As noted elsewhere, the guidance is that "residents have a means of completely withdrawing from public view, without staff assistance, while occupying their bed (e.g., curtain, moveable screens, private room)." Nursing home operators can use other, more definitive means to provide full visual privacy, with those means varying according to the needs and preferences of residents as well as their physical and cognitive ability to use them.

◇ Limited or Lack of Sensory Comprehension of Environmental Input

Care homes where sensory input is less understandable were found to be associated with higher levels of behavioral expressions classified as verbally aggressive.[159] In other words, when the sensory complexity of certain features in the physical environment exceeds the cognitive executive functions and perceptual resolution of residents with dementia, the residents may experience distress and lower ability to function independently; this is a rarely discussed form of excess disability in this population. The decorative features in some homes, such as carpets, wallpaper, chandeliers, and furniture, characterize hotels in their design rather than elder-friendly and dementia-friendly homes. As a person's dementia advances, increasingly higher doses of environmental stressors may contribute to the development of various distressing behavioral expressions, consistent with the principles of the Progressively Lowered Stress Threshold Model.[229]

It is important to recognize that many residents with middle- to late-stage dementia perceive and experience the physical environment in a fundamentally different way from people who are cognitively intact. Direct care partners and other interdisciplinary care team members need to pay attention to and regularly assess the "acoustic, visual, thermal, odor, and kinesthetic (i.e., bodily movement and position in space) environment in all spaces, and the degree to which these conditions may confuse or distress residents."[159] Once identified, they should work on developing ways to eliminate these types of stressors (when possible) or minimize their negative effects on the residents.

To the best of your ability, optimize the degree to which the ambient sensory environment is familiar and personally meaningful to residents. These efforts need to address domains such as smells, lighting, colors, heat, sights, sounds, and textures.[159]

◇ Noisy, Overstimulating, and Hectic Environment

Common environmental features in many care homes can often cause overwhelming sensory input for residents.[78] Several types of noise were reported as often being part of physical environments of residents involved in DHRRIs.[178] A study by Rosen and colleagues[14] found that calling out and making noise were reported most frequently by direct care partners as triggers of these episodes. Noise level is also related to poor sleep, distraction from completing a task, "agitation," and fear among people with dementia,[241] and research in nursing homes has found an association between noise levels and quality of life of residents with advanced dementia.[242]

Michael Ellenbogen,[243] a person living with early-onset dementia and a leading national educator and advocate, provides the following insight:

> Sometimes just having a noise in the environment can really set me off in many ways. It can really get me so aggravated. Luckily, today I am still able to control it but I wonder what it does to people who no longer have the capability of self-control. I believe that's the people [in whom] you'll start to see the behavior-type problems.

Noise is an "unwanted sound that is obtrusive or interferes with listening. Noise does not have to be excessively loud to qualify as interference. Loudness is a listener's subjective impression of the strength of a sound."[244] Although noise levels in nursing homes are highly variable, the levels probably vary between 30 and 75 dB (average values do not exist because most of the time the noise level fluctuates) (Steve Orfield, oral communication, September 19, 2013). Others have reported that nursing homes can have noise levels between 55 and 70 dB during the day, which is comparable to busy road traffic noise.[245] Every added 10 dB is equivalent to doubling of the perceived loudness.

However, loudness should be measured in more complex ways than simple decibel measurements. Measurement should include sound frequency, range, periodicity (i.e., a waveform pattern with clear cycles that repeat regularly in time), fluctuation, and precision (Orfield, oral communication, September 19, 2013). Another reason why decibel measurements are inadequate for measuring noise level has to do with levels of reverberation—the continued reflection of sound from surfaces within a room after its source has ended,[244] or the interference noted when a person hears sounds bounce off walls, solid surfaces, and floors. Specifically, if the reverberation time (RT/60) is low, then the noises will not be reinforced and will not travel (in other words, they will not bounce off the walls), which results in a lower negative auditory impact on residents compared with environments with high reverberation levels.

It is a good idea to observe and assess the levels of noise at different times of day, evening, and night. After identifying temporal and spatial patterns, proactively eliminate the noise from the source. Implement policies requiring quiet living environments; remember that residents with Alzheimer's disease and other forms of dementia, at all stages of disease, are very sensitive to noise. According to Orfield,

> Noise is split between background noise (such as heating, ventilating, and air conditioning system and other mechanical systems) and activity noise. . . . Activity noise can be limited by absorption in the space and by training the staff [in] quieter practices, such as speaking to staff at closer positions and not speaking in corridors next to residents' bedrooms, and closing residents' doors when sleeping, where this is safe" (e-mail communication, October 3, 2013).

Direct care partners should eliminate excess noise at its source as a routine practice.[246] Common sources of noise in care homes include kitchen machinery such as dishwashers; plates and silverware falling in the kitchen; direct and non-direct care partners or other care professionals speaking loudly during group activities or when calling a co-worker or resident; ringing phones and visitors talking on cell phones; squeaking of chairs, walkers, and medication carts; distracting public announcements; emergency call systems; and loud noise from vacuum cleaners, televisions, and radios. As explained by Grethe Berg[146] in the context of residents with dementia, "Too many [noise-related] distractions that cannot be sorted out lead to increased disturbance, restlessness, and a general decline in completing tasks." Even small noises, such as a dining room chair scraping along the floor, can cause irritation.[142]

Make sure that the areas surrounding organized activities are quiet; external noise can interfere with the ability of residents with dementia to concentrate on their activities. This problem was reported by a concerned direct care partner who was critical of some of her co-workers: "Some of them think that the residents, since they have Alzheimer's, it doesn't make a difference or matter to them if you speak loudly near a group activity because they do not understand what is going on anyway."[34]

Make available and train direct care partners to offer headphones to residents with dementia to enable them to listen to music or radio stations they like as a way to shield them from the various sources of distracting, frustrating, and annoying noise during the day and evening. This approach could also be used during rest or nap times or at night, when loud "night screams" can be heard from other residents.[247] Headphones can also be used with the television, allowing residents to watch TV and listen without disrupting their roommates.[14] Frequently offering or reminding residents with dementia to use their personal headphones with their favorite music on in general and during times of excessive noise is a recommended practice (for those who want it, can tolerate it, and enjoy it). That said, simply handing a set of headphones and a recorded music device to a resident with middle- to late-stage Alzheimer's disease without providing encouragement, cueing, guidance, assistance, and frequent reminders may not work because many individuals in these stages can have difficulty operating these devices. A simple task, such as increasing or lowering the volume of the music, that we all take for granted might be difficult or impossible for these residents to do or to recall how to do, even after receiving clear instructions.

It can be helpful to have your care employees view the inspiring documentary *Alive Inside: A Story of Music and Memory* during training programs, and to encourage and assist residents who are cognitively able or have early-stage dementia and family members of all residents to watch it. This inspiring and moving film demonstrates the powerful therapeutic value of using an iPod and headphones that enable nursing home residents with dementia and other conditions to listen to music that they enjoy and connect to deeply. The film follows social worker Dan Cohen, who brings iPods to nursing home residents. Listening to favorite music on an iPod can bring tremendous joy to the residents (such as by tapping into deep and personally meaningful remote memories), and it has a clear calming effect on many of them. Consider joining other residences across the United States and Canada (5,300 of them as of 2020) that have already been trained and certified as Music & Memory® Certified Care Programs. Directors of recreation therapies often find this program extremely valuable to their ability to provide personally meaningful engagement (through the thoughtful selection of personally preferred music) to residents with dementia. It enables these individuals to experience joy and a sense of calm, and it can help prevent various types of frustrations that are often caused by living in a noisy, overstimulating, and hectic care environment.

◇ Crowding

Congregation of a large number of residents with dementia in a small space can contribute to DHRRIs.[248] A study by Pillemer and colleagues[87] among 1,405 residents in several nursing homes in New York state found that higher levels of crowding increased the likelihood of DHRRIs. One resident said, "It's very hard to live here. It's like living in a big fishbowl."[35] Malone and colleagues[45] report on a resident who slapped another resident on the hand as she became frustrated in a crowded corridor. Berg[146] reports on a resident who became restless and began to shout when she took part in the Easter Sunday breakfast:

> Normally she had her meals with three other residents and a staff member. The large table with 15 people interacting together was too much for her. She was unable to enjoy the lovely Easter buns that the staff had arranged with the residents. When the residents began to sing, she became agitated, began to shout, and wanted to leave the table.

During my visit to a care home for veterans with dementia, a manager shared with me that the small size of the television lounge often led to overcrowding and DHRRIs.

Direct care partners should proactively monitor and to the extent possible regulate the number of residents with dementia present in the same room or area to avoid crowdedness, which often causes residents with dementia to feel overwhelmed and frustrated and in turn to engage in DHRRIs. Pay special attention to situations where residents with advanced dementia may be inadvertently invading the personal space of others in crowded spaces.

Do your best to have a sufficient number of direct care partners located in key areas in the care home where residents tend to congregate so they can provide adequate supervision and immediate response to early warning signs of distress and anxiety. During group activities, as a strict policy, there should always be at least one additional direct care partner inside or very close to the activity room. Although this will vary based on the room size and the number of residents participating in the activity, it is common to see group activities overcrowded with residents with dementia; this can be overstimulating to certain residents and lead to restlessness, invasions of residents' personal space, and DHRRIs. When this happens, the second direct care partner who is positioned in or near the activity room can quickly assist the group leader by responding to early signs of frustrations before they develop into DHRRIs. This approach allows the group leader to focus completely on leading and engaging the other residents in the activity with minimal interruptions; this approach also can help meet basic care needs, such as helping residents locate or use the bathroom if needed.

Crowding During Transition Times

A common situation that can contribute to DHRRIs occurs when a fairly large group of residents with dementia walk from one area in the care home to another. For instance, at the end of an activity, a group of residents may make their way from the activity room to the dining room. To ensure that the transition is done in a safe way, it must be carefully planned, orchestrated, and paced in a way that minimizes distressing and harmful interactions between residents—for instance, as mentioned earlier, "faster" residents trying to make their way around "slower" residents in order to reach their desired destination first. The number of direct care partners needed to accomplish this successfully depends in part on the number of residents in transit, their level of cognitive impairment and mobility, their use of walking aids (canes, walkers, and wheelchairs), their ability to wait patiently and follow instructions, and their history of engagement in conflicts with other residents in general and during transitions.

A creative way of leading these and similar transitions safely is to use an approach called "trailing music out." Music therapist Wendy Krueger,[249] director of Up Beat Music Therapy, regularly uses this approach to alleviate restlessness and anxiety among residents with dementia:

> If we leave the music group, in the living room, singing a song . . . like "When the Saints Go Marching In," something upbeat that they can march down the hall to, often if we sing a song starting in the living room and ending at the main activity room, the transition is a lot smoother . . . because it's not like we're ending music, now we are walking, now we are sitting . . . we're trailing music out.

I have seen Krueger and her colleagues doing this multiple times, and it has worked beautifully. It is a wonderful example of a proactive, "anticipatory" preventive strategy.

◇ Problematic Television Programs and Content

It is not uncommon to see disturbing, scary, and violent content on the TV in activity rooms of LTC homes, as well as on TV used by residents inside their bedrooms. Examples of the disturbing subjects include wars, accidents, injuries, fires, floods, pandemics (such as coronavirus), airplane crashes, terrorist attacks, and school shootings. At a certain point in their disease, many people with dementia have difficulty distinguishing the content shown on the television from what is happening to them in the room. These misperceptions often cause some people with dementia to experience great frustration and fear, which can contribute to negative inter-actions with other residents and direct care partners.

A veteran who had served in the South Pacific became distressed and shoved his friend while watching a documentary on World War II.[78] Another person with dementia who was watching a Western jumped up and lunged toward the TV, as if he intended to beat up the bad guy.[250] In my 10-month direct observation study[34] in two care homes for people with dementia operated in an assisted living residence, I observed that the television was a frequent source of distress and DHRRIs. Others have reported that images on the TV screen of warfare, car accidents, and acts of mayhem were causing nightmares in persons with dementia.[251]

It is important to regularly and carefully monitor the content shown on the television. As much as possible, avoid content that may trigger misperceptions and negative emotional states such as restlessness, anxiety, and fear.[186]

It is important for decisions about which programs will be shown on TV be based on the input and interests of residents (or their family members, for residents with advanced demen-tia). It is not uncommon to walk into a nursing home and see that the programs shown on TV are clearly for direct care partners' convenience and interests, and that residents have no interest in them. Residences should have clear policies in place instructing direct care partners to use the TV strictly for the enrichment and joy of residents.[252]

Consider using the television as an intentional and thoughtful therapeutic intervention. Show calming and soothing films (for example, nature series such as *Planet Earth*), enjoyable old films (e.g., *The Sound of Music*), and television shows suitable to the cohort of residents (e.g., *I Love Lucy*, for residents who enjoyed watching this show when they were younger).[186] Remember that many residents with dementia may benefit from watching thoughtfully se-lected short films that accommodate their short attention span. Observing each resident's re-actions to different types and lengths of films should inform your efforts to engage them in a meaningful and enriching ways in the future.

◇ Lack of Adequate Landmarks and Signage

More than one-third of people with Alzheimer's disease have been found to have disabling visuospatial disorientation,[253,254] which can limit their ability to reach desired destinations, a phenomenon called wayfinding difficulty.[255] Many residents with dementia, especially middle to late stage, experience difficulty finding their own bedrooms and instead enter other residents' bedrooms and bathrooms. In addition, residents having difficulty remembering or locating their assigned table and seat in the dining room may try to sit or actually sit in another resident's chair. Both of these difficulties, as discussed in Chapter 4, are frequent triggers of DHRRIs.

It is essential to use elder-friendly and dementia-friendly landmarks and signage to cue spatial orientation and compensate for wayfinding difficulties experienced by residents with dementia.[159] To increase residents' ability to locate their bedrooms and avoid walking into other residents' bedrooms, direct care partners may want to install shadowboxes with personal pictures and personally meaningful items outside residents' bedrooms.[195] To improve detec-tion, increase the contrast in the nameplate next to each resident's bedroom with the surround-ing background so it will stand out and be easier for residents to recognize (designers usually try to blend signage in, which reduces residents' ability to detect it).

Use large fonts and digits with high contrast for residents' names and room numbers (Or-field, oral communication, September 19, 2013). One resident with dementia was observed looking for her bedroom for 14 minutes. At one point, she stood in front of another resi-dent's bedroom, looked at the nameplate, and said, "606" (the actual number on the plate was "G06"). Then when she was directed to her bedroom and stood in front of her nameplate, she said, "This is 620" (the actual number on her plate was "G20").[34] This seemingly small example illustrates the importance of using elder-friendly and dementia-friendly signage in LTC homes. Direct care partners and other interdisciplinary care team members should be able to alert management of the need for changes in signage when they notice residents struggling like this.

Place orienting devices, anchors, and activity spaces along common paths in the care home.[159] Use large and simple landmarks (such as fountains or planters with large, nontoxic plants) because they can convey meaning to residents and over time are retained better in their memory (Orfield, e-mail communication, October 3, 2013).

It is helpful to use consistent seating arrangements in the dining room at all times (across shifts and weekends). Place a clear name tag on the table to designate each resident's location and help residents locate their seats. This can also assist in minimizing disagreements and conflicts in situations where residents mistakenly insist that a particular seat belongs to them.

Develop "mobility profiles" describing all the essential destinations a resident is cognitively able and unable to reach independently in the care home.[256] The mobility profiles should be developed for a select group of residents who regularly experience difficulty reaching their desired destinations. The profiles should be used to inform direct care partners' targeted efforts to cue, direct, guide, and lead residents to their destinations; to be useful, the profiles should be updated on a regular basis, as a resident's visuospatial orientation and wayfinding ability changes. Every effort should be made to developing individualized strategies for addressing this common problem. Not being able to reach one's desired destinations, especially when a need arises (such as the need to use the bathroom) can cause residents with dementia to experience a profound sense of frustration, sadness, fear, and embarrassment. It is a matter of dignity.

◇ Temperature Discomfort

Thermal comfort includes the cumulative effects of several elements, such as temperature, humidity, air velocity (too much creates draft; too little creates stagnant air), clothing, activity value (effort level of work required), and metabolic rate (Orfield, oral communication, September 19, 2013). The experience of temperature can be very subjective, so, of course, thermal discomfort can contribute to conflicts between residents with dementia. For example, it is not uncommon for roommates to experience significantly different room temperatures as personally comfortable and to demand that the temperature be adjusted to their preferred level (when they are cognitively able to verbally express this as a source of frustration). One roommate may insist angrily that the bedroom is too cold due to an open window, while the other resists closing the window ("I need some fresh air"). Similar tense disagreements may occur between residents in other parts of the care home, such as in activity rooms and dining rooms.

The fact that in the middle to late stages of dementia some residents lose the ability to dress appropriately for the season (for example, wearing a T-shirt or walking barefoot on a cold winter day) can make the experience of thermal discomfort occur more frequently and be more challenging to resolve. Direct care partners need to see that all residents with dementia dress appropriately in ways that enable them to experience an optimal thermal comfort. Knowing and documenting each resident's baseline sensitivity and preferences regarding thermal comfort should inform efforts to assist the individual in wearing adequate clothing. Sometimes, all it takes is offering a sweater to the person and/or assisting him or her to wear one. When the person is unable to convey her or his needs in words such as due to cognitive disability, paying close attention to the individual's body language (such as facial expressions) can often tell you whether she or he needs assistance to feel comfortable.

◇ Glare, Direct and Indirect

Many physical changes to several structures in the eye that come with increasing age result in elders being bothered by glare much more than younger people,[257] and more visually disabled by it.[259] For example, the most common cause of vision problems in adults 55 and older—cataracts—increases the person's sensitivity to glare; more than half of all Americans 65 and older have cataracts.[258] When elders develop Alzheimer's disease, and when it progresses into advanced stages, many individuals become more sensitive to glare, which may contribute to misperceptions, frustration, and anger. When these individuals live in a care home in close proximity to many other residents, this enhanced sensitivity to glare may compromise their and other residents' safety.[129,191] This may be especially true in buildings that are not designed to minimize glare.

"Direct glare is caused by light coming directly to the eye from a light source. Indirect glare is light reflected from a surface in the direction of the eye. Both can harm vision and cause visual discomfort or disability," according to Orfield and colleagues.[257] Brawley and Noell-Waggoner add, "Glare occurs when bright light interferes with the viewing of objects or surfaces that are less bright."[233]

It is important for direct care partners to regularly monitor and eliminate both *direct* glare from a directly visible lighting source, such as sun rays entering through a window and directly hitting resident's eyes, or an unshielded bulb, and *indirect* glare, which is a consequence of bright light bouncing off reflective surfaces, such as shiny floors,[260] television screens, microwave doors, shiny magazines, tables, and mirrors.

One nursing home resident with Alzheimer's disease was observed on several occasions to calmly get up from his chair, walk across the room, and hit another resident. Raia[261] began to keep a log of this resident's behavioral expressions and began to see that he would hit someone only in the activities room, but not every time he was in that room. Later, Raia noticed that the resident hit people only on sunny days, but not on *every* sunny day when he was in the activities room, and then, that he hit people on sunny days *only* if he was sitting on one side of the room. With the log, Raia was able eventually to determine that the resident hit people if he sat in the activities room and the sun was shining in his eyes. The intervention in this case was simple: Direct care partners made sure that the blinds were closed on sunny days when this man was in the activities room. Once the shades were closed, the behavioral expression discontinued. Thus, with patience and careful observation, documentation, and timely analysis the care team was able to avoid labeling the resident as aggressive and administering antipsychotic medication.[261]

◇ Challenges Accessing, Using, and Sharing Elevators

Elevators have been found to cause significant distress and anxiety among nursing home residents with dementia. Sometimes the waiting time exceeds a resident's attention span capabilities; residents also may have difficulty using the elevator, such as pressing the right command, getting in or out of the car before the door closes, and recognizing the correct floor to exit.[256] DHRRIs have often occurred in or near elevators as a result of violations of personal space, such as when access to or from the elevator is constrained.[72] Imagine a relatively small area leading up to a fairly narrow opening of an elevator car. Then, add to it seven quite frail residents with substantial cognitive disability; a few are using walkers and one is using a wheelchair. With only one care partner to orchestrate the task of entering, using, and leaving the elevator, it is not hard to see how things could go wrong, such as falls or invasions of personal space, leading to pushing.

The following tragic incident took place in a care home in Ontario, Canada. An 88-year-old woman and a 74-year-old man were involved in an incident by an elevator; both had dementia and a history of behavioral expressions labeled as aggressive. The woman was described as "yapping in the face" of the man, who was sitting down by the elevator. He got out of his chair and pushed her into the elevator. She fractured her hip and died from complications several weeks later.

It is important to carefully evaluate the physical features of the elevator by using direct observation (both when it is not in use and when it is in use by residents with dementia) to find out whether specific features may cause residents to experience misperceptions, frustration, and fear. For example, dementia expert Jan Garard reports, "I had residents who wouldn't step into the elevator because the floor of the elevator had a black carpet and I suppose they thought it was an open elevator shaft."[262] Once identified, some of these triggering features can be modified. In this case, using an elder-friendly and dementia-friendly carpet could have prevented residents' misperception and fear caused by the black carpet. In other cases, a glaring, distracting, and frustrating fluorescent or LED light inside the elevator should be replaced with one that makes residents feel more comfortable, such as shielded dimmer fluorescent or LED lighting (Orfield, e-mail communication, March 3, 2021).

When certain distressing features of the elevator cannot be modified, all care employees should be informed about these potentially risky features and proactively plan to use the elevator in safe ways. For instance, if the elevator door opens in such a way that frail residents and those using a walker can get caught in it and fall, or if it closes too fast, a care partner can continuously press on the "door open" button while physically blocking it from closing too fast until all residents have safely entered or exited.

An elevator car that is too small can contribute to overcrowding when too many residents use it at once. To prevent this from happening either inside or next to the elevator, it is helpful to plan ahead of time and carefully monitor and regulate the number of residents with dementia and serious mental illness who can use the elevator comfortably and safely at the same time. Direct care partners should be alert to scenarios where residents invade the personal space of other residents in or near the elevator, which can lead to push–fall incidents.

Never allow residents with middle- to late-stage dementia to use elevators without close supervision and hands-on guidance. As a policy, always have at least one direct care partner inside the elevator car when it is being used by residents and during residents' transitions into and out of the elevator. Depending on the number of residents and their levels of cognitive function, you may need two or more direct care partners attentively supervising these transitions. Depending on the residents' ability to operate the elevator safely, direct care partners may need to take over the operation of the elevators and assist the residents getting in and out at the desired floor.[256] That said, to avoid excess disability, direct care partners will need to use their best clinical judgment with regard to residents with early-stage dementia who are capable of operating the elevator (for instance, pressing the command button or the button for desired floor level) on their own. To alleviate residents' restlessness and anxiety, direct care partners will need to provide residents with frequent cueing, reminders, and reassurance throughout the process of using the elevator, including on the way in and out of it.

When possible and safe, it is best to avoid use of the elevators altogether. One 47-bed dementia care home in a VA Medical Center was experiencing a high rate of DHRRIs, which were clustered around mealtimes and were related to crowding on the elevators and in the hallways. When crowded, residents would push, shove, and slap at each other. Many of the incidents occurred when residents were going to or coming from the centralized dining room. In an attempt to resolve this problem, the administrators decided to change from having a centralized dining area located outside the care home unit to a dining area inside it (the latter did not require the use of the elevator). This change was implemented over a 3-month period. Two dayrooms in the care home were then used for dining, and residents were separated by functional ability during mealtimes. Beyond other positive effects on residents, including lower anxiety, and care partners, who reported feeling less rushed and having saved substantial time, the number of DHRRIs was reduced by half—from 40 incidents before the intervention to 21 during the 3-month period after the change was implemented. Eliminating the need to move all residents into the elevators six times each day (twice for each meal) reduced the number of invasions of personal space and thus the number of incidents.[72]

◇ Access to Sharp or Dangerous Objects

There have been numerous reports in the media of residents both with and without dementia using sharp and otherwise dangerous objects against fellow residents during incidents; the outcomes of these injurious episodes range from mild to severe injuries. Dozens of objects have been used by residents during physically harmful contact with other residents. In addition, my study showed that in 31% (27 out of 88) of fatal resident-to-resident incidents in which at least one of the residents involved had dementia, a physical object was used by a resident against another.[29] In other situations, a dangerous object has been used by a resident with dementia to threaten other residents, but these critical incidents did not result in physical harm (some of these incidents could be described as near misses). For example, in my earliest study on this phenomenon, one resident with severe cognitive impairment took a knife and a fork from a kitchen drawer and physically threatened other residents and direct care partners with them.[13] Direct care partners were able to de-escalate the incident without injuries to anyone involved.

Sometimes, even if a resident is not directly physically harmed by the object itself, incidents involving sharp objects can escalate to a dangerous level. The following tragic incident[263] illustrates this problem. A 76-year-old resident of a nursing home entered another resident's bedroom and took a paring knife and scissors from a drawer. He then walked into another room and thrust the knife and scissors forward at direct care partners and at his own neck. Police officers were called; when they arrived, they reportedly gestured to him to drop the knife and scissors (the resident did not speak English well), but when he thrust the knife and scissors at them and at his own throat, they tased him. As a result, the resident fell on the floor and sustained injuries to his head. He died 2 weeks later. Direct care partners stated that they were not aware that the resident whose bedroom was entered had the knife.

Remain vigilant and regularly take proactive measures to prevent access of residents with dementia (especially those with middle- to late-stage disease) to sharp and dangerous objects. Of course, every person and every form of dementia are different, and even certain individuals with early-stage dementia could place others at risk when they have access to these objects. There is no substitute for the best clinical judgment of your interdisciplinary care team. These efforts to limit residents' access to these objects should be based on an ongoing individualized assessment of each resident's history and current risk of harming others and him- or herself.

When your interdisciplinary care team and managers determine that it is necessary, lock knives and forks inside a drawer of the care home's kitchen. Avoid the use of unlocked drawers or cabinets, and lock scissors or other sharp objects used for nursing or recreation therapy in drawers or cabinets. Remember, though, that this is not only a matter of safety but also a matter of dignity. Not being allowed to use a knife during meals could potentially compromise one's sense of dignity. Striking a balance between these two competing needs often represents a serious and complex daily challenge for care employees and managers.

It is recommended that care homes reduce the use of sharp and otherwise dangerous objects during organized activities and that direct care partners make sure to collect all such items at the end of the activity (that is, maintain a checklist in a central location that details the exact number of these items to verify that all were collected). For example, some care homes for people with dementia offer woodworking activities. If specific residents are evaluated by the interdisciplinary care team to be able to use woodworking tools safely, recreation staff and other direct and non-direct care partners must carefully supervise participating residents at all times and make sure that all sharp or otherwise potentially dangerous tools are collected at the end of the activity; clearly marking each tool with a number and using a tracking sheet makes tracking such tools easier. In one care home for veterans that I visited, I noticed that several long, sharp nails and heavy woodworking tools were left on a shelf in a public space where residents with dementia had easy access to them. Although these did not lead to a problem in that home, a resident in another care home reportedly located long nails and then used a shoe to hammer two of them into her own skull (the nails were undetected for nearly a month). The woman, who had psychiatric disorders and history of self-harm, was hospitalized with serious injuries.[264]

It is important to implement a strict policy instructing all direct and non-direct care partners and family members to prevent at-risk residents with dementia or serious mental illness from having access to knives or other similarly dangerous objects. An individualized, ongoing interdisciplinary evaluation is needed, as most residents with early-stage dementia are able to use these objects safely and would not use them to harm another person; however, this may change as their brain disease progresses. Each form of dementia is different and some people, such as a subgroup of residents with the behavioral variant of frontotemporal dementia, may use sharp objects during incidents with other residents or direct care partners. As described above, one of the challenges has to do with the fact that certain residents with advanced dementia who should not have access to sharp objects (e.g., knives) may gain access to them by entering the bedrooms of other residents and taking these objects from their personal living spaces. Clear guidelines and requirements should be communicated verbally and in writing to residents and their families before and during the admission process and throughout the person's residency at the care home. Although access of at-risk residents to sharp and other dangerous objects can be difficult to avoid, when individualized risk assessment is conducted on a routine basis and serious preventive measures are taken, it is possible to reduce the majority of these situations.

To minimize the likelihood that at-risk residents will use objects to harm other residents, secure closet hanger rods, bed footboards, and towel bars; these and many other objects have been used by residents during injurious incidents with other residents. Think creatively about the types of objects residents could use to harm other residents. Similar measures should be implemented routinely in the public spaces of care homes serving residents living with dementia and serious mental illness.

Factors That Can Be Modified During Building Planning or Renovation

This section presents recommendations and suggestions for environmental designers and architects specializing in planning, building, and renovating LTC homes for elders living with dementia, as well as for owners and administrators to consider.

Planning and Design of Care Environments: Guiding Principles

The vast majority of people living with dementia are elders. Therefore, several fundamental principles need to be taken into consideration during the planning and design phases of care environments for elders in general, even before specific considerations related to cognitive disabilities caused by dementia. These general guiding principles are suggested by Steve Orfield,[259] founder and president of Orfield Laboratories, Inc. (Minneapolis, Minnesota).

- Focus on *"building performance."* In a nutshell, the building's design must be perceptually comfortable and clear (not confusing) for its users. Orfield explains that the science of building performance describes how to maximize factors that influence users' perception of comfort, such as acoustics, lighting, daylighting, temperature, and indoor air quality.[265]

- Focus on *occupancy quality*. Careful attention must be paid to the degree to which different features of the building cause its occupants to like or dislike it (occupants' preference). Examples of factors that affect occupancy quality include aesthetics, ability to navigate the physical spaces and reach desired destinations (i.e., wayfinding abilities and visuospatial orientation), and the occupant's lifelong and current preferences. The building needs to have "design resonance" for residents, which enables them to have a positive user experience reinforced by the aesthetic experience, an experience that enables the resident to meet her or his daily goals efficiently. The occupancy quality is also dependent on the extent to which features of the physical environment (such as elder-friendly signage) are easy to understand and use.

- Focus on *users, not façades*. There is a need for a paradigm shift toward a focus on the experience of the users—residents and care partners—and the areas of user focus in the interior, and reducing the emphasis on overly expensive façades and nonuser areas, such as the lobby. Façade design is often used for marketing and branding purposes, such as in hotel-like assisted living residences, but the solutions to problems in the user experience can usually be found on the inside, in the private and shared areas, such as bedrooms and bathrooms, frequently used daily by residents. Orfield suggests,

  > Strive for simpler environments that fit the lower perceptual resolution of many older adults. Prevent sensory complex and decorative environments consisting of fancy chandeliers in dining rooms, fancy lobby, carpets with fancy and large patterns, low contrast between surfaces (wall and floor), and visual textures. (Orfield, oral communication, September 19, 2013)

  Owners, administrators, and managers of care homes should think about ways to optimize the degree to which direct care partners can control auditory and visual "noise" and the degree to which such sensory complexity is controlled by design.[159]

- Accommodate for *changed perceptions*. Older residents need more cognitive and perceptual simplicity in their physical environment.[265] Design of care environments for older adults must take into account that they tend to have a narrower range of perception and lower levels of perceptual sensitivity; that they are far more sensitive to perceptual noise, such as background noise, visual glare, thermal discomfort, and offensive smells; and that they are likely to have slower cognitive processing of these more limited signals.

- Be aware of multiple possible *unintended implications of each design choice*. It is important to recognize that every decision an architect makes about the physical environment of a care home has multidimensional consequences for the user experience. For example, the choice of carpeting with specific characteristics and qualities affects several domains of residents' experience, such as acoustic, thermal, visual (pattern), tactile (roughness), and safety (e.g., fall risk due to friction and three-dimensional surfaces). Although this area of science in the specific context of residents with dementia is still largely in its infancy, empirical evidence from research studies in the coming years should inform and guide these decisions.

When considering plans for renovation, it is helpful to remember, as Benyamin Schwarz and colleagues[266] advise, that efforts in the physical space must be matched by the efforts of the organization. "Any modification in the architectural environment needs to be orchestrated with appropriate organizational, staff, and social changes to achieve the full potential of a physical design based on homelike characteristics."

◇ Larger Care Homes with a High Number of Residents

Residents living in larger LTC homes were found to exhibit more frequent territorial conflicts, invasions of personal space, and DHRRIs.[267] By contrast, smaller care homes with less crowding were found to be associated with lower levels of these episodes.[268] In addition, a study in 15 special care homes found that insufficient common spaces and inadequate total common space for the number of residents (that is, spatial density) was associated with residents' behavioral expressions labeled as aggressive.[159]

The following intervention study illustrates the importance of building and using small-scale spaces. A care home with a single large dining space that served 25–30 residents underwent renovations that included creation of three smaller dining rooms (each served 8 to 10 residents) and a less institutional ambience. A behavior mapping evaluation was conducted at three points in time (before the renovations, immediately after relocation into the renovated setting, and 3 months after the relocation). The change has led to fewer episodes classified in the study as "disruptive" and "agitated" in the new dining areas as compared with the larger dining space before the renovation. Direct care partners seemed to be having more sustained conversations with the residents in the new dining spaces than in the old one. The reduction of group size in the new and smaller dining areas reduced the likelihood of chain reactions of distressing behavioral expressions during mealtimes.[266] This finding is not surprising, especially given that restlessness and anxiety are known to be contagious among residents with dementia.

In planning for development or creation of a LTC home, or as a care employee working in one, it is useful to reflect on how you might feel if you had Alzheimer's disease and were forced to live in close proximity to 30 or more strangers all day and night, 365 days a year, for a few years. Ask yourself what features *you* would like to see in the physical environment if you were to find yourself living in a care home.

Whenever possible, to decrease crowding, overstimulation, and territorial conflicts, it is best to build small-scale care environments designed for a small number of residents (there is no "magic number," as each care home is designed differently, but a range of 7–15 residents is often recommended).[159] A study by Kovach and Calkins[269] suggested that a 12-resident household at a dementia care home provided direct care partners with more opportunities to become familiar with a smaller group of people through daily structured and informal interaction. This will obviously depend on the extent to which even small-scale care environments offer adequate staffing levels at all times. Examples of LTC organizations considered as leaders in dementia care that intentionally build small-scale home-like environments include the Green House (6–10 residents) and English Rose Suites (6 residents).

In addition, it is important to allocate adequate amounts of common and private space per resident during the planning and design phases of the care home. As mentioned in Chapter 4, British Columbia now requires newly built and publicly funded LTC homes to have 95% of the bedrooms and bathrooms to be built as private spaces and only 5% as shared ones.[141] This reflects a shift in recent years toward building and using private bedrooms and bathrooms as the standard of care in LTC homes. That said, the 95% figure should not be considered as a standard. The actual proportion will depend on the unique characteristics, care needs, and preferences of residents living in each care home as well as the resources allocated by owners and administrators to caring for them.

If renovations are not feasible, think about ways to make the care home *feel* smaller for the people who live there. For example, provide areas where a resident with dementia can rest and find solitude while ensuring adequate supervision by direct care partners in these spaces. Striking a balance between the right to privacy and the need for supervision and safety is an inherent daily challenge, but thoughtful and creative planning can often help to reconcile these competing needs (see "Private Away Spaces [Non-bedroom]" later in this chapter).

In the context of COVID-19, a 17-person panel of experts[270] reported that designing smaller, more homelike spaces would minimize the spread of viruses while promoting better health and quality of life for residents." The experts concluded, "The fact that smaller homes not only support better resident outcomes but are more resilient against infectious outbreaks should prompt policy makers to reimagine LTC infrastructure in a postpandemic world."

◇ Line-of-Sight Obstacles Reducing Ability to Supervise Residents

The physical layout or floor plan of most nursing homes, many of which were developed based on the design of acute hospitals, often limits direct care partners' ability to supervise residents with dementia effectively as they move around the care home.[159,268] Direct care partners often complain that the long hallways of the care home as well as certain layouts (such as an L shape or rectangular shape) limit their ability to see and immediately respond to early signs of distress, anxiety, and DHRRIs (beyond other situations, such as falls). Limited direct eye contact with residents with dementia caused by these design features is a common contributing factor to these episodes. One study in 10 nursing homes (33 care units) in Sweden showed that care units classified as having a high prevalence of "violence" had longer hallways than those with a low prevalence.[271] In addition, a study in 30 nursing homes in Germany described a "straight circulation system" layout, in which the whole corridor could be overseen from any point of the care unit, without shifts in direction; in addition to enhancing supervision, this layout could enable residents with dementia to find their way and reach their desired destinations more easily than other layouts.[272] Since wayfinding difficulties and unwanted entries into other residents' bedrooms are common triggers of DHRRIs, building designers should consider these alternatives and the research on them when planning new or renovated care homes.

Direct care partners need to be able to see the residents with dementia in their care. During a visit to a secure dementia care unit of a nursing home, I noticed two frail residents with dementia engaged in a tense argument over a chair at the end of a long hallway. They were pulling and pushing the chair; one wanted it there while the other wanted to drag it to his bedroom. Direct care partners were not aware of the episode as they gathered by the kitchen counter; they did not have direct eye contact to the end of the hallway. I notified them about it, and their intervention may have prevented a fall and possible injury of one or both of these residents. In another care home for elders with dementia, a TV screen was installed at the end of one long hallway. The intention was to create a quiet space where a small number of residents could watch TV away from the large and often crowded activity room and TV lounge. Unfortunately, the TV was placed in such a way that direct care partners could not have direct line of sight to supervise the residents while there. The TV had to be removed after multiple DHRRIs had taken place, with limited ability of care partners to detect them in time. If the managers of the care home had consulted with direct care partners before installing the TV set, it would have never been placed there.

Another common and challenging situation occurs when two residents with dementia engage in an episode inside a bedroom while direct care partners are busy providing assistance with care-related tasks to other residents in the public spaces of the care home. When bedrooms are located far from areas where direct care partners tend to complete their

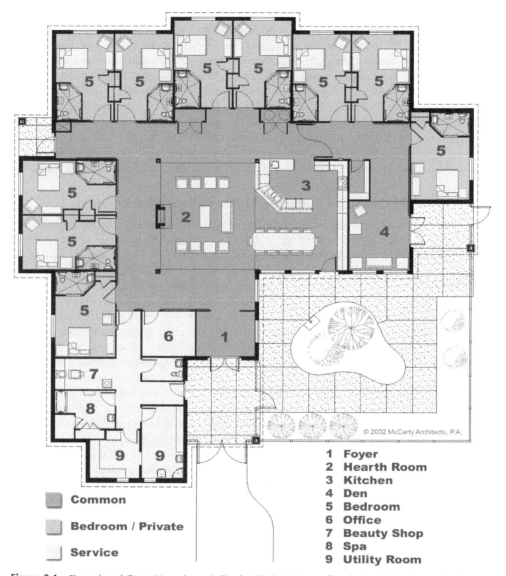

Figure 5.1   Floor plan of Green House home in Tupelo, Mississippi, a small-scale physical environment where ten residents live, each in a private bedroom with a private bathroom. Reprinted with permission.

care-related duties and congregate, they are less likely to see, hear, and respond in time to these episodes.

The reverse is also true. In many care homes, direct care partners are busy providing morning personal care to residents inside bedrooms, while no direct care partner can be found in the public spaces (such as the main activity room or TV lounge) where other residents congregate. During these vulnerable time periods, direct care partners are not well positioned to notice and quickly respond to early warning signs of DHRRIs.

To maximize direct care partners' ability to supervise residents with dementia effectively, care homes should be designed using helpful layouts such as those consisting of a small number of private bedrooms located around main shared spaces. A good example of a desirable layout is the floor plan of the first Green House home (Figure 5.1).[249]

◇ Institutional (versus Homelike) Qualities of the Residence

As noted earlier, historically, the majority of nursing homes in the United States were built and designed on the basis of the hospital model. Fewer incidents of behavioral expressions classified as verbally aggressive were found among residents living in special care units with physical environments that were more "residential" in nature compared with more "institutional" settings.[159] Residents with dementia are more likely to become irritated, frustrated, and angry and to be labeled as aggressive when living in a care setting that looks, feels, sounds, and smells like a hospital compared with one that looks, feels, sounds, and smells like a home. As stated previously, it is important to remember that nursing homes and assisted living residences are the *homes* of residents with dementia; they should look and feel like it. Would we want anything less for ourselves?

Care home leaders and planners should consider implementing residential qualities in the direct and non-direct care partners' dress and care setting's décor, linens, wall accessories, flooring, furniture, and lighting and encourage residents to use personal belongings and furniture. It is also helpful to eliminate hospital-related features such as nurses' stations and use of medication carts.[159] The Green Houses of The Eden Alternative represent an inspiring example of how institutional physical environments (aligned with and supported by deep changes in organizational operations) can be transformed into care settings that are truly residential and consistent with person-directed care practices.

◇ Private Away Spaces (Non-bedroom)

Lack of private away spaces or limited access of residents with dementia to these dedicated spaces can often limit residents' ability to meet their needs (such as the need for privacy) and thus can directly and indirectly contribute to the development of DHRRIs. Quiet, relaxing time alone can alleviate emotional buildups, such as those due to increased restlessness and anxiety and decreased tolerance of other residents.

It is important to build private away spaces (beyond bedrooms) to provide residents with dementia enough opportunities to spend time away from other residents. For example, outside each cluster of bedrooms at St. John's Green House in Penfield, New York, there is a small alcove, with seating available, before one reaches the common area where the living room and dining room are located. As Power[65] explains, "This enables people to choose how much they wish to engage with others, and it gives those who are a bit more hesitant a chance to 'scope things out' before plunging into the mainstream."

Design a sufficient number of quiet away spaces and place them thoughtfully in locations that enable direct care partners to see (in other words, maintain direct line of sight) and easily supervise residents with dementia who are using them. Close supervision should be directed toward vulnerable and frail residents with dementia who tend to experience negative emotional states, restlessness, anxiety, fear, self-neglect, and safety risks as well as complex healthcare conditions when they are on their own for significant periods.[161] Creative design and location of away spaces can help direct care partners maintain the balance between privacy and safety, as well as allow them to monitor those who require an enhanced level of supervision.

◇ Inadequate Outdoor Spaces

As noted earlier in this chapter, it is essential for residents with dementia to have regular access to an outdoor space, such as a garden or yard. Outdoor spaces must be designed in ways that maximize residents' safety and relaxation such as through the use of the following:

- Circular walking paths to avoid dead ends

- Benches for rest

- Flat but not slippery walking surfaces free of obstacles (to prevent falls)

- Adequate lighting, especially for evening hours

- Well-shaded areas with the use of pergolas as needed during hot summer days

- Walking paths completely clear of snow or black ice during the winter

- Nonedible plants to prevent poisoning

- Use of nontoxic strategies to repel biting insects

- A secured 8-foot fence

◇ Lack of Bedroom Privacy

The majority of nursing home residents are forced to share a very limited amount of living space with strangers. The decades-long normalization of shared bedrooms in care homes continues in many parts of the country despite strong evidence that elders overwhelmingly prefer private bedrooms over shared bedrooms in residential care settings.[273] "I don't want a roommate," said one nursing home resident. "If I'm off by myself, I won't have my feelings hurt and I hurt nobody else."[274]

Beyond an individual's preference or hurt feelings, of course, shared bedrooms and the accompanying lack of privacy can be dangerous in the context of dementia. One woman, whose father was beaten by his roommate, reported,[275]

> My father is in a ward room. It's a very small room actually with a total of three of them in the room, so there's not a lot of personal space in there. A lot of times, they're invading each other's space. It begs the question as to why people with known aggression are mixed with people who are quite frail and vulnerable. I believe having your own personal space and enough of it is critical in these facilities.

A 77-year-old resident in a nursing home who was severely beaten by his roommate, who had a history of violent behaviors, sustained a brain bleed requiring an emergency brain surgery and 20-day hospitalization. Prior to that incident, he told his daughter that he had discussed his situation with care employees: "I told them that if I have to spend one more night with this man, then I will kill myself. And they still ignored me." Power asserts,[65]

> Our elders in long-term living environments deserve privacy, no less than any of us. This means that the place where they sleep, use the toilet, conduct sensitive conversations, and express their sexual intimacy must be completely private. The only way to accomplish this is with a private room with a closeable door.

Although the words "private" and "privacy" are often used in the context of residents' rights, I believe that it is still worth remembering the following definitions. *The American Heritage Dictionary*[276] defines the word private as "secluded from the sight, presence, or intrusion of others," "designed or intended for one's exclusive use," and "belonging to a particular person or persons, as opposed to the public or the government."

A study by Terakawa[277] examined changes in satisfaction levels of residents who lived in shared bedrooms and then moved into a new building with all private bedrooms. Although almost 40% of the residents initially reported complete satisfaction with having a roommate and did not want to live in a private bedroom, by 8 months after the move, 100% of the residents were completely satisfied with having a private bedroom. Margaret Calkins explains, "People may tolerate and even accommodate to having a roommate, when it's necessary (making the best of it), but once they've had the opportunity to experience living in a private bedroom, that's what they preferred." Importantly for the prevention of DHRRIs, another study[268] found that transitioning from multiple-occupancy bedrooms to private rooms reduced the number of conflicts between residents.

Residents occupying multiple-occupancy bedrooms have been found to spend most of the day in their bedrooms or to establish territories in the hallways that they defend "aggressively" against intruders; residents who occupy private bedrooms are more likely to share the space in the hallway.[278] When planning or designing for a LTC home, it is important to make it a high priority to have the vast majority of resident bedrooms private to promote residents' privacy and reduce the number of conflicts between roommates.

While emphasizing private bedrooms, be sure to offer a few shared bedrooms as well, to accommodate those residents who prefer, enjoy, and benefit from having a roommate.[268] Some residents with dementia may even become tense or frightened by being alone (Judy Berry, e-mail communication, January 2016). In addition, a compassionate and supportive room-mate who is cognitively intact or has early-stage dementia could assist direct care partners by alerting them to situations experienced by a roommate that require their immediate attention (such as by using the call light). That said, Berry cautions that shared bedrooms must be large enough to allow for adequate personal space for each roommate, and once inhabited they may also require a higher staff-to-resident ratio for enhanced monitoring (e-mail communication January 2016).

In any design plans for transitioning a care home from multiple-occupancy to private bed-rooms, consider ways to maximize the ability of direct care partners to supervise residents living in these private rooms.[268] One way is to build all bedrooms in a circular configuration close to the main public areas (such as the living room) to increase direct eye contact with bedrooms.

Keep in mind that the Centers for Medicare & Medicaid Services' (CMS) regulations governing nursing homes state that bedrooms must "be designed or equipped to assure full vi-sual privacy for each resident."[32] According to CMS's interpretive guidelines of this regulatory requirement, full visual privacy means that "residents have a means of completely withdrawing from public view, without staff assistance, while occupying their bed (e.g., curtain, moveable screens, private room)."

Once again, direct care partners face a tremendous supervision challenge each and every day. On one hand, they want and are required to protect residents' privacy, but on the other hand vulnerable and frail residents such as those with advanced Alzheimer's disease require adequate supervision and frequent wellness checks to ensure their safety (many residents with advanced dementia are not able to verbally call for help or use a call light). Developing and implementing a thoughtful individualized care plan that aims to maintain this delicate balance between these competing needs for each resident is of utmost importance.

Aim for a minimum bedroom size of 125 square feet for a private room and 125 square feet per person in a shared room (exclusive of toilet room); Margaret Calkins recommends this area as a minimum,[279] although CMS's current minimum requirements are only 80 square feet per person in a multiple (shared) bedroom and 100 square feet for a single (private) bedroom. Adequate privacy in reasonably sized bedroom space should be the standard expectation in nursing homes and all other types of LTC homes. As Calkins explains,[279] "Ask any gathering of people—if they had to move into a nursing home tomorrow, would they want to share a room with someone they had never met before? Especially if the room looked like a hospital room with the beds separated by a piece of fabric? I have done this, and I can tell you, the answer is a resounding, 'No!'"

◇ Shared Toilets and Showers

The number of residents per toilet and shower was identified by Zeisel and colleagues[159] as an important indicator of the level of privacy among nursing home residents. The current reality, in which two or more roommates are forced to use a shared shower or toilet, is not only deeply disrespectful to these elders and a threat to their dignity but it is also a common trigger of DHRRIs. In a study by Teresi and colleagues,[144] almost one-fifth of cognitively intact residents felt bothered by a lack of privacy in using the toilet, often because their cognitively impaired roommate or neighbor would walk in while they were in the bathroom.[159] An alternative scenario occurs when residents with dementia enter the bathroom of *other* residents and use their toilet. Such unwanted entries often cause tremendous frustration to the residents to whom the bathroom and toilet belong. In the words of one resident, "A lot of them have Alzheimer's disease . . . It gets you mad enough though when someone is using your toilet, but you have to see where it is coming from. The guy himself doesn't know what he is doing."[152] The risk of conflicts is naturally higher when two or more residents with dementia need to use the toilet or shower at the same time.

Again, it is worthwhile to reflect on how you would feel if you were required to share a bathroom (toilet and shower) a few times a day with a stranger, possibly with dementia, in your own home. This structural design problem has been the norm in many LTC homes for decades. It is wrong, undignified, and it must change.

Even worse, in some nursing homes operating within very old buildings, a shower room is located in a centralized part of the care home, sometimes quite far from residents' bedrooms; many, if not all, residents in these care settings do not have showers inside or adjacent to their bedrooms. This old, outdated culture of structural design is a major source of humiliation to residents with or without dementia, and it can cause frequent daily conflicts between residents. It must be eliminated from any care home that is committed to providing person-directed care. Beyond being a safety issue, it is an issue of dignity.

It is important to remember that CMS–certified nursing homes must adhere to the federal nursing home regulations regarding bathroom facilities: "Each resident's room must be equipped with or located near toilet and bathing facilities. For facilities that receive approval of construction plans from state and local authorities or are newly certified after November 28, 2016, each residential room must have its own bathroom equipped with at least a commode and sink." (The regulations include a helpful definition of what "located near" means). For additional detail, owners and administrators of CMS–certified nursing homes need to consult with the relevant sections in the current CMS State Operations Manual (addressing the new federal nursing home regulations) and applicable CMS Interpretive Guidelines.[32] Beyond the importance of adhering to CMS regulations, the person-directed care design consisting of one private bathroom and toilet and one shower dedicated to each resident can substantially increase residents' sense of privacy and dignity, which, in turn, can minimize DHRRIs.

◇ Narrow Hallways

It is important to build wide hallways that allow residents easy two-way walking and flow.[159] Stephen Soreff reports that hallways that are not wide enough can contribute to DHRRIs,[78] and one study[248] reported that "traffic jams" in hallways led to outbursts of screaming, swearing, and hitting between residents. Hallways should be wide enough to allow at least two wheelchairs to pass by each other easily. According to the Ministry of Health and Long-Term Care of Ontario,[280] "At a minimum, the width of hallways should be at least 6 feet to 8 feet to provide adequate accessibility for persons using wheelchairs and other assistive devices."

◇ Dead Ends in Hallways

Dead ends at the end of hallways can contribute to conflicts between residents with dementia. For example, a few residents with middle- to late-stage Alzheimer's disease may walk in the hallway in the same direction. When they reach the end of the hallway, some of them may not have the cognitive abilities (such as visuospatial orientation or executive functions) to easily find their way out of the constricted area. Specific cognitive disabilities that may contribute to this problem include self-correcting difficulty or inability to think one's way out of a situation by visualizing an alternative route,[255] as well as difficulties in retracing one's steps; in other words, the person has to solve the problem of getting out of a dead end as if it were a new problem.[281]

Struggling to get out of this crowded situation, a resident with dementia may feel frustrated and/or threatened, which may cause him or her to push another resident away to create some space in an effort to leave the area. Alternatively, invasion of personal space of residents in such a small area could occur, which may trigger a resident's defensive physical response, leading to injurious "push–fall" incidents.

One way of avoiding the problem of dead ends is to build circular walking paths along the care home's perimeter that enable residents to keep walking freely. For this and other purposes (for instance, promoting physical activity), well-marked circular walking paths should also be built in the secured outdoor area or garden of the care home. As explained by a manager in one care home designed with circular paths, "The layout of the facility was designed specifically for people with Alzheimer's disease and memory loss. Both the indoor and outdoor walking areas are circular. This layout ensures that there are no 'empty endings' (i.e., 'dead ends); people can always keep walking and aren't set up for failure."[34]

If your residence is not able to reconstruct and renovate existing dead ends in the hallways, Elmståhl and colleagues suggest "avoiding dead ends in corridors by creating comfortable seating, activities (such as a life skill station), or signage at the end of the hallway to reorient residents with dementia and lead them back to activity areas."[282] That said, seating areas must be thoughtfully located in ways that do not create an obstacle for walking or even a safety hazard. In one secured care home for people with dementia, a resident with vascular dementia who was paralyzed on one side of his body and had limited vision on that side was observed walking in the hallway and bumping into a bench positioned against the wall where he was not able to see it.

◇ Outdoor Environmental Noise

A significant number of care homes are located in a noisy external environment such as near a construction site, major highway, busy road, or airport.[259] Other care homes may be going through construction and renovation processes. These constant sources of noise can be distracting, annoying, and upsetting, causing ongoing daily frustration among residents with dementia and direct care partners. The frustrating noise can have negative effects on residents' ability to hear and understand other residents and direct care partners and on the quality of their daily interactions. Many elders with dementia are highly sensitive to noise, and when the noise is frequent and when it takes place over an extensive period of time, it may lower their threshold of tolerance of other residents' verbal and behavioral expressions.

Orfield adds that outdoor noise may discourage direct care partners from opening windows in the summer—limiting fresh air—and they may decide to keep residents inside the care home, because it can be hard to hear clearly outside (e-mail communication, October 3, 2013). In addition to the stress of the noise itself, some residents with dementia who are unable to spend time outside in the fresh air to decompress, relax, and enjoy other psychological benefits of being outdoors are at increased risk of engaging in DHRRIs.

When possible, it is best to avoid building LTC homes in noisy areas and excessively noisy parts of neighborhoods. Instead, strive to build the residence in a quiet residential area. Beyond the important sense of belonging and inclusiveness realized when care homes are naturally integrated in residential areas (one good example is English Rose Suites in Minnesota), it could also save costs that you may otherwise need to invest in compensating for and reducing the effects of the external noise.

If your residence is already built, consider conducting an environmental noise assessment in order to determine what if any environmental features could be incorporated to compensate for the external noise, such as building better walls or acoustic ceilings tiles, roofs, and windows. Installing acoustic, sound-control glass can make a huge difference if your care home is located near a major highway or airport.

◇ Poor Indoor Sound Quality

Several factors in physical environments of LTC homes often cause excessive noise. These may include, among others, loud conversations; noise from the heating, ventilation, and air conditioning (HVAC) system; noise from the kitchen (such as from a dish washing machine; loud handling of plates, cups, and silverware), laundry machine, and dryer (when these are located within the care home as opposed to a central location in the building); squeaky wheel of a medication cart or activity cart; noisy handling of equipment and furniture (fast movement of chair in the dining room); loud overhead paging systems; call lights that generate alarms; and loud noise generated from the TV set or during organized activities.

Care home planners and designers can reduce sound issues before they become a source of frustration and anxiety, and thereby a factor leading to DHRRIs. Leaders of residences (either existing or in the planning phase) interested in improving their acoustic care environments should consult with acoustical consultants (acousticians) with expertise in gerontology. Orfield and Brand[244] suggest the following considerations when selecting acoustical consultants:

> An acoustical consultant is a professional, usually with an engineering or equivalent credentials, whose primary role is to provide advice on acoustical requirements and noise control in a variety of situations. These professionals come from a variety of areas and are generally not certified under any standardized certification process. Thus, experience, capabilities, and client references are very important to consider when engaging an acoustical consultant. Design firms must investigate the knowledge, abilities, experience, and testing and modeling capabilities of an acoustical consultant, as well as his or her general orientation to the holistic design process.

Orfield states, "There is a need to acoustically model the space for reverberation, background noise, and other aural interference"[259] and reduce background noise and reverberation levels. Elders usually understand speech far more easily in quiet spaces with low reverberation and low background noise levels.[265] It is best to design acoustically "dead" spaces (similar to a well-furnished living room) such as in dining rooms, activity rooms, and bedrooms (Orfield, oral communication, September 19, 2013). The use of sound-absorbent materials (carpeting, drapes, furniture) to reduce noise levels is recommended.[194]

Many nursing homes prefer using cleanable surfaces (for understandable reasons) and in the process reduce their sound absorption capacity. Designers should strive to use materials that are both easily cleanable and sound absorbent, such as cleanable absorptive ceiling tiles and cleanable perforated vinyl acoustic wall panels (Orfield, oral communication, September 19, 2013).

Additionally, HVAC systems are usually too loud in nursing homes and are considered a primary source of background noise (Orfield, oral communication, September 19, 2013). The HVAC system must be designed to have low background noise levels. It is important to note that building a quiet HVAC system is cheaper than trying to quiet it down after it has already been built. For more information and recommendations about noise and sound solutions, see the professional paper *Better Sound Solutions* from the American Society of Interior Designers, Orfield Laboratories Inc., and Haworth, Inc.[244]

◇ Inadequate Lighting and Daylighting[194]

"The typical nursing home lighting is inadequate to meet residents' lighting needs," according to Brawley and Noell-Waggoner.[233] Inadequate lighting in LTC homes may consist of inadequate artificial lighting, dim or dark areas, uneven lighting, low levels of natural daylight, and decreasing lighting in the winter. Previous research has shown some of the negative effects of inadequate lighting on residents living in LTC homes. Low lighting levels in the bedrooms of nursing home residents with severe dementia were found to be associated with negative affective mood,[242] and higher levels of "agitation" were found among residents with dementia in special care homes for this population.[167]

One study[283] in 53 nursing homes showed that the residences were often dimly lit, and illumination was rated as inadequate or barely adequate in 45% of the hallways, 17% of the activity areas, and 51% of the residents' bedrooms. Another study found ambient (general) light levels in residents' bedrooms that ranged from 50% to 65% lower than the recommended minimum light levels. When the light levels in the bedrooms were compared with the minimum recommended light levels for task lighting, the nursing homes provided only 20%–40% of the recommended minimum light[284]; task lighting is lighting that is installed specifically to light an area where a specific task (such as reading) is performed.[257]

This measurement does not account for dark finishes and glare. Orfield points out that using the foot-candle as a metric for evaluating light levels is inadequate (oral communication, September 19, 2013) because it does not describe lighting quality or the quality of the visual environment.[257] Specifically, knowing the lighting level (illuminance) without taking into account the effect of the light as it interacts and bounces back from surfaces (luminance, lighting glare) is clinically meaningless from the resident's perceptual point of view. Orfield explains,[259]

> When lighting is increased in senior housing in hopes of making the environment clearer for elders, often the result is lower visual performance (less visibility). Put differently, increasing the amount of foot-candles in a room can bring about a positive perceptual effect on residents only if one controls for glare (such as with appropriate color and gloss of finishes). What is needed are lighter and brighter luminance and glare-free environments (not just more foot-candles).

Daylighting is the term used to describe "that aspect of the architectural design of buildings that allows daylight to penetrate into interior spaces and which makes use of the available daylight in some fashion."[257] Orfield[259] argues that "designers often don't know that the failure to get sufficient daylighting reduces production of vitamin D and melatonin, thereby reducing the ability to sleep, and causing significant restlessness among residents with dementia."

Aging-related changes tend to exacerbate certain optical deficiencies (such as blurring of location and color, uneven acuity, and two-dimensional object ambiguity), so the negative consequences of poor lighting and daylighting design tend to increase with age.[257] The level of experience, knowledge, and expertise necessary for adequate planning of lighting in LTC homes is much deeper than can be addressed in this section.

To ensure careful design planning of lighting in your care home, include in your design team a certified and experienced lighting professional with a background in gerontology,[233] such as a member of the Illuminating Engineering Society of North America or the International Association of Lighting Designers (IALD). Design firms must "investigate the knowledge, abilities, experience, and testing and modeling capabilities of the lighting consultant, as well as their general orientation to the holistic design process."[257] Evidence-based research laboratories specializing in design of LTC homes tailored to the perceptual abilities and disabilities of elders in general and those with dementia should also be consulted.

Work closely with these lighting specialists to ensure the provision of necessary and high-quality lighting for older residents' eyes by implementing the following.

- Raising light levels substantially (to compensate for the decrease in light reaching the aging retina). This may improve independence, reduce late afternoon and early evening restlessness, promote better sleep, and stabilize mood.[261]

- Balancing natural light and electric light to achieve even light levels.

- Eliminating direct and indirect (reflected) glare.

- Eliminating shadows from outside such as by drawing the curtains, as these shadows can cause distress and fear among residents with dementia. The Alzheimer's Association states, "Reduced lighting and increased shadows may cause people with Alzheimer's disease to misinterpret what they see, subsequently becoming more agitated."[285]

Strategies for Enhancing Light

The best daylighting solutions use abundant natural light (for instance, taller ceiling and window openings to help daylight penetrate spaces).[233] The most common systems for bringing light into a building and distributing it evenly within the interior spaces incorporate windows, light shelves, skylights, and clerestory windows to prevent glare.[286] Orfield and colleagues[257] emphasize that windows located high on the wall are much more effective than windows lower down in terms of bringing daylight deeper into the space for a given surface area. Furthermore, these experts state,

> Daylighting designers sometimes add light shelves above view windows (i.e., at eye level) to bounce the incoming daylight onto the ceiling, which then reflects it down to the room so that the daylight distribution in the space becomes more uniform. Some manufacturers have recently started developing louver systems, which in effect do the same job as light shelves but do not protrude so far into the space.

A louver is a type of screen made of translucent or opaque material and geometrically designed to prevent lamps from being viewed directly at a given angle. Louvers are intended to minimize direct and indirect glare.

In addition, window framing, daylight shields, and other materials in the path of sunlight must be low in reflectance and matte (diffuse) in finish. Otherwise, they will become secondary sources of brightness and glare. According to Brawley and Noell-Waggoner,[233]

> Most glare can be controlled either by shielding the light source from direct view or balancing the light in the room. This can be accomplished by increasing the brightness of the surroundings with evenly distributed light on walls and ceilings, decreasing the brightness of the source, or both. The best solution for controlling glare is indirect lighting (e.g., indirect luminaries [light fixtures] which conceal bright light sources and spread diffused light over a broad area).

Fagan[194] suggests using light-filtering window coverings (such as sheers, blinds, or shades), and Orfield states, "The strategy to reduce the glare should include a secondary strategy to reduce the brightness when the light enters the room. This can be achieved with exterior light shelves, indoor automated shades (automated daylight control), and custom-made daylight louver (outdoors)" (oral communication, September 19, 2013). In addition, Orfield and colleagues[257] suggest using window films in situations where excessive sunlight is passing through the windows, causing harsh glare. When the amount of glare is a minor to moderate nuisance, typically a window film with a visible light transmission of 20%–40% is sufficient. However, when glare is extreme (such as with west- or east-facing windows where sunlight is directly shining through windows at low sun angles), window films with visible light transmissions of less than 20% are recommended. In severe glare situations that involve single-pane clear windows, it is usually necessary to use films with visible light transmissions of less than 15%.

Furthermore, Orfield and colleagues state, "with regard to gloss, the changes can be dramatic. If the finishes along a curtain wall include high-specularity (high-gloss) values, these finishes will mirror bright lighting sources, including the sun or the overcast sky. High-specularity window frames or window blinds will do the same. During certain seasons or times of the day, these surfaces will greatly increase glare or other visual distraction or discomfort."[257] For additional suggestions for eliminating glare, see the review article by Brawley and Noell-Waggoner.[233] The American Society of Interior Designers' report *Better Lighting and Daylighting Solutions* provides useful information and recommendations on lighting and daylighting (including daylighting control systems).[257]

Resources for Planning and Design of Care Homes

Innovative Designs in Environments for an Aging Society (I.D.E.A.S.)

Owners and administrators of LTC homes interested in learning more about the role of the physical environment in caring for residents with dementia and receiving guidance, training, and consultation could use the services provided by an organization that specializes in environmental design for elders, such as I.D.E.A.S. (Margaret Calkins, president; https://ideas consultinginc.com/).

Orfield Laboratories, Inc.

Orfield Laboratories is the nation's only independent multisensory design research lab consulting in architecture and product development. The lab has been developing building performance design standards (acoustics, audiovisual, daylighting, lighting, thermal comfort, and indoor air quality) for over 40 years. Orfield Laboratories has also consulted in occupancy quality research, including developing and administering occupancy studies, for over 30 years. For the past 20 years, the company has developed a worldwide specialty in perceptual and cognitive disabilities, and the first focus of this effort was on aging and dementia, which resulted in the first project, Western Homes in Iowa, being awarded the top research prize at the International Dementia Conference in Manchester, England. The company provides research-based consulting services using cutting-edge, holistic, and person-directed measurement focused primarily on increasing perceptual comfort and perceptual preference for the user. (https://www.orfieldlabs.com/)

6

Factors Related to
Direct Care Partners

Certified nursing assistants are the foundation
of the caregiving industry. I use the word foundation
because just like putting up a building, first you have a
strong foundation or else the building will not stand up.

Resident care assistant in an assisted living
residence for people with dementia[287]

This chapter identifies several factors related to direct care partners that can contribute to the development of distressing and harmful resident-to-resident interactions (DHRRIs). Owners, administrators, and managers of long-term care (LTC) homes need to be aware of these factors and should strengthen their commitment to providing ongoing support, acknowledgment, care resources, and dementia-specific training programs to direct care partners. The chapter also provides practical suggestions aimed at strengthening direct care partners' practices that, if applied consistently, could increase their ability to prevent and de-escalate these episodes. All the factors presented below (Table 6.1) are modifiable (◇).

◇ Low and Dangerous Staffing Levels

Federal regulations require that each nursing home must provide nursing services to meet the care needs of its residents:[288]

> The facility must have sufficient nursing staff with the appropriate competencies and skill sets to provide nursing and related services to assure resident safety and attain and maintain the highest practicable level of physical, mental, and psychosocial well-being of each resident, as determined by resident assessment and individual plans of care and considering the number, acuity, and diagnoses of the facility's resident population in accordance with the facility assessment . . . [32]

Despite the requirement in the regulations, an insufficient number of direct care partners per resident has been a major problem in U.S. care homes for decades. A review of dozens of research studies examining staffing levels in U.S. nursing homes found that half of the nursing homes have "low staffing levels and at least a quarter have dangerously low staffing."[68] This means that at the time these studies were conducted, approximately 350,000 residents received care from direct care partners who are dangerously understaffed, placing the residents at serious risk of experiencing neglect of healthcare and supervision and a whole host of other bad care outcomes.

This chronic problem persists despite the fact that a research study in LTC homes in Canada has shown that a higher number of nursing assistant care hours per resident per day

131

Table 6.1   Factors Related to Direct Care Partners

- Low and dangerous staffing levels
- Staff burnout
- New, inexperienced, and untrained direct care partners
- Inappropriate approaches, attitudes, and communication style
- Malignant social psychology
- Organizational tensions
- Inadequate reporting of episodes
- Labeling a resident, verbally or in writing
- Inattentiveness to early warning signs of distress and anxiety
- Language mismatch (care employee–resident)

was associated with higher overall quality of care—in this case, a composite score consisting of 12 indicators such as activities of daily living, "behavioral symptoms," antipsychotic medication use without psychosis, delirium, urinary tract infections, pressure ulcers, falls, and physical restraint use.[289] Other studies found that higher staffing levels, especially of registered nurses, were associated with improved care processes and a variety of improved care outcomes, such as better physical functioning, less weight loss, fewer pressure sores, fewer urinary tract infections, less dehydration, lower hospitalization rates, and lower mortality rates.[290,291]

Certified nursing assistants (CNAs) and nurse aides are, indeed, the backbone of the LTC industry. They serve as the primary care partners in nursing homes and assisted living residences (providing about 80% of the hands-on care to residents).[292] According to Irvine and colleagues,[293] a typical workload for a nurse aide in a nursing home is 11 or 12 residents during the day and evening shifts and 45 residents during the overnight shift.[292] Although staffing levels vary greatly across nursing homes, this ratio is disturbing because it is often extremely difficult, if not impossible, for a single CNA to care for such a large number of frail and vulnerable residents—the majority of whom have Alzheimer's disease and other forms of dementia—in an effective and safe way. As reported by Schnelle and colleagues, "the average nurse aide staffing levels reported by nursing homes falls below the level of staffing predicted as necessary to provide consistent activity of daily living care to all residents in need."[294]

It is a cruel situation for these dedicated and caring direct care partners, who try to do their best when caring for residents despite challenging and distressing working conditions, low pay, and often insufficient recognition for their tremendous daily efforts. Judy Berry, president of Dementia Specialist Consulting, reflected on the critical role of adequate staffing levels in preventing DHRRIs. She reports that in 16 years her specialized dementia care homes had only two serious DHRRIs, a low rate that was due to the high staff ratios, specialized staff training for prevention, and a robust meaningful engagement program.[27,60] As one resident care assistant said, "We know each and every one of our residents intimately. We love working with the residents. It gives us joy that we can assist them in the evening of their lives. We truly care for the residents and that honest care shows in the work we do."[287]

According to Stephen Long, expecting a nursing assistant who helps a large number of residents with their activities of daily living to also be effective at following best practices in addressing residents' psychological, behavioral, or mental health needs[295] "may not be realistic."

An insufficient number of well-trained direct care partners on the floor (especially nurse aides) causes work overload and decreases their ability to engage and supervise residents with dementia effectively.[296]

Numerous studies have found major gaps in the supervision of residents with dementia, as well as links between those gaps and DHRRIs. Lachs and colleagues[87] found that lower staff-to-resident ratios increased the likelihood of DHRRIs. Low staffing results in lower supervision and attention to residents. According to Rosen and colleagues, "Staff only witness a portion of resident interactions, and absence of staff may actually precipitate incidents and allow them to escalate."[38] A pilot study using 24/7 video cameras in the public spaces of a dementia unit using CareMedia technology showed that nearly 40% of episodes of physical resident-to-resident "aggression" were not witnessed by direct care partners.[297,74] Furthermore, my study found that 62% (52 of 84) of fatal resident-to-resident incidents were reported as not witnessed by direct care partners.[29] Understaffing was often noted as a contributing factor in these deadly incidents. Another study, examining the circumstances surrounding deaths resulting from resident-to-resident incidents in U.S. nursing homes, reported that of 50 deaths for which there were data available to determine it, staff were reported as not having been present in 38 (76%) of these incidents.[30] As Miranda Ferrier, president of the Ontario Personal Support Workers Association, said, "It all comes down to not enough staff on the floors."[7]

In one example, a resident with Alzheimer's disease entered the bedroom of another resident with dementia. Some time later, the resident whose bedroom it was came in, saw the other resident there, and beat him severely with his cane. The condition of the resident who had entered the wrong bedroom deteriorated, and he died a week later. An investigation conducted by the office of ombudsman for LTC found that there was a shortage of staff at the time of the incident, after 9 p.m.[57] As discussed in Chapter 4, evening hours represent a vulnerability period when staffing levels are typically lower, meaningful engagement programming is less available, and active presence of managers is often low.

One international study[298] compared levels of behavioral expressions classified as "violence" toward direct care partners in LTC homes in three Canadian provinces (Manitoba, Nova Scotia, and Ontario) with four Nordic European countries (Denmark, Finland, Norway, and Sweden). The study found that Canadian direct care partners were nearly seven times more likely to experience daily "violence" than their counterparts in Nordic countries. More than other factors, working short-staffed was found to be a major contributing factor for the difference. Working short-staffed is typically much less common in the Nordic countries than in North America.

To avoid a high risk of DHRRIs, LTC homes must provide sufficient staffing levels on all shifts and at all times to decrease direct care partners' workload strain[299] and enable them to supervise residents effectively and meet their psychosocial and physical needs. Having enough direct care partners on all three shifts, including weekends and holidays, increases the likelihood that they will be better positioned to proactively identify and address early warning signs of distress, anxiety, unmet needs, and situational triggers before they escalate into DHRRIs.

Many owners, administrators, managers, and care professionals in nursing homes and assisted living residences report that the ability of care homes to provide adequate staffing levels at all times would be strengthened with increased government funding.[296] As would be expected and required in childcare settings, our society (particularly federal and state government and regulatory agencies) needs to provide sufficient funding and implement adequate reimbursement mechanisms to LTC homes to ensure that sufficient numbers of direct care partners (including nursing assistants, nurses, social workers, and recreation therapists) will be on duty to meet residents' varied care needs as well as to prevent DHRRIs and recognize them in time to promptly and skillfully de-escalate them.

An encouraging initiative called the Payroll-Based Journal System (PBJS) is now required in all nursing homes certified by the Centers for Medicare & Medicaid Services (CMS). This system, which was required by the Affordable Care Act, went into effect in April 2018 and has brought about significant positive changes in CMS's ability to track accurate staffing levels more reliably than the previous nursing homes' self-report system. Significant discrepancies in nursing homes' reporting on staffing levels have already been demonstrated in the first year of the new program; 70% of more than 14,000 nursing homes submitting payroll records had lower staffing than they reported using the old method.[300]

This CMS initiative is encouraging because it allows for more rigorous research studies on the role and effects of staffing levels on various care outcomes and phenomena including DHRRIs. This, in turn, may allow researchers to generate solid empirical evidence that could be used by care advocacy organizations to ensure that appropriate staffing standards are required in U.S. nursing homes.[301] Similar payroll-based systems should be required in assisted living residences—the fastest-growing residential care option for elders in the United States—where 40%–50% of the residents have a diagnosis of dementia.

Be aware, though, that simply hiring more direct care partners may not necessarily translate into improved care and supervision of residents and reduction in DHRRIs. As Berry states, "Higher ratios of appropriately trained staff are critical to proactive care management and prevention of these types of incidents." Direct care partners must be given ongoing dementia-specific training in recognition, prevention, and de-escalation of DHRRIs.

◇ Staff Burnout

Caring for residents with dementia can be a stressful, physically and mentally exhausting job, especially when training, support, and adequate staffing levels are not provided. Over time, this often leads to feelings of burnout among direct care partners. All direct care partners are at risk of burnout, defined by Maslach and Leiter[302] as "a psychological syndrome emerging as a prolonged response to chronic interpersonal stressors on the job." These authors report that the three key dimensions of this response are "an overwhelming exhaustion, feelings of cynicism and detachment from the job, and a sense of ineffectiveness and lack of accomplishment."[302]

When direct care partners are burned out, they are less likely to be in a position to proactively seek to identify residents' unmet needs, frustrations, early warning signs of distress and anxiety, and situational triggers leading to DHRRIs. Physically and emotionally exhausted, they are also less able to adequately respond to and de-escalate them once these episodes have begun. When direct care partners feel burned out, they are also more likely to experience and exhibit emotional distress; this limits their ability to be calm, present, and centered, which is critical to being able to skillfully de-escalate emotionally charged and scary episodes. Feeling stressed, these dedicated care employees are less able to genuinely validate the emotional states of residents with dementia—emotions that often underlie residents' behavioral expressions. Many residents with dementia are able to sense the core emotional states of direct care partners, which further interferes with their attempts to de-escalate these episodes.

Owners and managers should work proactively to address and decrease direct care partners' burnout because it has a measurable effect on quality of care. Previous research examining direct care partners' responses to residents with dementia and behavioral expressions classified as "challenging" has found that burnout was associated with less willingness to assist residents, low optimism, and negative emotional responses to residents' distressed behavioral expressions.[303] Another study found a relationship between direct care partners' burnout and the quality of their interactions with residents with dementia.[304] Specifically, those who reported lower levels of personal accomplishment on the Maslach Burnout Inventory (MBI, measuring

feelings of competence and successful achievement in one's work) had lower quality of interactions with residents.

Relevant examples of questions from the eight-item personal accomplishment subscale
of the MBI include "Can easily understand patients' feelings," "Deal effectively with patients'
problems," and "Deal with emotional problems calmly." The importance of understanding the
feelings of residents with dementia is a core principle not only in working with, supporting,
and caring for elders living with dementia during routine times; it is also a key principle in
prevention and de-escalation of DHRRIs.

Finally, a study by McPherson and colleagues[305] of 188 direct care partners and managers
in 16 LTC care homes found a strong relationship between their perceived levels of psychological distress and residents' "aggressive" behaviors over one week. Distressed direct care partners
were more likely to report on lack of support from others at work and to shout back at residents exhibiting these behavioral expressions. It is important to provide a formal Employee
Assistance Program for nursing assistants and other care professionals working in care homes.
Social workers and psychologists should typically lead this effort but others, such as chaplains,
can also assist on this important front.

If you are a manager or supervisor, provide direct care partners with frequent guidance,
emotional support, role modeling, and "experiential learning" (i.e., hands-on guidance on the
floor) during all work shifts, including evening hours and weekends. Provide specialized training to direct care partners on working with and caring for residents with cognitive impairment;
when this has been provided, it assists care employees in dealing with burnout and perceived
job pressure.[306] Studies have found that supervisors' support of direct care partners predicts
the perceived "management difficulty" of residents' behavioral expressions,[307] and increased
supervisory support in healthcare organizations was found to decrease the odds of physical
and nonphysical patient "violence."[308] Taken together, these studies highlight the importance
of a strong commitment by care home owners, managers, and supervisors to proactively and
routinely supporting direct care partners on all work shifts. Routinely recognizing direct care
partners' daily care efforts is an integral part of such critical support.

One study in 24 care homes found that direct care partners tend to receive more support
from their peers (through informal communication) during and after DHRRIs than they do
from supervisory staff.[40] These authors report a history of insufficient support from supervisory
staff after these incidents.

Supervisors need to strengthen and support direct care partners' sense of self-efficacy related to dealing with care-related challenges. Self-efficacy is defined as "a person's belief that
they can be successful when carrying out a particular task."[309] Specifically, low self-efficacy has
been found to predict staff burnout, and high self-efficacy, to act as a buffer against it.[310] One
intervention program was successful in increasing self-efficacy and decreasing burnout among
direct care partners working with people with dementia by offering practical advice on understanding and addressing behavioral expressions and by facilitating interactions with residents'
families.[311] Other suggestions include the following:

- *Time to decompress.* Provide direct care partners with frequent (at least weekly) structured opportunities to decompress distressing emotional buildups and express their
  anger and frustration in a supportive and discrete forum, such as a support group
  led by a social worker, psychologist, or chaplain. Be prepared to provide your care
  employees one-on-one or group support sessions also on an as-needed basis (stressful and even traumatic events may be experienced by care employees unexpectedly in between the regularly scheduled sessions). It is critical to the psychological
  well-being of direct care partners to receive structured, predictable support as well as
  support on an as-needed basis. Remember, the quality of care provided to residents

with dementia can only be as good as the quality of support provided to their direct care partners.

- *Teamwork.* Continuously encourage and nurture a sense of teamwork among direct care partners and between them and other employees, such as nurses, recreational therapists, and managers. Teach by example; routine role modeling by supervisors and the administrator on *all* work shifts is critical for effective teamwork.

- *Respect for direct care partners.* In every interaction you have with them, treat direct care partners as the most important employees in the organization, which they are. They provide the vast majority of the hands-on care to residents with dementia and are typically at the highest risk of experiencing burnout. The more respected they feel for their physically and emotionally hard daily care work, the less likely they will experience burnout. One way to show them respect is to regularly listen to them and their suggestions for improvement in care, including ways to address DHRRIs, and to provide them with hands-on guidance and specialized training as well as emotional support. Strive to build and nurture a workplace culture that places a high priority on honoring their needs and contributions to realizing the care mission of your organization.

- *Celebration of successes.* Regularly acknowledge and celebrate employees' successes. Offer an Employee of the Month program, in which the efforts and accomplishments of individual employees (direct and non-direct care partners, including housekeeping staff) are prominently featured on a beautifully designed poster containing high-quality photos of the employee in the main lobby and entrance of the care home. Sometimes a single inspiring act of extraordinary kindness, compassion, or creative solution to a challenging care-related problem may warrant such recognition of a care employee.

- *Caring about employees' lives.* Pay attention to the extent and quality of social support received by a direct care partner from her or his family and friends, as these factors outside of the job can affect an employee's work stress[306] and ability to provide adequate care.

- *Support for a healthy lifestyle.* Educate, encourage, and assist direct care partners to engage in healthy lifestyle behaviors (e.g., physical activity, meditation, yoga, healthy diet, sleep hygiene, and smoking cessation). Provide them with flyers, information about programs, and awareness-raising events to promote these healthy behaviors.

- *Good wages.* An integral but often overlooked part of a healthy and balanced lifestyle is making sure direct care partners are paid a living wage. Such a commitment to your care employees can also assist in reducing their overall workloads, as many direct care partners work double shifts or work in two or three jobs to make enough money to live on. Inadequate pay has been reported to contribute to increased staff turnover. Direct care partner Culix Wibonele shares, "Many CNAs do not get paid enough . . . You have a lot of responsibility taking care of members . . . when you are not earning enough money to make ends meet, many people leave to find better pay."[312]

- *Healthcare coverage.* Make sure that direct care partners have easy access and affordable healthcare coverage; 11% of direct care workers in nursing homes nationally did not have any health insurance in 2017[313] or paid family and medical leave.[314] The latter could assist care employees address the difficult dilemma of how to care for themselves (when experiencing a serious medical condition or when they need to be with and care for a newborn) or their family members (when they experience a serious medical condition) without losing wages or even their jobs. Without adequate paid family and medical leave, this terrible dilemma and stress caused by these situations could contribute to increased burnout of these dedicated care employees.

- *Measuring burnout.* To evaluate the level of direct care partners' burnout at your residence, consider using structured and validated instruments such as the MBI.[315] For other suggestions for minimizing staff burnout, as well as the nine-item questionnaire, "Warning Signs of Burnout" and the 14-item "Evaluation of Self-Care Strategies," see Rasin.[316]

◇ New, Inexperienced, and Untrained Direct Care Partners

Well-meaning, compassionate direct care partners who are new or inexperienced in caring for and communicating with people with dementia may inadvertently use ineffective approaches that contribute to development or escalation of DHRRIs. A study by Zeller and colleagues[317] among 814 nurse aides and nurses in 21 nursing homes in Switzerland found that younger care employees were at substantially higher risk of experiencing behavioral expressions classified as aggressive from residents. For example, direct care partners under 30 years of age were twice as likely to experience physically aggressive behaviors (such as slapping, pushing, and shoving) and threats (such as warnings of intent to injure another person) compared with their co-workers who were over 45 years of age. Less experience in working with and caring for residents exhibiting these behavioral expressions early in their careers was suggested as an explanation for the difference.

It is important to recognize, however, that, in practice, there are many exceptions to these research findings. For example, it is not uncommon to see young direct care partners who are very compassionate, insightful, and successful in building and maintaining close trusting relationships with residents with dementia and effective in preventing and de-escalating DHRRIs (many of them use creative approaches older and more experienced direct care partners do not think about). Alternatively, some individuals start working as nurse aides when they are older (such as in their mid-40s), and therefore they do not have experience caring for elders with dementia.

Before any direct care provider's first day at work with residents with dementia, it is essential that the LTC home require and provide comprehensive specialized dementia care orientation training. Beyond many other topics, the training should include at least 1 hour on understanding (risk and protective factors), recognizing, preventing, and de-escalating DHRRIs. In addition, at a minimum, 1 hour of in-service "refresher" training on prevention and de-escalation of DHRRIs should be provided to direct and non-direct care partners at least once a year and on an as-needed basis (such as when certain direct care partners clearly struggle in their approach when trying to prevent and de-escalate these episodes). This phenomenon is currently considered at least as common[16] and harmful[318] as care employees' abuse of residents, and thus such minimum training is warranted.

In addition, it is often very helpful to offer peer mentorship programs in which an experienced, compassionate, and effective direct care partner pairs with a new direct care partner to provide her or him with hands-on guidance, emotional support, supervision, and advice. An excellent example is the 6–10 days of individual mentoring of new direct care partners as they interact with and care for residents with dementia, an initiative that was an integral part of the Lakeview Ranch Model of Specialized Dementia Care developed by Judy Berry.[60]

◇ Inappropriate Approaches, Attitudes, and Communication Style

Many direct and non-direct care partners and managers use approaches and communication styles with people who have dementia that reflect ageist, dementist, and biomedical approaches. These approaches and styles are described as custodial, task-oriented, controlling, authoritative, confrontational, and demanding.[319] They are fairly common and often harmful, and belong to the old culture of care of elders living with dementia.

A common example of this type of approach is called "elderspeak," consisting of a patronizing tone or language; "baby talk"; infantilizing terms that are inappropriately intimate and childish, such as "Honey" or "Good girl"; using "we" instead of "you" to address the person (for example, "Are *we* ready for *our* bath?"); and controlling, dominating, or bossy communication.[320] Many elders with dementia can hear and understand elderspeak for what it is, and they may respond by rejecting care as a way of indicating their need for respectful, caring, less patronizing, adult-to-adult communication.[321] Research using video recordings of interactions between direct care partners and residents with dementia during personal care—bathing, eating, dressing, and oral care—has shown an increased likelihood of "resistiveness to care" following direct care partners' use of elderspeak rather than normal talk or silence.[321]

Cognitively intact elders, of course, also have negative perceptions of elderspeak. One study found that elders who listened to directions for completing a task using this type of language reported that the communication was patronizing and demeaning and made comprehending the instructions difficult.[322] Elderspeak may "challenge the personae or face presentation of self, constructed and maintained through interactions with other people."[323] In other words, residents' dignity and personhood are at stake. It is worth considering what the term *personhood* actually means. Tom Kitwood defined it as "a standing or status that is bestowed upon one human being, by others, in the context of relationship and social being. It implies recognition, respect, and trust. Both the according of personhood, and the failure to do so, have consequences that are empirically tested."[64]

One can imagine how residents with dementia might react when these demeaning communication styles are used by direct care partners before, during, and immediately after DHR-RIs. These episodes represent critical times for building—not compromising—trust with residents by recognizing and genuinely validating their distressed emotional states and situational frustrations and promptly and skillfully meeting the unmet human needs underlying them.

One important way to minimize the use of the elderspeak communication style and maximize trust with residents with dementia is through training programs. For example, a communication training program on elderspeak and its potential negative effects on residents (one-third with dementia) delivered in five LTC homes to CNAs has been shown to reduce their use of elderspeak and increase the use of more effective person-directed communication strategies. In addition, the emotional tone of direct care partners' speech with residents was rated as less controlling and more respectful after the training program.[320]

◇ Malignant Social Psychology

Inappropriate, disrespectful, and demeaning attitudes, approaches, and communication toward residents with dementia can extend and/or manifest in more serious and harmful ways. A series of these acts have been identified and characterized by Kitwood[64] as malignant social psychology (MSP). Under some circumstances, these approaches could be characterized as mistreatment, such as verbal or physical abuse and neglect of healthcare, and they can sometimes contribute to (if not directly cause) residents' behavioral expressions that are inaccurately labeled as aggressive.

Well into their disease, many residents with dementia remain capable of sensing who is a trusted care partner and who is not. Feil calls this remaining ability in elders with Alzheimer's disease "intuitive wisdom." When their verbal capacity declines, residents with dementia often recognize and respond to disrespectful approaches in ways that are often labeled as aggressive, but when looking closely, these expressions are understandable attempts to preserve their dignity and personhood. Harmful acts of MSP toward elders with dementia may include any of the following:

- Deceiving the person
- Infantilizing the person
- Instilling fear or threatening the person
- Stigmatizing the person
- Hurrying the person beyond her or his normal pace (*outpacing*)
- Not validating the person's emotions
- Rejecting the person
- Objectifying the person
- Ignoring the person
- Forcing the person to do something against her or his will
- Not providing the person with a choice
- Refusing to give the person something he or she needs
- Blaming the person for doing or not doing certain things because of her or his lack of ability or understanding
- Laughing at the person
- Humiliating the person
- Devaluing the person
- Sending messages to the person that damage her or his self-esteem

When direct care partners do any of these things during routine care or during DHRRIs, it can exacerbate and perpetuate residents' frustrations, anger, and behavioral expressions. Al Power asks us to consider, "How much of the 'challenging behavior' that we experience is actually created or inflamed by our own challenging behavior and words?"

Care homes must educate direct and non-direct care partners about the far-reaching negative impacts of MSP's acts on residents' emotional states and distressing behavioral expressions. Using real examples, demonstrate to direct care partners the various ways in which such acts can exacerbate resident-to-resident incidents and resident–staff conflicts. Share successful examples to demonstrate the effectiveness of person-directed approaches in promoting residents' emotional and psychological well-being.

Instill in direct care partners the value underlying the golden rule: "Do unto others as you would have them do unto you." In other words, treat the residents the way you would want to be treated if one day you will develop dementia and live in a care home.

It is very important that managers send a strong and consistent message of zero tolerance of such harmful and frankly abusive and neglectful acts.[324] Consider discontinuing employment of direct care partners who, despite repeated guidance and training on respectful and effective communication approaches, do not adhere to this expectation. Some people are simply not suited to working with and caring for elders in general, especially those living with a serious brain disease. Strong policies and screening procedures are critical to hiring the right people for this sacred but physically and emotionally demanding job—one that requires compassion, sensitivity, and emotional intelligence—with some of the most vulnerable and frail members of our society.

◇ Organizational Tensions

It is not uncommon to hear that the quality of the working relationships and daily communications between managers and direct care partners hinders the latter group's ability to provide effective and safe care to residents and prevent behavioral expressions labeled as aggressive. These tense relationships may contribute to critical breakdowns in care-related daily communication that can directly impact the care home's ability to prevent DHRRIs. For example, picture a team leader who doesn't get along with her manager. The team leader may not inform her manager about a serious resident-to-resident incident due to concern that she will be criticized or even disciplined by the manager. The tension between the two employees will contribute to a lack of important communication and reporting, which may result in lack of immediate and thorough internal investigation of the root cause of the episode. This lack of action can represent a missed opportunity for learning and prevention, which creates fertile ground for these incidents to recur and places residents with dementia at risk of harm.

In addition, direct care partners, who typically provide about 80% of the hands-on care in LTC homes, are often insufficiently encouraged by their managers to regularly participate in and contribute to the daily decision-making processes related to the care they provide. One study of nursing home administrators and directors of nursing examined the association between leadership style and quality of care.[325] Leaders were categorized into four groups: consensus managers, consultative autocrats, shareholder managers, and autocrats. The study found that a consensus manager leadership style was strongly associated with better quality of care. Managers using this style regularly ask for and act on input from their care employees. In some excellent care homes for people with dementia, direct care partners are empowered—in actions, not only in words—to be at the heart of almost all care-related decision-making processes. Care employees in these homes provide input on development of policies, procedures, day-to-day operations, care practices, and strategies for resolving care-related challenges, and have a key and valued role during individualized care plan conferences. As the most important care employees in the care home, their perspective, thoughts, and suggestions for change are heard and cherished.

If you are a manager, it is important to examine your working relations with your direct care partners and, where needed, make efforts to improve them. Bill Thomas, founder of The Eden Alternative, shares, "The most important part of our work when Edenizing a facility is teaching the managers how to rebuild their relationship with the staff."[326] The quality of care is largely determined by the ongoing support and education received by direct care partners from managers and co-workers. Put succinctly by Thomas, "As managers do unto staff, so shall the staff do unto the elders." Recognizing the importance of this fundamental principle, one administrator said, "If we treat our employees right, they'll treat the residents right. But, we have to model the behavior that we want them to have."[327]

A shift is needed from top-down bureaucratic authority to placing as much decision-making authority as possible in the hands of the elders (residents with mild, or no, cognitive impairment or early-stage dementia) and those closest to them (direct care partners and family members). As Thomas[326] explains, "Flat social structures . . . rely on deeply personal relationships as the basis for decision making and mutual responsibility." However, he warns, "perfect flatness would create a dangerous anarchy. The struggle in this case is not to eliminate hierarchy but to create an organization in which it is far less steep and far less slippery."

Jayne Clairmont, former owner of English Rose Suites, took this idea one step further, inverting the traditional organizational chart "to place herself at the very bottom and the residents at the top."[328] The general sequence from top to bottom includes residents, CNAs, team mentors, registered nurse, quality-of-life coordinator, administrator, vice president of operations and marketing, and owner and chief executive officer (Clairmont, e-mail communication, March 24, 2015).

Whatever the structure of your organization, it is important to involve direct care partners in decision processes related to the care they provide to residents. Invite them to all resident care plan meetings, meetings with family members, and management meetings. Make sure they feel comfortable sharing their opinions during those meetings and send a clear message that their opinions are valued and that their suggestions are seriously considered and regularly incorporated into the individual residents' care plans. As suggested by Cindy Kincaid,[166] a regional LTC ombudsman in Charlotte, North Carolina, "[Work] to really encourage involvement with front line aides or care staff. They know the residents better than anybody. They have dealt with the residents the most and often times have the best information to offer." As mentioned earlier in this chapter, direct care partners are the foundation and backbone of the LTC industry; they must therefore always be treated as such.

◇ Inadequate Reporting of Episodes

Problems with information transfer between direct care partners, between direct care partners and managers, and between employees from different departments and disciplines is a persistent problem in many LTC homes. Such communication lapses and breakdowns may occur, for example, within shifts as well as across shifts, days (such as between weekdays and weekends), and during holidays. The inadequate or lack of transfer of essential information often leads to missed opportunities for prevention of DHRRIs.[13] CMS encourages state surveyors of nursing homes to consider during their inspections the communication between disciplines, across shifts, and between weekday and weekend staff, as well as between nursing staff, medical teams (prescribers of antipsychotic medications), pharmacists, behavioral health teams, and family members. According to CMS,[329] "This is an essential component of dementia care; failure of the team to communicate effectively must be considered and appropriately cited as deficient practice."

Inadequate Communication Among Care Employees

Events and behavioral expressions occurring during one shift often have direct effects on behavioral expressions occurring during subsequent shifts. Consider the following episode, which took place during my early study on DHRRIs. A recreation assistant entered a secure care home for people with dementia to lead a group activity. In the course of leading the activity, she directed two residents to sit next to one another. Shortly after the activity started, resident A began burping, and resident B became upset and angry, shouting and cursing at resident A, and physically threatened to hit her.[34] The recreation assistant was unaware that resident A had been known to burp frequently during group activities for several months before this day, and that earlier in the day, resident B had verbally and physically threatened to harm resident A. If the recreation assistant had been informed of this prior episode and the trigger (burping), she would have guided resident A to a seat where she would be less likely to trigger the episode.

It is important for the LTC home to have structured mechanisms (policies and procedures) in place to ensure effective communication in real time—among all employees—to decrease the likelihood that "information slippage" becomes a contributing factor to DHRRIs. Below are some suggested strategies.

Communication Log, Preferably Electronic

Require all "direct contact" employees (those who come into direct, regular contact with the residents) to read the daily communication log at the beginning of each shift, including after leaving and returning to the care home during the work shift, and a few times during the shift.

The log is a critical learning and risk management resource that should be used to systemati-cally document the circumstances surrounding and situational triggers of behavioral expres-sions and the unmet human needs and frustrations underlying them.

It is recommended that the communication log be electronic where possible. Many direct care partners for whom English is not the first language (about one-fifth of direct care work-ers) have difficulty reading handwritten logs, which can lead to lapses in communication.[330] Not being aware of previous episodes often translates into lack of timely implementation of measures necessary to prevent them from recurring in similar circumstances. An electronic log that is used systematically and effectively—by all direct and non-direct care partners, all other interdisciplinary care team members, and managers—can increase the likelihood that key in-formation is shared and understood by all who need it. It can literally help prevent residents' injuries and deaths.

Shift-Change Meetings

Consider requiring that the shift-change meeting between team leaders last anywhere between 15 and 30 minutes; the actual time needed should be determined based on the number of res-idents within each care home, their healthcare needs, behavioral expressions, and the resources available to care for them (such as staffing levels, training, and skill set). Some readers may think this suggestion is unrealistic because certain owners of care homes will never be willing to pay for the extra time such overlapping shift changes require. Implementing this suggestion, however, would not only improve the care provided to residents but it could also enable care employees to keep them safe. One coroner, who regularly reviews deaths due to resident-to-res-ident incidents, recommends a 30-minute shift change. He recommends that the resident's chart be read and reviewed at the start of each shift, and that all reports place particular em-phasis on new admissions and on instructions for monitoring residents who require additional observation.[117] The practice has been used in innovative care homes many years.

Bob Woods reflects on one of the components of the training and development strategy he and Kitwood developed for a UK care home in the 1990s:[69]

> A key organizational change was to set up rotas so that morning and afternoon shifts had a period of overlap, so that all staff (including direct care staff) could be included in hando-vers, thus enhancing communication between staff at all levels.

Time for transition meetings should be included in every direct care partner's regular work schedule, and all direct care partners must be paid for their time in contributing to this im-portant step in improving care and the prevention of DHRRIs. The types of information transferred during these shift change meetings could obviously help address and prevent many other care-related needs, problems, and safety issues, as well.

Written Procedures

Have a clear written procedure in place requiring employees in key positions, such as charge nurse and team leader, to inform *all* direct care partners (including float, per diem, outside agency, and weekend staff) about previous DHRRIs. Also, have structured mechanisms in place to improve communications between employees across departments, such as between CNAs and recreational therapists.

Underreporting of Episodes

The majority of DHRRIs remain unreported.[331] In one study[332] examining CNAs' re-sponses to resident-to-resident incidents in five nursing homes, only 4 out of 97 CNAs re-ported making an entry in the behavioral expressions log about these episodes. Accordingly, other studies show that 60%–80% of incidents classified as aggressive in nursing homes are underreported.[13,333] Underreporting of DHRRIs limits direct care partners' ability to understand the root causes of these behavioral expressions; identify underlying unmet needs, situational frustrations, and triggering events; and anticipate and prevent future incidents.[13] This lack of reporting is important generally but also because many of these behavioral expressions are recurrent.[40]

Even when reporting is done correctly, the lack of a strong commitment from some managers to routinely review and use the information to inform prevention is another persistent barrier for change. In a study[334] of 11 nursing homes based on 19 focus groups, many of the 138 nurse aides perceived a persistent lack of action by nurses and managers in response to their reports of resident-to-resident incidents. One aide said, "We have filled boxes of them and nothing is done, not even medications." Another said, "We have quit [reporting] because nobody listens—just quit." Still another said, "Record, record, nothing ever changes." Many nurse aides in the study noted that they had given up reporting because they felt blamed for the incidents, and their formal reports had had no effect.[334]

The first step in bringing a fundamental change in the chronic problem of underreporting of DHRRIs is to fully recognize—and encourage all care employees to recognize through ongoing education and training—that these behavioral expressions should not be normalized (in other words, should not be perceived as inevitable and therefore not able to be addressed or resolved). It should be made clear to all those who come into direct regular contact with residents with dementia that dangerous normalization of these episodes often results in serious psychological or physical harm to residents and direct care partners.

Hirst observes, "If a nurse does not perceive abuse as occurring, then a behavior will not be reported and an older resident may be left at risk."[335] Although the vast majority of DHRRIs in the specific context of residents with dementia should not be considered as abuse, ongoing educational efforts are urgently needed to prevent care partners from minimizing these episodes in this population. The decades-long dangerous normalization of this phenomenon has already led to the injury and death of scores of elders.

Require *all* employees (including non-direct care partners, nurses, recreation therapists, social workers, and managers) to report in writing on every DHRRI; this requirement should be explicitly specified in the policies and procedures of your residence. To be effective, the report itself needs to be done using a Behavioral Expressions Log (displayed and described in detail in the downloadable resources accompanying this book at https://healthpropress.com; see p. viii for access information),[336] which should be completed immediately after (or if not possible, shortly after) the episode ends. Waiting to fill it out at the end of the shift is likely to compromise recall accuracy of important details that are essential for future prevention efforts.

Teresi and colleagues[17] have developed an 11-item instrument (Table 6.2) for research purposes and to assist interdisciplinary care teams in recognizing and documenting DHRRIs in LTC homes. The instrument was designed to collect data on staff recollection of resident-to-resident incidents during the preceding 2-week period; this period is often used in psychiatric and behavioral measures addressing underlying latent constructs that may be rare. Nursing homes using this instrument after receiving a training program were found to document six times as many incidents per resident per year as did the control nursing homes.[331] Recognition and detection of this phenomenon is the first step in addressing it.

As much as possible, owners and administrators of care homes should encourage systemic change to support as full as possible reporting of DHRRIs. Most direct care partners are likely to perceive DHRRIs as a challenge, but various systemic factors at the organization level, such as those discussed throughout this chapter, can substantially limit their ability to report on incidents. One of the recommendations made by the Chief Coroner of Ontario, Canada, after two roommates were killed by a third roommate with dementia (who had been admitted to the nursing home only 7 hours earlier during the weekend) may be useful:[117]

Table 6.2   Eleven-Item Staff-Reported Resident-to-Resident Elder Mistreatment Instrument[17]

1	Use bad words toward another resident
2	Scream at another resident
3	Try to scare, frighten, or threaten (another resident) with words
4	Boss around/tell another resident what to do
5	Hit another resident
6	Grab or yank another resident
7	Push or shove another resident
8	Throw things at another resident
9	Threaten another resident with a cane, fist, or other object
10	Other physical behavior like kicking, biting, scratching, or spitting at another resident
11	Going into another resident's room without asking or taking/touching/damaging or breaking other residents' "personal" things

Care employees' recollection of resident-to-resident incidents during the preceding 2-week period.

Residents' characteristics, care needs, and nature of behavioral expressions, as well as the language used by direct care partners to describe and document them vary greatly across LTC homes. Therefore, based on local needs, LTC homes could use the items as they appear in the structured instrument, or they could modify the wording and, if needed, add other items reflecting the type of behavioral manifestations occurring in their care setting.

The developers of the instrument recommend adding a twelfth item on sexual DHRRIs such as "Saying sexual things and inappropriate touching of another resident." Because of the low rates of occurrence in their study, this salient item was omitted from the original analysis during the development of the instrument.

> Ensure that those RNs who are assessing the charting of the behaviours have sufficient time to actually assess and record the behaviours. In addition, all staff that the RNs are supervising must also have the training and time to report the behaviours.

It is essential for all care employees to commit to the systematic and consistent reporting of verbal, physical, and sexual DHRRIs; this could enable direct care partners to improve identification of situational triggers and behavioral patterns, which are the fundamental basis for development of effective individualized preventive strategies. As explained by Teresi and colleagues, "Nursing staff need to be encouraged to complete the required documentation on all aspects of resident-to-resident elder mistreatment so that patterns of behavior can be identified and care strategies implemented."[331] Furthermore, all injuries must be reported to the supervising nurse to ensure proper follow-up care.

Also important is to ensure that learning and improvement in prevention are the main goals of reporting. Using direct care partners' documentation and reporting of DHRRIs as a punitive tool against them (such as evidence that they do not fulfill their duty to protect residents from other residents) will, in many situations, lead to reduced reporting and loss of precious opportunities for learning and prevention. Training CNAs on documentation leads to significant gains in their knowledge related to risk factors, recognition, and management of DHRRIs.[331]

Repeated or otherwise harmful incidents that are not resolved through care planning may require formal, external reporting to the state survey agency; reporting requirements vary for CMS–certified nursing homes versus assisted living residences that are regulated at the state level.

Poor Documentation Quality of Episodes

The quality of written documentation of DHRRIs in a large number of LTC homes is often far from what is needed for developing effective individualized prevention strategies. For example, a common type of report made by direct care partners, such as "Mr. Smith hit Mrs. Cohen in the face this afternoon," does not include enough detail about the circumstances, sequence of events, and situational triggers leading to the hitting.

A key principle in understanding the person exhibiting behavioral expressions considered aggressive is the "effort to understand the *meaning of the sequence* that led to the aggressive behavior."[337][emphasis mine] As mentioned in the preceding section, the lack of essential information in daily written reports made by direct care partners and other interdisciplinary care team members represents a missed opportunity for learning and prevention of DHRRIs. It also reflects the important distinction between using written documentation, in effect, as a tool for labeling residents versus as a learning and prevention tool.

It is important to cultivate a culture of learning. Learning organizations are fully committed to systematically and consistently using detailed written documentation of behavioral expressions to guide their individualized care practices and as an integral part of their risk management program and DHRRI prevention and de-escalation. Written reports in these care organizations often include detailed descriptions of the situational circumstances and sequence of events leading to or directly causing the behavioral expressions, beyond a description of the expressions themselves and what key actions and events took place after the expressions discontinued. When the actions and events taking place immediately after an episode ends are unhelpful, they often function as reinforcers of the behavioral expressions and thus they further decrease the resident's trust in care partners (trust that care partners will need in future care interactions with the resident, including during subsequent DHRRIs). Care homes that excel in their documentation policies, procedures, and practices know that documenting the actions and events immediately after these episodes is a crucial strategy for learning from them in ways that help them build trust with the residents involved. Timely identification of patterns underlying behavioral expressions among people with dementia is the fundamental basis for individualized prevention.

In addition, despite the prevalence and harm caused by resident-to-resident incidents, the Minimum Data Set 3.0 (the largest federally mandated clinical dataset in CMS–certified nursing homes, which is often used in large-scale research studies) does not enable nursing staff to report on them (in the Behavior E Section).[12] This major gap in tracking this phenomenon in over 15,000 nursing homes nationwide represents a persistent barrier for learning from these incidents and informing prevention efforts. Furthermore, reports on DHRRIs to state survey agencies are often devoid of critical pieces of information that otherwise could have informed better prevention efforts. In their groundbreaking study using complaints and incident reports on injurious resident-to-resident incidents in nursing homes in Massachusetts, researchers Shinoda-Tagawa and colleagues[26] reported that they were unable to characterize or quantify the circumstances of the incidents due to insufficient reporting details that were almost always devoid of information about the resident reported to be exhibiting the physical contact resulting in an injury. This is yet another barrier for research, learning, and prevention.

◇ Labeling a Resident, Verbally or in Writing

As has been mentioned previously, the act of labeling a resident with a serious brain disease and his or her behavioral expressions can lead to further negative outcomes for that individual. Examples of labeling terms in the context of residents with dementia are "violent," "abusive," "out of control," "the pincher," "the grabber," "the wanderer," "the crazy one," "wacko," "they are the only ones that appear to be normal," and "they are all suspicious."[34] As mentioned previously, even the term "aggressive" should be avoided in most situations in the context of elders with dementia because this term implies intent to harm or injure another person; in most situations in this population this is not the case.

Additionally, there is an inaccurate, misleading, and dangerous misconception by which DHRRIs are seen as an inevitable outcome of brain pathology due to dementia, when in most situations the cause or situational trigger for the behavioral expression can be identified with close observation of the person's physical and social environment.[338] Of course, these causes and triggers intersect with the resident's cognitive disability, and together they contribute to DHRRIs, but brain pathology alone typically accounts for only a small portion of the series of factors leading to these incidents. The focus, as this book has shown repeatedly, should be first and foremost on residents' unmet human needs as the main set of factors contributing to these episodes. Among these, unmet emotional and psychological needs are often the most common factors contributing to the development of DHRRIs.

Some leading educators, care advocates, and LTC providers are moving away from even using the term "behaviors" in the context of people living with dementia. Power, for example, now uses the term "personal expressions." Several authors have written about various harms inherent in labeling language. Sue and colleagues[339] explain,

> A label can predispose people to interpret all activities of the affected individual as patho-logical; it may lead others to treat a person differently; it may lead those who are labeled to believe that they do indeed possess such characteristics (labels can become self-fulfilling prophecies), which may have a profound effect on the person's self-image; and it may not provide the precise functional information that is needed.

Herbert and Bradshaw[39] warn that attributing risk factors for DHRRIs to people rather than to the care environment tends to isolate people as problematic and lead to their stigmatization. Åkerström asserts, "The very process of identifying someone or some acts as 'violent' is inher-ently exclusionary. Underlying the term 'violence' is a welter of images, feelings, and assump-tions. Wording holds important consequences."[340]

Labeling residents with dementia limits direct care partners' ability to identify unmet human needs, frustrations, circumstances, sequences of events, and situational triggers under-lying DHRRIs, which are all considered the basis for individualized prevention.

In addition, the largely unhelpful term "unpredictable" is often used by care employees to describe various forms of behavioral expressions of elders with dementia, including DHRRIs. Slone and Gleason[341] observe,

> An important team dynamic becomes apparent when caregivers report a behavior as being "unpredictable." Although there do appear to be occasions when there is no discernable trigger, in most cases, time and experience with the resident will reveal one or more triggers. It is important to keep caregivers open to observation for triggers, even if this process takes some time.

Most importantly, it is critical to cultivate an attitude of respect during all interactions with residents and communications about them—an attitude that is often reflected in our words. Edmond Chiu suggests, "Be sensitive to the possible damage that we can do to our residents by every act we perform and every word we speak in the transmission of information."[342] A CNA and a manager were discussing a resident who would soon be moving to a home with a higher level of care for people with dementia. "She is difficult," commented the CNA. The manager responded, "You just sent the wrong message, because everyone works differently."[34] The manager was clearly aware of the potential negative impact of labeling the resident in the minds of other direct care partners even before she moved to her new care home.

Make every effort to avoid using labeling terms that push residents with dementia "outside the boundary of normalcy and continued acceptance."[340] Achieving this goal, however, can be challenging because, as pointed out by Erving Goffman, author of the groundbreaking book *Asylums* (a seminal book identifying striking similarities across different types of total institu-tions), "normalcy is never recognized by the attendant in a milieu where abnormality is the normal expectancy."[343] Ongoing training of all employees who come in direct regular contact with residents with dementia is key.

As part of orientation and ongoing in-service training to direct care partners, stress that the majority of behavioral expressions among residents with dementia that are labeled as aggressive have meaning, purpose, and an important function, even when residents' cognitive disabilities prevent them from articulating them in words. Care partners should always seek to identify the unmet human needs and situational frustrations underlying these behavioral expressions by closely observing the circumstances and sequence of events leading to their manifestation, and adequately documenting these. The insights gleaned from these observations often show that there is a good reason why residents with dementia exhibit the behavioral expressions.

Because written labeling and stigmatizing words can contribute to emotional and social harm to residents with dementia,[342] encourage and make sure that all care employees use the communication log as a learning and prevention tool, and not as a labeling tool. Written labeling words have a tendency to leave a lasting stigmatizing legacy on residents with dementia. How would you feel if you were living with a serious brain disease in a nursing home and were labeled as an aggressive and violent person?

◇ Inattentiveness to Early Warning Signs of Distress and Anxiety

In a care home dedicated to caring for people with dementia, a male resident with dementia pushed a female resident against the wall. When the new direct care partner was asked why she did not intervene to de-escalate the episode, she said, "I was doing dishes." The episode lasted about 3 minutes, and there were at least two observable warning signs when the man was clearly frustrated and shook his fist at the woman before pushing her. After reviewing the in-house security video footage of the episode, the CEO shared, "I am frequently told that these resident-to-resident aggressive episodes happen fast, but it didn't happen fast. It is something that is brewing up before it happens." She added, "It was so obvious what was missing . . . Staff attention."

Although distressing behavioral expressions among residents with dementia can certainly develop within a few seconds or even a split second, a growing body of research sheds light on the typical trajectory. Observable early warning signs, situational triggers, and antecedent events have been found to precede the majority of behavioral expressions classified as aggression,[344,345] rejection of care (for instance, resistance during bathing),[346] and DHRRIs in the context of dementia.[13] Accordingly, Eller and colleagues state, "Anxiety is often the first observable level of agitation"[347] in people with dementia. Anxiety is defined as a feeling of distress, subjectively experienced as fear or worry, and objectively expressed through autonomic and central nervous system responses. Anxiety is always a response to a real or perceived threat.[255] As Volicer and Mahoney advise, "Caregivers must identify and treat anxiety before it channels the person's energy into defensive behaviors."[348]

Paul Raia, a national expert in use of psychosocial strategies for prevention of behavioral expressions in people with dementia, warns, "If emotions are ignored, they fester and can lead to violent behavior."[122] Slone and Gleason[341] add that although behavioral expressions may occur suddenly at times, more often the behavior represents the high point in a cycle of agitation, and therefore intervention strategies are typically more effective when applied earlier in the escalation cycle. Taken together, these research studies and experts' opinions suggest that the majority of DHRRIs are preceded by early warning signs; therefore, they are usually preventable.

As noted previously, it is important to train direct care partners in the observational skills necessary to recognize early warning signs of distress and anxiety, such as physiological signs of anxiety, general signs of anxiety, facial expressions signaling anxiety, tense body language, hand signals, signs of anger, and frightened facial expressions. Proactively detecting and addressing residents' initial signs indicating that they are worried and/or fearful, for instance, through timely provision of emotional support and reassurance, could go a long way in reducing the incidence of DHRRIs.

For further detail and concrete examples from each of these seven domains of distress and anxiety, see Table 8.1. Regularly encourage and support direct care partners, with adequate staffing levels at all times, as well as specialized training, to use a proactive "anticipatory care approach"[349] as opposed to the all-too-common and much less effective reactive approach. Specifically, direct and non-direct care partners should proactively seek to identify early warning signs of distress and situational triggers leading to DHRRIs. Detailed descriptions of common circumstances and situational triggers of DHRRIs in the context of dementia are presented in Chapter 4.

If you are a supervisor and/or trainer, consider gathering real-life, compelling examples— detailed descriptions of episodes of DHRRIs representing both success and failure in understanding their root causes and preventing them—and discuss these with direct care partners during routine care planning meetings; the episodes discussed could be those that occurred in your care home or others. The primary goal of these discussions should be to reflect on effective and ineffective prevention policies, procedures, and strategies for prevention of similar episodes in the future. It is important to avoid blaming direct care partners for mishandling certain episodes or using disciplinary or punitive measures against them unless, of course, neglect or abuse of residents has been substantiated.

As mentioned previously, instilling an atmosphere of open and constructive shared learning is essential for this approach to be successful. Because contributing factors and the origins of DHRRIs can often be found at the systemic level and multiple levels of the care organization, illustrative examples should also include successes and failures stemming from internal policies, procedures, and care practices directed by managers and owners. Such a "teach by example" approach can go a long way in nurturing direct care partners' trust and openness to new learning and approaches. This in turn can have tremendous potential in improving person-directed care practices and prevention efforts.

◇ Language Mismatch (Care Employee–Resident)

In 2017, approximately one-fifth of nurse aides in U.S. nursing homes were foreign born; among these, 8% were not U.S. citizens and 13% were U.S. citizens by naturalization.[312] When direct care partners' first language is different from that of residents, it can lead to challenges in communication with residents, adding to the existing communication challenges caused by residents' cognitive disabilities. Language mismatch can contribute to and exacerbate DHRRIs and create barriers for effective prevention and de-escalation strategies.[78] In addition, many elders with advanced Alzheimer's disease revert to using their native language, which can lead to yet another source of language mismatch, further complicating routine care and efforts to prevent and de-escalate DHRRIs.

To improve communication with a resident with advanced dementia who speaks a different language from care employees, it is helpful to ask a care professional, such as a social worker, to meet with the resident's close family members and friends to learn from them key words and phrases in the person's language. Some essential words or phrases should be documented that could assist in facilitating provision of care or engagement in personally meaningful activities, or that might tend to calm the person when she or he becomes upset. Also important is to learn about words that tend to upset the person, so those words can be avoided. This information should be added to the resident's care plan so that other direct and non-direct care partners can have easy access to it. Make sure all care employees in direct regular contact with the resident know these helpful and unhelpful words and phrases.

Recruit and train volunteers who speak the resident's language. The active presence of an attentive and compassionate visiting companion who speaks the resident's language could in itself have a calming effect on the resident. Understanding the person's unique culture, customs, and traditions, and translating her or his verbal expressions can assist direct care partners in quickly detecting situational frustrations and proactively meeting any unmet needs that could lead to DHRRIs. If the resident has early-stage dementia, the volunteer could simply ask her or him what upsets as well as what tends to calm her or him. Documentation of these words can inform prevention and de-escalation strategies.

Care homes may want to consider creating and using creative approaches such as the one developed by Cameron Camp and his colleagues, who noticed direct care partners struggling to communicate with Russian-speaking nursing home residents. He and his team developed the InterpreCare System™ (ICS) intervention.[350] In this system, English words central to specific care tasks were phonetically translated into Russian, including phonetic pronunciation cues (e.g., "Thank you" translated into "Spah-see-bah"). These were printed on lightweight, portable, and adaptable display boards used by care partners during personal care tasks. The intervention led to substantial reductions in both verbal and physical behavioral expressions considered as aggressive in a resident with advanced Alzheimer's disease who was legally blind, spoke only Russian, and was physically rejecting care partners' attempts to assist him with eating. Later adaptations of the intervention led to increased positive staff–resident interactions and communications. According to the developers of the intervention, "Hearing even a few phrases in their own language often has a dramatic, positive emotional impact on residents." The same technology could be applied to other languages as well. For suggestions on how to create and use ICS display boards, including material used, recommended sizes of boards and letters, see article by Camp and colleagues.[350]

Part III

Prevention and
De-escalation Strategies

One understands behaviors as meaningful responses to
disability and to an environment that an individual may perceive
as threatening, uncomfortable, confusing, or uncontrollable.
Uncovering these meanings as a basis for preventive intervention
requires examination of patterns of behavior.

E. K. Mahoney and colleagues[255]

This section provides detailed descriptions of dozens of psychosocial strategies for prevention and de-escalation of distressing and harmful resident-to-resident interactions (DHRRIs) in the context of residents with dementia. The strategies are based on an extensive practice and research literature, as well as on my own long-time experience as a nurse aide, social worker, educator, consultant, care advocate, and applied researcher in long-term care (LTC) homes for elders with dementia.

Chapters 7–10 present procedures and strategies at the organizational level, proactive measures, immediate strategies during episodes, and post-episode strategies. These chapters correspond to the four levels in which these strategies need to be applied in an individualized (i.e., whole-person), holistic, well-coordinated, and consistent manner in order to achieve the highest possible and most sustainable preventive effects. If one of these four levels is not adequately addressed, the overall preventive impact will likely decrease, and residents' safety will remain at risk. In other words, if one brick (i.e., level) is removed from the care home's overall prevention program, the others will likely fall down as well. Equipping all employees who have direct regular contact with residents with a comprehensive (multilevel) set of strategies for prevention and de-escalation of DHRRIs—through orientation training, in-service training, and hands-on guidance from skilled supervisors and co-workers during episodes—can enable them to have a strong foundation when addressing these episodes.

7

Procedures and Strategies at the Organizational Level

Up to now, the issue has been one of indifference,
that these are old people and they're going to die anyways.
Somehow in a collective setting like a nursing home,
the abnormal becomes normalized.

Gloria Gutman[351]

To effectively address the phenomenon of resident-to-resident incidents, there needs to be a focus on the broader care system level. Creating a climate of safety requires a multifaceted approach with a strong organizational commitment to implementation of best practices in operations at all levels. This chapter describes standards, practices, reporting mechanisms, and safeguard measures. When these practices are implemented adequately, routinely, and consistently, they can strengthen the care home's ability to prevent and reduce distressing and harmful resident-to-resident interactions (DHRRIs) and keep residents and direct care partners safe.

Organizational Culture

Avoid Normalization of DHRRIs

Very little has been done to date to track, study, and learn from DHRRIs in long-term care (LTC) homes, in part due to attitudes toward older adults living with dementia. A study in 11 nursing homes conducted by Morgan and colleagues[334] has shown that residents' behavioral expressions considered as "aggressive" were frequently normalized by nurses, supervisors, and managers. One nurse aide said, "You are trained that it is part of your job, you deserve it because you work with old people and that is how they are." Another said, "If I work 6 days, the first few days I put up with it, but then [I] think, 'How come we have to put up with it every time we work?' We go to management and we are told it is part of the job, put up with it." Frequent normalization of different forms of these behavioral expressions in LTC homes (including resident-to-staff incidents and DHRRIs) was also found in a large-scale study by Daly and colleagues.[352] As concerning is the fact that some residents themselves may normalize the occurrence of DHRRIs as something to be expected when living in LTC homes. In a study conducted on this phenomenon in a care home in Canada, one resident referred back to his school days, and said, "We all got beat up at school."[152]

As mentioned previously, when residents' distressing and harmful behavioral expressions are normalized, it is less likely that serious efforts will be made to understand the root cause of these episodes and develop individualized psychosocial strategies to prevent and de-escalate them. To break the chronic and dangerous cycle of normalization of DHRRIs, owners, administrators, and managers of LTC homes must take the lead in the following efforts and initiatives.

Acknowledge Human Rights

Leaders must routinely acknowledge and instill among all care employees the notion that it is the human right of residents with dementia and direct care partners to live in safe care homes. Owners and administrators must ensure that every possible measure will be funded and implemented to protect residents from the harmful effects of these episodes.

Understand Ageism and Dementism

Leaders of care homes must understand the harmful effects of deeply ingrained ageist perceptions toward elders in general and perceptions characterized as dementism toward individuals with dementia. Dementism is defined by bioethicist Stephen Post as "prejudice against the deeply forgetful." It reflects "a deep cultural sickness that combines a bias against old age (ageism) with a bias against impaired cognition (cognitivism)."[353] Care professionals in care homes need to recognize that the negative attitudes elders with dementia experience are often as disabling as the brain disease itself.[123]

Ensure That Managers Are Actively Present on the Floor

Making sure managers spend sufficient time on the floors with direct care partners throughout the day, evening, and night will enable the managers to better understand and appreciate the many challenges care partners face in their daily efforts to address these episodes. As suggested by a nurse aide, "Start by having management work a few shifts as an aide; they have no idea what we do, what we take."[334] Active presence of managers who are well aware of widespread misconceptions about behavioral expressions—including DHRRIs—among elders living with dementia can help guide direct care partners in minimizing the harmful normalization of these episodes and the perception that they are inevitable.

Listen to Direct Care Partners

Care home leaders must actively seek the input of direct care partners, consulting with them on a regular basis regarding ways to improve residents' care and safety and including them in *all* decision-making processes at all levels of the care organization related to the care they provide. In addition, managers need to remain open to learning from direct care partners about the innovative approaches they often develop in their hands-on work and care for residents with dementia. Routinely adopting and incorporating these approaches into residents' care plans can go a long way toward improving the quality of care and the safety of residents, as well as keeping direct care partners safe. Encouraging and adopting direct care partners' creative approaches can help prevent various forms of behavioral expressions, including DHRRIs.

Empowering direct and non-direct care employees to develop creative approaches and strategies can often demonstrate that many of these episodes are preventable, which helps minimize the normalization of this phenomenon. An older woman with advanced Alzheimer's disease was frequently involved in incidents with other residents in a secure care home for people with dementia. A young and insightful direct care partner began taking her twice a week to exercise in the fitness center, a room with equipment adapted to elders and designed to simulate what they do in their daily functions, in a different part of the building. Exercising with weights had been a lifelong activity and source of joy for the resident. When exercising with the guidance of the fitness instructor and cueing and praise from her care partner, the resident was calm and happy. The very fact that she was not inside the secure care home in close proximity to 30 other residents with dementia reduced her involvement in these episodes. She also benefited physically from these exercise sessions. Her son, who would take her for lunch every week, reported, "The exercise improved her strength . . . you can see it in her walking and when she gets out of the car, she can do it by herself." See further discussion and examples in the section "Encourage Creative Approaches" in Chapter 8.

Stay Informed

It is important to keep as up-to-date as possible with guidelines, best practices, and key findings from research studies on DHRRIs in general and psychosocial strategies for their prevention in the context of dementia. For instance, approximately half of fatal resident-to-resident incidents have resulted from "push–fall" contact. The integration of these findings from three research studies enabled us to know this fact, and this knowledge should have far-reaching implications in guiding individualized prevention strategies.

It is also important to learn from the rich experience of other care homes that have demonstrated success in reduction of these behavioral expressions. Consult with leading dementia experts such as Judy Berry (Dementia Specialist Consulting and developer of Lakeview Ranch Model of Specialized Dementia Care™), Dr. Allen Power (geriatrician, author, and leading educator), Jayne Clairmont (consultant and former owner of English Rose Suites), and Teepa Snow (Positive Approach® to Care).

Help Direct Care Partners Develop Their Understanding

Regularly share with your direct care partners case examples demonstrating that it *is* possible to prevent the majority of these episodes. Brain pathology and cognitive impairment account for only a small portion of behavioral expressions in this population. Distressing factors in the social and physical environment and, as importantly, contributing factors operating at the highest level of the care organization (such as unsafe staffing levels) account for the majority of these behavioral expressions.

Address Resident-to-Resident Incidents in Policies and Procedures

The policy and procedure documents of LTC homes should state a zero-tolerance policy for harmful resident-to-resident incidents and should outline the procedural, proactive, and immediate measures that must be taken to prevent and de-escalate these episodes, including post-episode strategies. Teresi and colleagues[331] emphasize the need to make sure that direct care partners and all other employees know and follow their care home's policies and procedures related to DHRRIs. An excerpt of a policy identified by Lachs and colleagues[178]—simplified, shortened, and modified—is presented here for illustration:

> The care home will ensure that all residents have the right to be free from physical or verbal aggression, unwelcome sexual behavior or advances, psychological mistreatment and misappropriation of property by other residents—all considered resident-to-resident incidents. The care home is responsible for protecting residents; educating staff in prevention and identification of resident-to-resident incidents; and for investigating, documenting, and immediately reporting resident-to-resident incidents to the nursing management and administration. In cases when it is determined that a resident has been emotionally or physically harmed by another resident, there will be a planned intervention or corrective actions taken, and reporting to [*name of applicable state survey agency*] immediately upon achieving a reasonable cause threshold of resident-to-resident incidents, which should not exceed [*reporting time periods as required by federal and/or state regulations governing your care home*].

Internal policies are important because they set the standard of expectations for all employees, residents, and their family members regarding residents' rights, care, and safety, whereas the procedures describe the ways in which the policies should be implemented to achieve their goals. They can also be useful to state surveyors during state survey agency's annual inspections and complaint investigations related to DHRRIs.

Promote Empathy and Compassion Between Residents

A community-wide, coordinated, and ongoing effort is essential for creating a care environment in which residents' expressions of empathy and compassion are highly valued. Routinely encouraging and instilling these expressions in your care home's policy and daily practices can eventually lead to a substantial reduction in DHRRIs and safer care environment. As explained by Robin Bonifas,[354] who studies bullying and DHRRIs in LTC homes:

> This requires, among others, a culture of respect where everyone is willing to stand up for what is right, and a high level of trust. Acknowledge members of the community who go out of their way to welcome new residents and those who are perceived as "different." Institute a "Caring Squad" whose job is to notice acts of kindness and reward them. Hold a "Peace Learning Circle," a group event to help recognize problematic behaviors and present simple strategies to call attention to them when they occur building on bystander intervention concepts.

In addition, each quarter, one resident who has gone out of her or his way to assist another resident or has engaged in an outstanding and inspiring act of compassion or kindness toward another resident could be publicly recognized, such as by placing a high-quality framed picture of the resident in a central location in the care home with the caption, "In Recognition of Exceptional Acts of Kindness and Compassion." Over time, such tradition could help reinforce the expectation of a compassionate, caring, and supportive community not only between care employees and residents but also between residents.

Stay Informed and Attend to At-Risk Residents

Regularly document residents' characteristics that may put them at increased risk of harm due to engagement in DHRRIs and make sure that *all* employees who come in direct regular contact with them (including float staff and external agency staff) are informed about them on time. That said, even during the risk-management process, it is important to remember to avoid stigmatizing residents with dementia by labeling them with the terms such as "violent" and "abusive." Making such information easily accessible in a timely manner to all employees can increase their awareness and vigilance, placing them in a better position to anticipate and proactively recognize, prevent, and de-escalate these residents' engagement in harmful episodes.

Know the General Characteristics of Residents with Dementia Who Tend to Be Harmed

There is limited empirical evidence from which to generalize the characteristics of those who are typically harmed during resident-to-resident incidents, but the research has revealed some preliminary patterns. One of my studies found that residents who died as a result of resident-to-resident incidents were, on average, nearly a decade (9.3 years) younger than exhibitors (75.2 versus 84.5 years old, respectively),[29] and a study by DeBois and colleagues found the difference in age to be, on average, nearly 13.5 years (83 versus 69.5 years old, respectively).[30]

My study also found that male and female residents died as a result these incidents at an equal rate, a finding that is fairly consistent with the one found in the study by Murphy and colleagues in nursing homes in Australia,[28] as well as in a recent study on fatal incidents in U.S. nursing homes.[30]

Shinoda-Tagawa and colleagues[26] examined visible physical injuries sustained during resident-to-resident incidents in nursing homes in Massachusetts and found the following:

- Male residents were almost twice as likely to be injured as female residents. Research is needed to explain the discrepancy in the gender-related findings between this study on injurious episodes and the aforementioned studies on fatal ones.

- A lower level of cognitive function was associated with increased likelihood of being injured by another resident. Compared with residents who were cognitively intact, the likelihood of experiencing injuries was about five times higher for residents classified as having borderline or mild impairments, eight times higher for those with moderate impairment, and 12 times higher for residents with severe cognitive impairment. The study showed that, in general, as cognitive function declines, the risk of being injured increases significantly.

- Residents who were physically injured were more physically independent than residents with no injury. In other words, needing extensive help and being severely dependent in activities of daily living (ADLs) was associated with lower levels of being injured. One possible explanation for this finding is that residents who are more physically independent are also generally more mobile and thus, with substantial cognitive impairment, they may be more likely to inadvertently instigate episodes (e.g., by invading others' personal space) than residents who are not independent in walking and tend to stay in one location for extended periods of time.

- Injured residents were also found to be more verbally and physically "abusive," exhibit socially "inappropriate" and "disruptive" behavior," engage in "wandering," and resist care than their counterparts without injury (none of these four biomedical and stigmatizing labels should be used today in the context of residents with dementia). The findings suggest that residents with dementia exhibiting behavioral expressions may be more at risk of being injured in resident-to-resident incidents. These expressions can act as situational triggers to other residents' physically injurious responses, such as when they attempt to protect their personal space or reach a breaking point after repeated and frustrating verbal expressions by other residents.

Direct care partners interviewed in a study by Sifford-Snellgrove and colleagues[83] described distinct characteristics of residents that made them particularly vulnerable to being harmed during resident-to-resident incidents. These characteristics, which are consistent with those found in the study by Shinoda-Tagawa and colleagues, include:

- Good physical mobility status, enabling them to move around and invade the personal space or bedrooms of other residents—two very common triggers of DHRRIs.

- A higher level of "confusion" than exhibitors (we should generally avoid this unhelpful term that was used in the cited study and instead describe the specific types of cognitive impairments experienced by the resident).

- Impaired communication, including problems with either sending or receiving verbal messages, repetitive verbal communication patterns, inability to use the right words to express a thought, mumbling or stuttering speech, or having severe hearing impairment. This finding aligns with what we know about the common situational misunderstandings between residents with dementia, which often contribute to interpersonal distressing situations and resident-to-resident incidents.

In addition, preliminary findings from my early study showed that residents involved in these episodes tend to be either the exhibitors or on the receiving end of the behavioral expressions, but less likely to be both. That said, some residents with dementia can certainly be both exhibitors and on the receiving end across different episodes.[13]

Taken together, the findings from these studies should guide owners, administrators, and interdisciplinary care teams' efforts to develop individualized prevention and de-escalation strategies aimed at protecting the most vulnerable residents with dementia from other residents. Research studies are needed to identify other factors associated with residents who are at risk of being psychologically harmed and physically injured during these episodes.

Learn to Distinguish the Roles of Residents During Episodes

Distinguishing who is the exhibitor and who is the resident on the receiving end during DHR-RIs is not always simple.[355] This important fact is often overlooked in many discussions, care practices, research studies (including mine until recently), and policies related to this phenomenon. This is particularly the case in the context of residents with dementia who experience situational misunderstandings, misperceptions, lower tolerance for frustrations, poor safety judgment (such as invasion of another resident's personal space or bedroom), and problems with impulse control. The difficulty or inability to determine a resident's willful intent to harm, injure, or kill another resident, especially among residents with middle- to late-stage dementia, further complicates this task. One study suggests that resident-to-resident incidents should be conceptualized as a process rather than an aggressive event, given the dynamic, interactional, reciprocal (bi-directional process), often multistage, and multilayered circumstances surrounding most of these episodes.[355]

Take, for example, a situation in which two residents with dementia struggle to obtain possession over a walker (each claiming that it belongs to himself/herself). The two pull and push each other and the walker for 30 seconds until the resident who is more physically frail loses balance, falls, hits the floor, and breaks her or his hip. To what extent can we truly tell who is "the exhibitor" in this episode?

In certain situations, behavioral expressions classified as "physically aggressive" might actually be a resident's defensive (self-protective) response, as in the case of a reaction to another resident's repeated and upsetting intrusion into another's personal space. For example, one female resident explained her defensive acts toward a male resident as follows: "There's this guy. He made advances to me all the time. I did not want his advances. Many times I had to take my grabber and actually strike him to get him to leave me alone."[48]

Furthermore, "contagious anxiety" can lead to what Raia calls the "billiard effect," which can make efforts to identify instigators, exhibitors, and residents on the receiving end more challenging. Sometimes, several residents can be involved in an unfolding episode throughout a trajectory consisting of a few segments or phases (the whole incident could last less than a minute to more than half an hour) where, at each point, a different number or combination of residents is involved. When one looks closely at the episode in its entirety, it is often possible to notice a thread connecting and driving all segments or phases throughout its duration until it ends; the thread typically consists of emotionally charged events and situational triggers that lead from one segment or phase to another, and the process repeats itself until the entire incident discontinues. The simplest and at times shortest scenario occurs with only three residents; here, the resident instigating the episode is a different person from the two residents ending up being involved in the harmful incident itself.[33] Picture the following episode. Resident A says something threatening or hurtful to resident B. Concerned for the safety of resident B, resident C approaches the two and tries to protect resident B by getting close to him (from behind) and trying to physically redirect him away from the area. Frightened and now startled, resident B instinctively pushes resident C away, causing him to fall and hit the floor.

Employment Policies

Employ the Right People and *Support Them*

A hundred hours of specialized dementia care training may not change the fact that a direct care partner is not suitable to care compassionately and effectively for elders living with dementia. As Andrea Moser, associate medical director of Baycrest Geriatric Centre (Toronto, Ontario, Canada) says, "It's not only the issue of the number of staff, but it's the right staff, the staff who have the right training, the right attitude, and the right approach."[356] When direct care partners with a natural inclination, motivation, and passion for caring for elders with dementia are carefully selected and continuously trained and supported, they are more likely to know each resident as a whole human being with a rich lifelong history, understand her or his unique care needs, and actively seek to identify the causes and triggers of their behavioral expressions. These individuals are typically in a better position to recognize early warning signs as well as prevent and de-escalate these residents' engagement in DHRRIs. In addition, feeling supported and recognized for their efforts, these direct care partners are also more likely to stay on the job. However, literature reviews conducted by the Paraprofessional Healthcare Institute show a substantial staff turnover rate (between 40% and 60%) among direct care workers.[357]

Kitwood[3] addresses the process of hiring suitable direct care partners:

> If the organization is to function well, it is essential that it has a sound process for selecting its employees. If the employees are unsuited for their jobs, limits will very soon be reached. Great discernment is needed in the selection process. In many respects, attitudes are the key. It is relatively easy to help a person to gain in knowledge and skill, but attitudes are often difficult to change (such as pathologizing and distancing attitudes). Ageism, rigidity, and that arrogance which bespeaks a lack of openness to new learning are particular drawbacks. In the process of selection, it is often possible to discover a person's attitudes by asking them to describe examples of good and bad practice.

Certain care homes that specialize in caring for people living with dementia use different hiring approaches (some use a 90-day trial period) as an integral part of the hiring process of direct care partners. Kitwood[64] explains, "From observation of their mode of interaction with the clients, it is often possible to discover who has a real aptitude for this kind of work. People with dementia generally have a clear sense of who has real concern for them, and so have their own selection procedures."

With some exceptions, residents' reactions to direct care partners and their care and communication approaches should generally be perceived as one helpful barometer regarding a direct care partner's suitability for working and caring for the person and possibly her or his fellow residents. The exceptions typically occur when a direct care partner who is caring, compassionate, and skilled simply reminds the resident of someone else in her or his life with whom she or he experienced a negative (traumatic or abusive) event or relationship. Some residents with middle- to late-stage dementia misperceive certain people interacting with them in the present as other people from their past. In other cases, the care employee may be suitable for caring for elders with dementia but does not receive adequate specialized training, orientation and ongoing, in order to care effectively for this population.

Supervisors interested in conducting an evaluation of direct care partners' skills in coping with residents' behavioral expressions should consider using or building on the 14-item Basic Skills Evaluation Form developed by Stephen Long.[295] For an excellent discussion of the issue of direct care partners' suitability in caring for elders with dementia, see Chapter 8, "Requirements of a Caregiver," in Kitwood's book *Dementia Reconsidered: The Person Comes First*.

Power[65] reports on care homes that use enlightened and innovative approaches. In one home, elders are included in group job interviews of prospective direct care partners. At the end of one such interview, after all team members had approved the applicant, a resident with dementia said, "I wouldn't hire her." She explained that it had to do with the candidate's nonverbal signals. The woman said all the right words, but her posture, tone of voice, lack of eye contact, and other body language belied her answers. The applicant was an expert in interviewing but seemed insincere to the resident. She was not hired.

Once an appropriate applicant has been hired, it is important to provide training and support in their critically important role as a direct care partner. Kitwood suggests, "Drawing the right people into caring for elders with dementia entails designing the jobs in such a way as to make them both challenging and attractive. For example, well-motivated people are encouraged to become care assistants if there is a route for promotion and opportunities for personal development."[64] The Paraprofessional Healthcare Institute compiled an excellent report in 2018 entitled *Growing a Strong Direct Care Workforce: A Recruitment and Retention Guide for Employers*. The ten strategies addressed in detail in it include:

1. Recruit the right staff;

2. Improve the hiring process;

3. Strengthen entry-level training;

4. Provide employment support;

5. Promote peer support;

6. Ensure effective supervision;

7. Develop advancement opportunities;

8. Invite participation;

9. Recognize and reward staff; and

10. Measure progress.

Finally, it is critically important that policy makers and legislators at the federal and state levels fully recognize and address the complicated challenge of recruiting and retaining suitable direct care partners to work in LTC homes given the major workforce shortages in a large number of communities across the country—shortages that existed for many years even prior to the COVID-19 pandemic. Examples of steps these entities can take on this crucial and urgent front include, among others, ensuring the provision of a living wage, affordable and accessible health care insurance, paid family and medical leave, adequate training, psychological support programs, and requirements related to safe staffing levels at all times in nursing homes and assisted living residences.

Resident-Related Procedures

Consider Admission Criteria

Admission criteria should be compatible with direct care partners' ability to meet admitted individuals' health care and psychological needs, and to provide meaningful engagement and a safe care environment, including the ability to prevent and de-escalate various forms of behavioral expressions. Raia suggests the following examples of issues to consider when developing admission criteria (e-mail communication, November 29, 2010):

> . . . the staffing level, the talent and skill of the staff, the mission of the unit, and the current composition of the residents. First, determine the mission of the unit. Is it palliative care, therapeutic, custodial care, aging in place or an early or later-stage unit? Do the staff have the capacity (the specialized knowledge, skill, and training) to effectively care for residents with certain types of dementia and not others? The mission will in part drive the admission policy. Other practical considerations are: How many challenging residents do you

currently have on the unit and how many more challenging residents can your staff handle? How many are ambulatory and how many are bed bound? Is your activity program sufficiently robust enough to handle residents in the earlier stages? Do you want to maintain a set ratio of males versus females on the unit?

It is important to avoid admitting a resident simply because there is a bed available for him or her. According to the Office of the Chief Coroner in Ontario, Canada,[117] "At no time should residents be admitted to fill an empty bed if that facility is not appropriate for the resident." Similar concerns have been voiced in the United States by Toby Edelman, senior policy attorney for the Center for Medicare Advocacy. She reports that some nursing homes are "admitting people they have no business admitting. They don't have the staff who are trained to take care of the residents."

Another recommendation of the Office of the Chief Coroner in Ontario[117] is that all LTC homes should have an "admission team" consisting of the administrator, director of care, chief medical administrator, and one experienced and highly trained registered nurse. When possible, social workers should also serve on the admission team, as their training and skill set can often be very helpful in ensuring adequate psychosocial evaluation and a whole-person admission process consisting of lifelong history, family history, personality, coping style, abilities and disabilities, likes and dislikes, preferences such as for meaningful engagement, behavioral expressions, safety issues, and so forth.

Conduct Thorough Preadmission Behavioral Evaluations

Admission and adjustment to a new life in a care home can often be very stressful for many elders with dementia and their close family members. When a person has exhibited distressing and harmful behavioral expressions in her or his prior care setting (whether in one's home, previous LTC home, rehabilitation center, or hospital), admission to a care home can often be a high-risk time for that person and for the other residents.[358] Challenging behavioral expressions may intensify at this time; a significant number of residents with middle-stage dementia, for example, may try to leave the LTC home unattended and go back to their previous home within hours, days, and weeks after admission.

It is critical to assess candidate residents in their current living environment and/or adult day health program to inform the decision as to whether or not to admit the person to the LTC home, including a detailed history of any behavioral expressions considered as aggressive or prior convictions of violent behavior. Although this may not always be possible—for instance, if the person lives in another state—every effort should be made to implement this best practice. In the long term, the benefits of conducting this evaluation often outweigh the time required to complete and review it. Being informed about the resident's history and triggers often takes much less time than the time required to address them when they are discovered during a crisis situation after admission. A thorough assessment allows the new care home staff to proactively develop an individualized psychosocial strategy for prevention of safety risks for the incoming person as well as for everyone else in the home. Identifying people with dementia who have a history of behavioral expressions reported as aggressive is very important; behavioral expressions before admission to a nursing home may predict similar expressions postadmission.[77]

Meeting the person in his or her living environment and meeting close family members often yields essential information and important insights about health conditions and care needs related to the individual's functional, cognitive, emotional, psychological, behavioral, social, cultural, ethnic, and spiritual states. A careful and timely review and integration of the information can assist the admission team with their best estimate, based on their best clinical judgment, regarding the extent to which the care setting is or is not capable of meeting the varied care needs of the person and keeping her or him, other residents, and direct care partners safe. In addition, there is often a need to improve collaboration and timely transfer of complete, updated, and reliable information between community-based nurses, physicians, social workers, hospitals, and other agencies (such as adult day health centers) and the LTC home during the preadmission evaluation process.

During the preadmission evaluation, the admission team will need to use a preadmission behavioral expressions review form to identify and document the behavioral concerns for each person with dementia who is a candidate resident. To my knowledge, no such tool has been published to date; therefore, it will need to be developed by the interdisciplinary care team, if it does not already exist.

Review of the filled-out form could assist the admission team in deciding whether or not to admit the person to the care home (i.e., whether or not the care team would be able to meet the individual's care needs, including the psychological, medical, and other needs underlying any behavioral expressions, and to do it in a way that is safe for the person and others). If the person ends up being admitted to the LTC home, all employees in direct regular contact with residents should be required to initial that they have read the form before caring for the person. Key information from the evaluation form will need to be incorporated into the care plan of the newly admitted resident, and the care plan should identify the measures and strategies planned to address the behavioral expressions identified. An example of one component series of questions that can be used during the preadmission behavioral expressions evaluation is described in the section "Learn What Causes a Resident to Lose His or Her Temper" in Chapter 8. Other questions should be developed by the interdisciplinary care team of the LTC home and incorporated into the form.

Key domains (and some examples of items) for inclusion in the form include the following:

- Issues related to the person with dementia attempting to leave or leaving the home/care setting unattended

- Wayfinding difficulties/getting lost within and outside the home/care setting

- Rejection of care, such as during assistance with bathing, toileting, dressing, transferring, eating, and medication administration

- Behavioral expressions perceived as aggressive (including whether these expressions are considered to pose a threat to others and/or the person)

- Other forms of behavioral expressions (such as collecting and/or hiding items excessively) and distressing verbal expressions (such as screaming)

- Self-injurious acts

- Eating inedible objects

- Urinating or defecating in public spaces (not in toilet)

- Smearing feces or food

- Making sexual comments or advances that are uncharacteristic to the person's usual behavior prior to dementia onset and perceived by the family care partner or others as inappropriate

- Exposing or touching one's sexual parts in public, making strange noises, repeatedly screaming or shouting

- Self-neglect

- Sleep problems and other challenges during the night

- Fears, such as of harm, theft, spousal affair, imposters, abandonment

- Delusions and hallucinations

Items within each domain should be rated using a scale indicating the frequency in which the primary family and/or paid care partner believes that they occurred during the past 7 days. For example: 3 = occurred daily; 2 = occurred 4–6 times; 1 = occurred 1–3 times; 0 = did not occur. A column entitled "Comments" should be included to provide the evaluator with a space to add what would be important to take into consideration when the admission team reviews the completed form.

If it is not possible to conduct a preadmission visit and evaluation (such as due to remote geographic residence of the person), the admission team should collect a comprehensive medical, functional, cognitive, psychological, social, and behavioral history of the person remotely. This can be accomplished through gaining access to this background information from the person directly when cognitively capable, close family members, and health care providers.

When the admission team determines that direct care partners at the LTC home will *not* be able to meet the person's healthcare and psychological needs or keep her or him safe—when there is a history of behavioral expressions that are beyond care partners' ability, skill level, and training to handle, or beyond the resources and supports allocated by the care home to them—the team should do its best to assist the resident and/or his or her family in identifying another care home capable of meeting those care needs.

It should be emphasized that admitting even one resident with tendencies that cannot be handled effectively and safely by direct care partners can have far-reaching negative consequences on the person and on the lives of a large number of residents and direct care partners for extended periods of time. I've seen it have a profound negative impact on an entire care home. In one home for elders with dementia, a single resident with Alzheimer's disease engaged in approximately two-thirds of all DHRRIs documented over a 10-month period. Most of the care employees had only limited ability to address his behavioral expressions effectively and safely. It was extremely painful and scary for everyone involved, including the resident himself and his family.

If the admission team decides to admit the person, the information gathered during the preadmission evaluation must be shared with all direct care partners and all other interdisciplinary care team members as early as possible before the admission day. At the same time, the team will need to develop a thoughtful plan to protect the person's privacy and confidentiality when handling and sharing sensitive personal and medical information among all care employees, for instance, when a resident has a history of being sexually abused.

In crisis situations such as those caused by unsafe and dangerous aggressive behaviors directed toward family members at home, care homes may be asked to admit people with dementia on an emergency basis within a very short period of time. A predesignated, experienced, and qualified on-call team at the care home should always be ready to conduct a preadmission behavioral assessment of the person in his or her current living or care environment. The goals of the evaluation are the same as for a non-emergency admission, described above. If the team determines that the LTC home does not have the necessary resources to keep the person and others safe, they will need to refer the person and/or his or her family to a different (i.e., suitable) LTC home or to a temporary care setting that specializes in evaluation, care, and treatment of people with dementia with behavioral expressions considered aggressive.

The following recommendation is based on the extensive experience of the Office of the Chief Coroner of Ontario, which regularly reviews deaths due to resident-to-resident incidents in LTC homes:[117]

> At a minimum, standards must be set to ensure that complete and accurate information is obtained prior to decision making about an applicant's eligibility and admission, despite the fact that the family is in crisis. The policy should ensure that no decisions regarding eligibility and placement are made without all relevant information.

This coroner's recommendation may seem unrealistic to some LTC home owners, administrators, managers, or directors of admissions. However, it is important to note that this recommendation was "written in blood"; that is, it is based on traumatic and tragic incidents that could have been prevented if care homes had not admitted residents whose history they did not know, and for whom they were unable to provide appropriate care.

Lack of proactive and thorough preadmission behavioral evaluation during crisis situations can lead to inappropriate admission of residents with dementia or those with serious mental illness (such as schizophrenia, personality disorder, or antisocial personality) with a history of harmful behavioral expressions. Many of these admissions result in a physical injury or death of another resident within days, weeks, or several months after the person moves in. In one case, a 74-year-old man with cognitive impairment was admitted to a Toronto nursing home around noon. At around 7:30 p.m., the resident grabbed a piece of metal from a wheelchair footrest and beat to death his two roommates, then proceeded to another bedroom and attacked another resident (who survived head injuries) before housekeeping staff intervened and disarmed him. Before the move to the nursing home, the person had been described as "physically aggressive" at home and impossible for his family to manage. He was admitted on an emergency basis on a Saturday, which meant that a full preadmission behavioral assessment was not completed.[117]

After the tragic deaths, the president of the nursing home commented on the need for timely and high-quality information transfer with community-based care agencies before all crisis admissions. He said the most important factor is "completeness and accuracy of the information" provided to his nursing home. He added, "That's the way the process works. We are part of the process, but we're at the end of the process."[359]

Early Postadmission Phase

The need for enhanced attention to the initial period (hours, days, and weeks) after admission is also supported by research. One study found that approximately half of the first incidents labeled aggressive occurred either on the day of admission or the next day, and more than three-quarters of the events occurred within a week of the admission to LTC homes.[360]

These findings also suggest that assessment of potential risk for engagement in DHRRIs among newly admitted residents must be conducted during the initial period after residents' admission to the care setting; of course, this assessment must continue throughout the residency. Care homes should conduct assessment of newly admitted residents' risk of engagement in harmful behavioral expressions within 24 hours after admission.

Preadmission behavioral assessment must still be conducted to inform the development of the person's initial care plan, if admission is warranted, and because physically harmful incidents often occur within the first hours after admission. One instrument that could be used for this purpose is the six-item Aggressive Behaviour Risk Assessment Tool for Long-Term Care (ABRAT-L). This instrument has been demonstrated to have a fairly good ability in predicting newly admitted residents' "aggressive behaviors" within 30 days after admission to 25 LTC homes in three provinces in Canada. Behavioral expressions in the study consisted of physical attacks, threats of physical attack, verbal abuse, and sexual harassment directed against other residents or staff. For further detail and instructions for using the ABRAT-L, readers should consult with the research article by Kim and colleagues (2017)[361] as well as the confirmatory follow-up study that validated the usefulness of the instrument.[360] Using this simple and easy-to-use risk-assessment tool could assist care homes in early identification of residents' risk of engaging in DHRRIs. Such early identification is critical and should be used by interdisciplinary care teams to inform the development and implementation of proactive individualized biopsychosocial prevention strategies aimed at keeping residents safe.

Assign Roommates Carefully

In an exploratory study, I examined the circumstances surrounding the deaths of elders as a result of resident-to-resident incidents among those with dementia in LTC homes (majority nursing homes but also a significant number of assisted living residences). The study showed that 33 out of 77 fatal incidents (43%) for which data were available to determine the relationship between the residents occurred between roommates.[29] A recent study in U.S. nursing homes examining fatal resident-to-resident incidents found that, out of 71 deaths for which relationship data were available, one-quarter (18 deaths) occurred between roommates.[30] These findings suggest that careful attention needs to be dedicated to the roommate selection, supervision of the relationship between residents sharing a bedroom and bathroom, and the process of reassignment, when it is warranted. According to Zeltser,[153]

> When roommate pairing is tailored to each individual, it conveys respectfulness, lessens distress and uncooperativeness, and can increase trust between residents. Overall, roommate pairing helps residents maintain control over their outward actions and inner feelings. . . ."

This author cautions, however, that "like any relationship, it takes time to work and will not happen overnight!"

To increase the likelihood that a roommate-pairing process will be successful and that the residents will get along, a review and careful consideration of the following factors should be conducted before any roommates are matched:

- Individual life histories

- Childhood background

- Cultural, racial, and ethnic background

- Personality traits

- Demeanor

- Cognitive function level (for example, stage of dementia) and specific cognitive deficits (such as short-term memory or executive functions)

- Serious mental illness, such as schizophrenia, personality disorder, and bipolar disorder

- Psychological well-being

- History of behavioral expressions

- Toileting and bathing needs

- Sleeping habits

- Strengths and remaining abilities

- Likes and dislikes

- Sources of irritability

- Noise tolerance

- Typical times of television viewing, if a TV set is installed in the bedroom[44]

In addition, each person's history of sharing a bedroom with another resident(s), including challenges and problems, should be reviewed and inform the roommate selection process.

After the roommates are paired, it is important to continue to monitor and document any arguments, tensions, and conflicts between them and make timely proactive changes in roommate assignments on an as-needed basis. This is true in general, but also due to cognitive changes caused by the progression of dementia.

In addition, it is critically important to listen and promptly act upon the concerns and complaints of residents and families regarding problematic and potentially risky roommate assignments. A 77-year-old resident in a nursing home in Minnesota[362] complained about his roommate, who had a history of psychiatric problems and violent behaviors—including a conviction for assault—as well as altercations between the two. The roommate was reported to have thrown objects across their shared bedroom, slammed doors, and regularly taunted the 77-year-old resident. He and his daughter begged administrators to assign him a different roommate. The resident was reported as saying, "I told them that if I have to spend one more night with that man, then I would kill myself. And they still ignored me." Sadly, the resident's fears materialized. He was attacked by his roommate and sustained a severe brain injury. The injured resident said, "He nearly beat the life out of me." He never regained his physical independence after his emergency brain surgery. After the injury, the daughter reflected on her father's and her requests to replace the roommate, "How many times were we supposed to warn them?"

Many people with mental illness do not pose a risk to others, but some have such histories, and these must be considered seriously when assigning roommates. The following tragic story demonstrates the need to thoughtfully assign and carefully monitor certain residents with serious mental illness who share a bedroom with other resident. As importantly, it speaks to the importance of listening to residents when they express concerns, fears for their safety, and complaints about their roommates. In the spring of 2014, just before midnight in a Houston, Texas, LTC home, a 56-year-old resident with schizophrenia and a history of psychotic episodes beat to death his two roommates (74 and 50 years old, respectively) with a wheelchair armrest. According to one report, he believed someone was trying to poison him. The daughter of the 74-year-old resident said that her father had long complained about the resident, as he was scaring him. "My father said to me . . . please, can they move this man out of this room?" After she reported her father's complaints to officials at the nursing home, she was told that she could move her father to a different facility. In her words, "They said that in order for people to move that person, he has to commit a crime or something—and now two people are dead."

Consider a "Buddy System"

Cognitive disabilities and behavioral expressions among people with dementia are among the leading reasons for admission to LTC homes.[363] As discussed earlier, the transition and adjustment to these care homes can increase the person's risk of developing psychological distress and anxiety,[364] as well as frustration, anger, fear, and feelings of abandonment. One randomized controlled trial used physiological assessments of stress among 116 residents one week before, one week after, and four weeks after relocation to a LTC home. Morning salivary cortisol levels were found to be highest during the first week of relocation. By the fourth week, the cortisol level started to decrease, suggesting the possibility that the resident was "settling in" to the care setting—at least as indicated by this physiological marker.[365] As explained by Vernooij-Dassen and colleagues,[366] "Having to start a new life in a place you have not deliberately chosen, under difficult physical and social circumstances, presents a major challenge to many residents."

The negative emotional states experienced during residents' initial adjustment to living in a care home can contribute to their engagement in DHRRIs. In fact, one study[367] found that nearly one-quarter (79 of 339) of residents were involved in DHRRIs within the 3-month period after admission to three LTC homes in Ontario, Canada (the behavioral expressions examined in the study caused "physical injury or psychological/emotional harm" to other residents). Residents involved in the episodes were more likely to have a diagnosis of dementia than those who were not involved in them. For these reasons, Tilly and Reed[190] assert, "Newly admitted residents with dementia require close monitoring."

The following innovative program was developed by Judy Berry to proactively address and decrease these common and anticipated postadmission challenges. Berry's model specializes in caring for people with dementia at risk for engaging in behavioral expressions reported as aggressive. The model has shown substantial reductions in behavioral expression–related hospitalizations and psychotropic medications among new residents with dementia compared with the year before the admission.[31]

An essential feature of this model was an innovative "buddy system" intervention, designed to assist new residents with dementia during their period of transition and adjustment to the residence. Berry reports that the intervention also showed a reduction in residents' adjustment period to the residence compared with the time period before the introduction of the system (Berry, oral communication, February 6, 2013). In the buddy system,[60]

> Each new resident is assigned a "buddy" from the time she or he arrives at the residence and for 6–10 days as needed to start building a trust relationship, [to] reduce the resident's anxiety and fear that is often present during transition, and to learn about the resident's individual needs.

The buddy was a highly trained volunteer; some of the volunteers had previous experience in providing direct care to people with dementia. The buddy would usually greet the new resident at the door upon his or her arrival at the care home and accompany her or him for 8 hours or until bedtime. Before the arrival of the resident, the buddy would learn about the person from the family, including occupation, favorite foods, medical history, and so forth. Among other tasks, the buddy would introduce the new resident to other residents, try to keep the person occupied by engaging in meaningful activities or simply sitting with the person and encouraging her or him to talk about her or his interests, join the person for a cup of coffee and a cookie or going over a family album together, distract the person when she or he is uneasy, alleviate fear, build a trusting relationship, and make her or him feel wanted and at home (Yvonne Morehouse, oral communication, March 1, 2013).

This anticipatory intervention is just one example of proactive measures taken by care homes to assist residents with dementia during adjustment periods to living in LTC homes. It is important to recognize that for some residents with dementia, the transition and overall adjustment to a move and life in a LTC home is not as difficult and distressing as it is for other residents.

Other, more common, examples of helpful measures include a welcome committee composed of carefully selected and dedicated residents who are cognitively intact or with early-stage dementia, as well as one-to-one peer mentoring programs both providing emotional support and practical guidance to the newly admitted resident during the days, weeks, and months after the move to the care home.

Such initiatives are critical in enabling newly admitted residents with dementia to experience the highest practical psychological well-being during the initial period after their move to the care setting. These initiatives are also likely to reduce the newly admitted resident's risk of engagement in DHRRIs and thus keep her or him and other residents safe.

Hold Regular Resident Council Meetings

The federal Nursing Home Reform Law requires that residents living in CMS–certified nursing homes have "the right to form and hold regular private meetings of an organized group called a resident council." The nursing home must consider the views of a resident council and act promptly upon grievances and its recommendations concerning issues of resident care and life in the care home. It also must demonstrate its response, and the rationale for its response, although it does not mean that nursing homes are required to implement every request of the resident council. In addition, the resident council meetings "are closed to staff, visitors, and other guests. For staff, visitors, or other guests to attend, the resident council must invite them."[368]

Resident council meetings held at least monthly enable cognitively intact residents and those with mild cognitive impairment and early-stage dementia to voice their appreciation and concerns about the quality of care provided to them and their fellow residents, at times voicing the concerns of those with more advanced dementia who are unable to participate in these meetings due to advanced cognitive impairment. Among other purposes, these meetings enable residents to discuss and offer suggestions for improvement in the nursing home's policies and procedures affecting residents' care, treatment, and quality of life.

Previous research has shown that, when the right dementia-friendly conditions are created, people with mild to moderate dementia can be reliable informants about their own quality of life.[369] These research findings highlight the importance of thoughtful and meaningful inclusion of residents with early-stage dementia in council meetings; that is, to avoid including only cognitively intact residents. A subgroup of residents in middle-stage dementia could also meaningfully participate in and contribute to these meetings, although some of these latter residents may need assistance such as with cueing, reminders, or encouragement.

Resident council meetings are also urgently needed in assisted living residences. Toward the end of a 45-minute-long resident council meeting held at a secure dementia care home for people with early-stage dementia in Massachusetts, an older woman with Alzheimer's disease said, "I think a meeting of this type should be held on a regular basis. The meeting is important. It gives us a chance to voice our opinions . . . as long as we know that someone is listening." This was the first time that a resident council meeting had been held in the assisted living community since it had opened a decade earlier. A few months before that meeting, another resident with early-stage Alzheimer's disease said, "We are cut off. Nobody inquires about how things could be improved. If they would only ask us, things could be improved." Still, a couple of weeks later, the same resident said angrily about management, "Nobody ever asks us what we think. Why the devil they don't ask us what we're thinking? They could benefit from it. I really don't understand why they don't ask us." Occasional informal attempts to seek residents' opinions about ways to improve the care were made by certain care employees and managers at the care home. In addition, family council meetings were held regularly at the assisted living residence. However, the need for a structured forum in the form of a resident council was made clear by several residents with early-stage dementia who attended the meeting.[370]

Resident council meetings also allow residents to express their concerns regarding psychological harm and safety risks resulting from distressing behavioral expressions, including DHRRIs (results of unsafe staffing levels and gaps in direct care partners' specialized training in understanding, recognition, prevention, and de-escalation of these episodes).

It is important to carefully plan resident council meetings and document concerns expressed during them. It is not uncommon for certain LTC homes to hold these meetings but not to document and/or follow up on residents' concerns voiced in them. When planning and holding meetings, it is also important to reinforce a culture of respect, sensitivity, empathy, and compassionate tolerance of residents with cognitive impairment, some of whom will participate in the council. As mentioned earlier, cognitively intact residents or those with early-stage dementia may have difficulty tolerating residents with more advanced cognitive impairment in general and during these meetings.

Hold Regular Family Council Meetings

The federal nursing home reform law of 1987 states, "The resident has a right to have family member(s) or other resident representative(s) meet in the facility with the families or resident representative(s) of other residents in the facility." Under the revised nursing home regulations (November 28, 2016), family members are still permitted to organize a family council, "but it is now the *resident* who has the right to have his or her family meet with other families, rather than the family having the right as was the case in the prior regulations" (i.e., the right of family members to participate in a family group is a result of and subordinate to residents' rights). CMS explains that there could be situations where a resident would not want to allow a family member, such as an estranged spouse, to join the family council. In addition, the new regulations expanded the resident's right to include her or his representatives.

In addition, care employees are required to consider families' views and act upon their grievances and recommendations. They must consider these recommendations and attempt to accommodate them, to the extent practicable—such as developing or changing policies affecting resident care and life. The nursing home should discuss its decisions with the family group and document in writing its responses to requests and rationales for changes.[32]

These family council meetings, when held regularly, offer a structured forum for family members to express their appreciation and concerns about the quality of care at the LTC home, including to discuss problems and safety concerns related to DHRRIs and the strategies that could be used to address these episodes. Family members often hold invaluable information about their relatives' life background, current abilities, disabilities, preferences, likes, and dislikes, which can be key for development of personalized biopsychosocial approaches that work in reducing DHRRIs and keeping residents safe. For example, close family members may know about remote triggers from their loved ones' distant past such as childhood physical or sexual abuse, profound traumas experienced during the Holocaust, or combat-related traumas experienced by war veterans. When direct care partners become aware of residents' deeply personal traumas, not only may they become more sensitive and empathetic to the resident with dementia but they can also be in a better position to recognize and understand the unmet emotional needs underlying any engagement in DHRRIs. For example, an older woman who was sexually abused as a teenager now fears for her life when men with dementia mistakenly enter her bedroom at night. Proactively validating and addressing these emotional traumas and ensuring that adequate protective measures are implemented could assist in preventing her engagement in DHRRIs, such as when she tries to physically prevent someone from entering her bedroom, and ensuring her safety.

Reporting and Documentation

Develop and Implement Reporting Policies

As mentioned previously, research has shown that the majority of incidents classified as aggressive, and DHRRIs in particular, are not reported in many nursing homes.[331,13,178,333] Lachs and colleagues[178] found that although verbal DHRRIs were the most frequent type reported by direct care partners, these behavioral expressions were not recorded in the residents' charts. The lack of reporting of yelling and insulting remarks by residents toward other residents is a source of concern because these verbal expressions can quickly escalate into injurious and fatal incidents between residents. In fact, a recent study examining fatal resident-to-resident incidents in nursing homes found that arguments were reported as the trigger in 44% (24 out of 54) of the incidents for which data were available to determine it.[30]

Care homes must address the chronic and common problem of underreporting of episodes in order to help identify their root causes and situational triggers and develop personalized psychosocial interventions to reduce them and keep residents safe. Specifically, care homes must institute and implement a residence-wide policy by which *all* employees are required to report to supervisors (such as a charge nurse) *all* episodes of verbal, physical, and sexual threats and "aggression"; one way is by using the Behavioral Expressions Log presented in the downloadable resources available with this book.[34] Beyond filling out an incident report for episodes with potential for or actual emotional or physical harm, care employees need to thoroughly document and report on episodes that could be characterized as "near misses." For example, a cognitively intact resident sits in the hallway and intentionally sticks his leg or cane out in order to trip a frail resident walking by. His attempt fails but, if witnessed by a care employee or reported by the target resident, it must be reported to supervisors (verbally and in writing), as some episodes have a tendency to recur over time.

The detailed written (preferably, electronic) reports should be completed immediately or, if not possible, shortly after the episode ends. Direct care partners, nurses, and social workers should make every possible effort to avoid waiting to fill out the report at the end of the work shift, as this may compromise their recall accuracy of key details from the episode. Omission of important details about causes and situational triggers will likely minimize their and their co-workers' ability to recognize and prevent subsequent episodes with similar causes and situational triggers that may occur in the hours, days, and weeks following the episode.

Supervisors, managers, and educators need to regularly demonstrate to direct care partners that behavioral expressions tend to manifest among individual residents in recurring patterns (such as time of day, location, events, causes and situational triggers, people, environmental factors, and objects), which is the fundamental basis for developing individualized and effective psychosocial strategies. Direct care partners must be provided frequent opportunities to see the clinical and preventive value of filling out reports on distressing and harmful behavioral expressions (such as by discussing exemplary case studies of successful and unsuccessful strategies used).

As discussed earlier, managers must regularly demonstrate to direct care partners that reports are meant primarily for learning and improvement purposes, not to blame judge care partners or criticize their job performance, or to use the reports for punitive or disciplinary measures against them. Using the latter approaches commonly increases direct care partners' mistrust, reluctance, and fear of reporting, which in turn decreases the scope, frequency, and quality of reporting of DHRRIs—a crucial basis for effective prevention.

In short, if direct care partners, who are commonly understaffed and overworked, do not believe in the preventive value of filling out these reports, they will simply not do it or they may do it but not as thoroughly. They need to see that the reports are taken seriously by *all* employees, that they are being reviewed and analyzed regularly by managers, and that the clinical insights gleaned from their analyses are routinely incorporated into individual residents' care plans and thus their care, as well as into direct care partners' training programs (orientation, in-service, and experiential learning through hands-on guidance by supervisors when episodes occur in real time).

Most importantly, direct care partners need to regularly see that these reports help them in understanding risk and protective factors, identifying, preventing, reducing, and de-escalating DHRRIs. They need to see on a regular basis that such a significant time investment on their part is clearly helpful in creating a safer care and work environment for residents and themselves, respectively. The key for success on this front is provision of adequate staffing levels at all times and specialized training including ongoing guidance from managers in skilled and detailed documentation and reporting of the causes and triggers of DHRRIs. This should be the expected standard of care in all LTC homes no matter where they are along the journey to become a true learning organization.

Improve *Quality* of Documentation

As mentioned in the previous section, all direct care partners and other interdisciplinary care team members need to understand the importance of complete documentation to the prevention of DHRRIs. Previous research has shown that the quality of direct care partners' documentation of DHRRIs in many nursing homes is poor.[13] For example, a common report, such as "Mrs. Rogers spilled a cup of water on Mr. Barry during dinner" is largely unhelpful because it does not include critical detail about the circumstances and the sequence of events, situational frustrations, and triggers leading up to the episode. In the words of Jiska Cohen-Mansfield,[337] who conducted the largest number of studies on behavioral expressions among residents with dementia in LTC homes, "The most important principle in treating the aggressive person is the effort to understand the meaning of the sequence that led to the aggressive behavior." Written reports must therefore include a detailed description of the sequence of events leading up to the incident, where that is known. See the section "Routinely Use a Behavioral Expressions Log" in Chapter 10, as well as the log itself in the downloadable resources available at health-propress.com (see p. viii for access information).

Maintain a Master List

Using a master list of *all* DHRRIs at the LTC home[78] is an important risk management and learning tool that enables direct care partners and administration to track, analyze, and identify patterns underlying residents' distressing and harmful behavioral expressions (e.g., temporal, spatial, factors in the physical environment, triggering events, and people), which are key to effective prevention. Care homes must have quality assurance and improvement mechanisms in place to analyze DHRRIs and to identify trends, risk, and protective factors within and across care units throughout the LTC home. Over time, insights gleaned from routine analysis of the circumstances surrounding these episodes can inform development of individualized measures to prevent further incidents. The clinical rationale for keeping a master list is that behavioral expressions among people with dementia, including those classified as aggressive and DHRRIs, tend to manifest in distinct patterns.[122] Recognizing this fact represents an important opportunity for prevention of DHRRIs. Keeping a master list should be considered an integral part of any behavioral risk management and quality improvement programs in LTC homes.

8

Proactive Measures

We are not trying to get rid of behavioral distress.
What we're trying to do is to create well-being.

G. Allen Power[48]

This chapter describes a series of proactive, anticipatory practices and measures that direct care partners, interdisciplinary care teams, and managers should implement routinely in long-term care (LTC) homes. Strong and ongoing support and adequate resource allocation by owners of care homes are key for successful implementation of these measures. Systematic implementation of these practices and measures will assist in the following ways:

- Minimize the likelihood that distressing and harmful resident-to-resident interactions (DHRRIs) will develop in the first place, for example, by building and maintaining close trusting relationships with residents living with dementia, by proactively meeting their emotional and medical needs, by providing them with a structured daily routine and personally meaningful engagement, and by ensuring a timely information transfer between care employees, with all direct and indirect care partners being informed in a timely manner about previous episodes and "at-risk" residents (both exhibitors and residents who could potentially be harmed during these episodes).

- Maximize direct care partners' ability to anticipate these episodes, for instance by being aware of individual residents' unmet needs, physical discomforts, triggers in the physical or social environment, and ongoing risk factors (both at the individual resident level, any dyads repeatedly engaged in these episodes, and at the group level).

- Maximize direct care partners' ability to identify episodes early, by knowing the life history of residents and what may upset them, being able to recognize early warning signs of distress and anxiety, enabling care employees to respond promptly and effectively to these episodes as early as possible (e.g., working as a team and being adequately trained in using dementia-specific communication techniques such as those developed in the Validation Method).

The chapter also describes key resources—assistive technologies—that could help direct care partners in strengthening their ability to supervise residents with dementia, as well as suggestions for reducing residents' access to objects they could use to physically harm other residents during episodes.

In a nutshell, when well-trained direct care partners provide care under conditions of safe people-to-people ratios (staffing levels) at all times, they are much more likely to succeed in proactively and routinely fulfilling the varied psychological and medical needs of residents with dementia. One of the direct outcomes of such strong commitment from owners of LTC homes is that residents could experience the highest practicable well-being and thus a substantial re-duction in DHRRIs. Both residents and care employees will be safer.

Daily Habits to Cultivate Among Direct Care Partners

Remain Alert and Watch Residents Vigilantly

In a focus group study conducted in a nursing home, direct care partners reported that re-maining alert and vigilant is a key strategy they use for prevention of DHRRIs.[14] Verbal and physical DHRRIs among residents with dementia may sometimes develop within seconds (such as in situations of invasion of personal space), so, to the best of their ability, direct care partners must remain vigilant and respond immediately and skillfully to early warning signs of residents' distress and anxiety, before they escalate into verbally and/or physically harmful episodes. As explained by an insightful director of recreation therapies[34] during a training program she led for direct care partners, "You almost have to be a mind reader . . . if you can stop a situation before you think it's going to happen, you always have to be two steps ahead of yourself with somebody that has an aggressive behavior . . ." More importantly, anticipating these situations and proactively preventing them from occurring in the first place (primarily by meeting residents' emotional and other needs) is often the most effective and efficient strategy.

It should be recognized, however, that this kind of vigilance will be difficult to achieve without adequate staffing levels at all times; specialized training in recognition, prevention, and de-escalation of these episodes; and managers' guidance and supervision of direct care partners, including well into the evening hours and during weekends.

Federal and state governments urgently need to require adequate nursing staffing levels including allocation of adequate funding and resources to ensure that a sufficient number of well-trained direct care partners and nursing supervisors (such as registered nurses) will work on all care shifts in nursing homes.[371] In addition, the establishment of strong standards and requirements of safe staffing levels in assisted living residences and secured dementia care homes operated within this fast-growing LTC setting are also urgently needed. Put simply and succinctly by Tom O'Hanlon, Office of the New York State Attorney General, Medicaid Fraud Control Unit, who regularly investigates elder mistreatment in LTC homes, "Understaffing is neglect."[372] Indeed, in contrast to common beliefs, most of the injurious and deadly resi-dent-to-resident incidents in the context of dementia are the result of neglectful care practices and not resident "abuse" of other residents.

Identify Residents' Unmet Needs and Address Them Proactively

As has been discussed, unmet needs and frustrations in various domains underlie the vast majority of behavioral expressions labeled as aggressive in residents with dementia. Following is a compilation of the primary quality indicators of needs of people with dementia living in specialized LTC homes, as identified by researchers.[373]

- Autonomy

- Privacy

- Dignity

- Social interaction

- Meaningful activity

- Individuality

- Enjoyment versus aversive stimulation

- Safety and security

- Spiritual well-being

- Clarity of structure

- Functional competence

Proactively meeting these various needs for each resident will go a long way in terms of direct care partners' ability to anticipate and prevent DHRRIs. During a training program on prevention of behavioral expressions in residents with dementia, a director of recreation therapies[34] made the following helpful suggestion, "Be responsive to what their needs might be. It's all about our approach. It isn't us. It isn't them. It's about their needs."

A study by Snellgrove and colleagues[151] found that when CNAs were asked whether they believed that unmet needs of the residents influenced development of resident-to-resident "violence," they unanimously denied it. However, when viewed objectively, each of the trigger categories related directly to one or more residents' unmet needs. The researchers explained, "The disparity in recognizing triggers as unmet needs may be explained by the way in which CNAs conceptualize them. They may view the existence of unmet needs of the residents as a failure on their part to sufficiently care for the residents." Ongoing educational efforts are needed to overcome this barrier in addressing DHRRIs.

In one case, reported by Power (citing social worker and leading educator Cathy Unsino),[48] every day around 6:00 p.m., a resident was observed slamming drawers at the nurse station and throwing books across the room, while screaming, "I need a line, I need a line, I need a line." The direct care partners could not understand what he meant. Review of his life history revealed that he had been a businessman who traveled all over the country for his work. No matter where he was, he would call his wife every evening to tell her "Good night" and "I love you." As an intervention, shortly before 6:00 p.m., a direct care partner began assisting him with calling his wife. The behavioral expression was eliminated, he was calm, and the use of psychotropic medications was avoided.

Carefully Observe Residents to Identify Early Warning Signs

Residents with dementia typically show signs of distress, irritability, restlessness, frustration, anxiety, anger, or fear *before* engaging in harmful resident-to-resident incidents. Observable early warning signs, situational triggers, and antecedent events have been found to precede the majority of behavioral expressions classified as aggressive in elders with dementia[344,345] and in DHRRIs in the context of dementia in particular.[13] Eller and colleagues[347] state that anxiety in people with dementia is often the first observable level of "agitation" (the biomedical term commonly used in the literature to describe a host of behavioral expressions including those labeled aggressive). Jitka Zgola, author of the book *Care That Works: A Relationship Approach to Persons with Dementia*,[59] asserts, "In most cases, the person with dementia is telegraphing her feelings long before the outburst occurs." According to Dr. Roger Skinner, chair of the Ontario Coroner's Geriatric and Long-Term Care Review Committee, who regularly reviews fatal resident-to-resident incidents in the context of dementia in LTC homes (the committee has published annual reports on these deadly incidents for over 25 years),

> Usually there's an escalation of that behavior prior to the incident. Most of the incidents involve initially a verbal altercation and then a physical altercation in which one individual is pushed and falls and either suffers a fracture like a fractured hip or suffers a head injury.

Therefore, it is important for all care employees to carefully observe residents' body language (facial expressions, gestures, posture, eye movement, and tone of voice) and other early warning signs indicating that the resident is about to engage in a potentially harmful interaction with

Table 8.1   Recognizing Early Warning Signs of Distress and Anxiety in People with Dementia

Domain	Observable Early Warning Signs
Physiological signs of anxiety	• Abnormally rapid heart rate • Rapid, noisy, or irregular breathing • Difficulty breathing (shortness of breath even when not exerting) • Hyperventilation • Feeling hot • Dizziness or light-headedness (complains as if going to faint) • Sweating (not due to heat) • Flushes (face) or chills • Trembling or shakiness • Increased muscle tension • Dry mouth (not due to medications) • Sinking feeling in the stomach • Higher urinary frequency • Tingling or numbness of fingers and toes • Indigestion or discomfort in abdomen • Fainting or feeling faint • Being unsteady
Tense body language	• Clenched fist • Knees pulled up tightly • Strained, inflexible body position • Hunched shoulders
General signs of anxiety	• Irritability (more easily annoyed than usual, short tempered and with angry outbursts) • Nervousness • Fidgeting • Unable to relax • Restlessness • Inability to sit still • Squirming or jittery movements • Leg jiggling • Wobbliness in legs • Repeated or agitated movement or motions • Asking repeated questions • Rapid, disconnected speech • Voice changes • Anxiety about upcoming events • Poor attention span (worse than baseline) • Pacing • "Shadowing" others • Trying to leave the area to avoid the source of distress, anxiety, or fear • Withdrawing from other(s) without anger

Table 8.1 Recognizing Early Warning Signs of Distress and Anxiety in People with Dementia *(continued)*

Domain	Observable Early Warning Signs
Facial expressions signaling anxiety	• Grimacing • Line between eyebrows • Lines across forehead • Eyes widened • Tight facial muscles • Poor eye contact • Wariness • Sighing • Frowning: face looks strained • Stern or scowling looks • Displeased expression with a wrinkled brow • Corners of mouth turned down
Hand signals of anxiety	• Hand wringing • Forceful touching, tugging, or rubbing of body parts • Tremor
Signs of anger	• Drawing eyebrows together • Furrowed brow (with other anger signs) • Clenching teeth • Pursing lips (downward curve) • Narrowing eyes • Making distancing gesture • Lower jaw out
Frightened facial expression	• Terrified, scared, or concerned-looking face • Strong feelings of dread (e.g., thinking she/he is going to die) • Looking bothered, fearful, or troubled • Alarmed appearance with open eyes and pleading face • Tearfulness • Crying

Compiled from the following sources: Mahoney and colleagues[255] (Clinical Indicators of Anxiety); Beck and colleagues[374] (Beck Anxiety Inventory); Lawton and colleagues[375] and Lawton and Rubinstein[376] (Observed Emotion Rating Scale); Hurley and colleagues[377] (Discomfort Scale in Dementia of the Alzheimer's Type); and Shankar and colleagues[378] (Rating Anxiety in Dementia Scale).

another resident. As suggested in an even more nuanced way by Naomi Feil,[63] developer of the Validation Method, who has over 50 years of experience working with elders with dementia,

> Carefully observe the physical characteristics of the person and the way in which she/he moves. You should observe the person's eyes, facial muscles, breathing, changes in color, chin, lower lip, hands, stomach, position in the chair, position of the feet, and the general tone of the person's muscles . . .

Table 8.1 contains detailed descriptions of body language and facial expressions that direct and non-direct care employees and managers should pay close attention to in order to proactively and effectively recognize, prevent, and de-escalate DHRRIs. The information contained in the table could also be used during direct care partners' training programs to increase their awareness to these important emotional states that often precede harmful episodes.

In addition, the educational video *Recognizing and Responding to Emotion in Persons with Dementia*[379] (Terra Nova Films) could be used during direct care partners' training programs to strengthen their knowledge and skill in recognizing early warning signs of residents' distress, anxiety, situational frustrations, and impending DHRRIs. The 22-minute film can improve care employees' ability to understand and decipher facial expressions, vocal signs, and body language indicating distress in residents with dementia. Although the film is old, the real-life second-by-second illustrations presented in it (such as subtle changes from baseline emotional state at the individual resident level) can still be very useful today.

Be Proactive Instead of Reactive

A study in five nursing homes found that the vast majority of strategies used by 97 direct care partners to address DHRRIs were reactive in nature and involved de-escalating an existing episode rather than using proactive strategies to meet residents' needs and preventing future episodes.[332] Zgola[59] calls on care homes and direct care partners to "stop the vicious cycle of reactivity" that typifies the care provided to people living with dementia in many of these settings. Instead, there is a need to shift to an "anticipatory care approach." Anticipatory care[349] is defined as "actions taken before the usual time of onset of a particular need or problem in order to prevent or moderate the occurrence of the problem." According to Christine Kovach and colleagues,[349] "Failing to understand the source of or solution to a problem compromises the caregiver's ability to know how to prevent the problem from recurring."

The following story[295] illustrates the practice of anticipatory care. Several residents in wheelchairs would leave the dining room at about the same time and slowly move through the hallway, creating a "traffic jam" of wheelchairs outside the dining room. Each day, one of the women in the wheelchair group was among the first to leave the dining room, but she always found herself in the middle of the jam as others caught up to and bumped into her. After being bumped a few times, she would curse and punch the next resident who bumped into her. The more she got bumped, the louder she would curse and the more she would hit. Other residents cursed back at her, told her to stop, and threatened to hit her back. She would only get more distressed, yelling and hitting even more, at times even using an ethnic slur against another resident.

The cursing and hitting stopped only when a nurse aide proactively took the woman out of the situation. The aide realized that the trigger was the overcrowded hallway and that others yelling back, threatening, or telling the woman that her words and actions were inappropriate was reinforcing them. The nurse aide implemented an individualized anticipatory care intervention. She watched for the woman to begin to leave the dining room after lunch, and she made sure to assist her in getting beyond the area that usually got clogged. The woman's shouting and hitting—and the frustrated, angry, and potentially harmful reactions from the other residents—discontinued.

Other examples include the need for direct care partners to ensure that two residents with a history of DHRRIs are not left alone unsupervised in the same area, such as in the television lounge or dining room, or to see that they will not sit one next to the other during a group activity. Of course, choosing a seat in the television lounge is a personal choice, but that needs to be thoughtfully balanced with the risk of harm that could potentially result from such proximity between residents with a serious brain disease who do not get along.

In my early study on DHRRIs in an assisted living residence for people with dementia, I observed discreet, simple, and timely information transfer between recreation staff that was used as a proactive and effective preventive strategy in the context of problematic seating during group activity time. For example, a director of recreation therapies[34] used the positions on a clock face to indicate specific residents to an expressive therapist who had just entered the secured care home to lead a group activity. She quietly told her co-worker, "Pay attention to 6 o'clock and 12 o'clock . . . they don't get along." Armed with this information, the expressive therapist took proactive measures to prevent verbal conflicts between the two residents during the activity.

Since it is not uncommon for transitions of a group of residents with dementia from one area in the care home to another to result in verbal and physical conflicts between residents, a proactive and creative approach can make the difference between a successful transition and a distressing and harmful one. You may recall the example from Chapter 5 of music therapist Wendy Krueger, who invites residents to sing a song together as they are about to leave a room at the end of an activity; they keep singing until they arrive, calmly and safely, at their destination.[13]

Direct care providers can also proactively eliminate congested areas by limiting the number of residents served per area (e.g., waiting to see the nurse for a physical examination or to be weighed, or waiting for the elevator).[78] A resident who tends to repeatedly become anxious or engage in behavioral expressions at the same time of day (say, around the 3:00 p.m. shift change) can be engaged in a personally meaningful activity (such as therapeutic gardening, music therapy, walking group) shortly *before* the expected time of anxiety; this can assist in meeting the resident's needs (such as the need for purposeful engagement and meaning) and thus prevent or alleviate the distressing emotional states (such as those caused by boredom). The interest and joy experienced during these diversional engagements can often divert residents with dementia away from the source of distress experienced during these vulnerability time periods. A warm invitation for a walk together in the secured outdoor garden can often also achieve this effect. Singing at just the right time can also be helpful, as Jolene Brackey[205] suggests,

> Prior to the time the person becomes most anxious, I want you to do something the person loves. While I was an activity person, the one thing I could always count on to get through the confusion of shift change was singing. A half an hour before the first shift was over, I would start to sing the old familiar tunes and we would continue to sing until the second shift was in place.

Assess and Treat Physical Discomfort and Medical Needs

Physical and even medical conditions are common triggers of behavioral expressions among elders with dementia, but, because of their internal nature, they can be more difficult for the direct care provider to detect.[261] Common examples include thirst or dehydration, hunger, constipation, pain, skin problems, acute illness, fever, urinary incontinence, being wet due to incontinence and/or the need to use the bathroom, infections (such as urinary tract infection), delirium, delusions, hallucinations, dental problems, hearing loss, low vision, and sleep deprivation. Due to scope considerations, only a few conditions will be addressed in this section for illustrative purposes. To do justice to the complexity underlying other medical conditions and needs, in-depth and specialized attention is warranted elsewhere.

It is important to engage in routine individualized assessment, early detection, and timely treatment of physical discomforts, medical and physiological needs, and functional difficulties of residents with dementia. Besides the suffering they may cause, these conditions can sometimes contribute to the development of DHRRIs.

Discomfort

In at least one study, distressing behavioral expressions (classified as "agitation") were associated with discomfort.[380] Discomfort is defined[377] as "a negative emotional and/or physical state subject to variation in magnitude in response to internal or environmental conditions." One tool for assessing discomfort is the Discomfort Scale in Dementia of the Alzheimer's Type (DS-DAT).[377] Under the supervision and guidance of the nurse in charge, direct care partners should routinely be on the lookout for any of the following seven negative dimensions covered in the DS-DAT scale:

- Noisy breathing

- Negative vocalization

- Sad facial expression

- Frightened facial expression

- Frown

- Tense body language

- Fidgeting

When these manifestations of discomfort are noticed over an extended period, especially when they seem to be out of baseline/character for a resident, they should be reported immediately to nursing supervisors, and nurses and direct care partners should make an effort to identify and treat the underlying unmet need, such as skin rash or acute illness. This, in turn, can reduce the likelihood that residents with dementia experiencing discomfort will become restless, frustrated, or anxious—all distressed emotional states that could decrease their tolerance to other residents around them and thus increase the risk of engagement in harmful episodes.

Constipation

The following story[381] illustrates the importance of identifying and treating the root cause of residents' physical discomforts in alleviating their emotional distress. A resident was often heard yelling, "Help me, help me, help me!" When direct care partners would ask how they could help him, he was unable to explain. Instead, he began digging in his rectum and smearing feces around (throwing it on the floor and against the window). Care partners tried to redirect him and invite him to use mittens, and even treated him with antipsychotic medications, but these interventions failed. After they implemented a strict toileting plan, rectal exams, enema if stool was present, and administration of laxatives, the yelling decreased, the smearing discontinued, and all antipsychotic medications were discontinued. The unmet need causing the behavioral expression was constipation, defined as infrequent, incomplete, or painful evacuations of feces. The authors reported on 14 other people who also smeared their feces; all were found to have constipation, which was resolved with laxatives. Constipation can cause behavioral expressions labeled as aggressive in residents with dementia, but also a resident's yelling can trigger angry responses from other residents.

Constipation may be caused by various diseases and conditions, including cancer or cancer-related conditions; endocrine, gastrointestinal, metabolic, neurologic, and psychological disorders; and low-fiber or high-fat diet, among others.[382] In addition, not drinking enough liquids (poor hydration), drinking large amounts of alcohol, certain medications (known to have constipation among the adverse effects), and lack of exercise may contribute to constipation.

Delirium

Delirium is characterized by an acute onset of mental status change (fluctuating course, decreased ability to focus, sustain, and shift attention; and either disorganized thinking or an altered level of consciousness).[255] Predisposing factors for delirium may include advanced age (>65), severity of dementia, functional deficits (activities of daily living, or ADLs) such as immobility, depression, number of medications used, exposure to high-risk delirogenic drugs, sleep deprivation, visual impairment, hearing impairment, severe illness, multiple comorbidities, alcoholism, and history of delirium.[383-386]

Precipitating factors include acute illness, surgery, pain fever, dehydration, malnutrition, sepsis, electrolyte disturbance, urinary retention, fecal impaction, behavioral expressions, use of physical restraints, understimulation (such as lack of engagement in meaningful activities), and inadequacy of the physical environment (e.g., lack of orienting objects, excessive noise, and inadequate lighting levels).[384]

The prevalence of delirium among LTC residents is estimated to range from 6% to 14%.[387] A review of the research literature has found that having a diagnosis of Alzheimer's disease or other forms of dementia is a risk factor for developing delirium,[388] and LTC residents with moderate to severe cognitive impairment are at particularly high risk for this condition.[389]

Previous research among elders in 16 hospital wards has found that developing delirium substantially increases the likelihood of engagement in incidents classified as "serious aggressive behaviors" (consisting of risk of harm to the patient or others).[390] Key manifestations of delirium that could potentially contribute to a resident's involvement in DHRRIs include changes and fluctuations from baseline cognitive function (examples are difficulty keeping track of conversation, being easily distractable, and using the wrong bedroom), perception (for instance, visual or auditory hallucinations or misinterpretations), physical function (such as restlessness or sleep deprivation), and lack of cooperation.[391]

The Confusion Assessment Method (CAM) can be used to detect delirium. This is a standardized evidence-based tool that can enable clinicians to identify this condition quickly and accurately.[392,393] For details about the CAM and how to use it, see the *Try This* guide from Hartford Institute of Geriatric Nursing, New York University.[386] Delirium can be resolved if the precipitating medical causes (such as infections, dehydration, metabolic disorder, or pain) are identified and treated and when medications causing adverse effects are changed.[255]

In addition, in a study among 272 elder residents (63% with dementia) in seven LTC homes, environmental factors were found to predict changes in severity of delirium symptoms over a 6-month period; residents with dementia were found to be more sensitive to the effects of these factor.[394] Among these factors was the *absence* of any of the following:

- Reading glasses, for visually impaired residents who need them to be able to see well

- Aids to orientation, for instance, a calendar, clock, or watch

- Contact with a family member

- A glass of water within reach of the resident

These aids and supports should be proactively provided to residents with dementia as part of an overall effort to prevent the onset of delirium. In the absence of contact with family, volunteers could be recruited and trained to serve as residents' supportive companions. Other aids and supports that were used in a multicomponent intervention by Inouye and colleagues[385] to prevent delirium in hospitalized older adults should be provided. These include the following:

- Magnifying lenses and large print books for residents with visual impairment

- Hearing aids, portable amplifying devices, and earwax disimpaction

- Early recognition of dehydration and volume repletion (i.e., replenishing fluid volume) and encouragement and monitoring of fluid intake

- Familiar objects, board with day's schedule, communication to orient to surroundings, interpreters

- Daily exercise and engagement in meaningful activities for an adequate level of cognitive stimulation

- Implementation of individualized sleep care plan, such as a non-caffeinated warm drink at bedtime, relaxation techniques, tape or music, back massage, and uninterrupted sleep in quiet and low-level lighting

- Avoidance of *excessive* daytime napping; although naps are helpful to many individuals with dementia, excessive frequency and duration of naps during the day could result in negative effects, such as difficulty sleeping at night

- Maintaining resident's mobility and self-care ability, minimal use of immobilization equipment such as bladder catheters

Finally, when safe to do so, avoid physical restraints, Foley catheters, intravenous lines, psychoactive and sedative agents (or reduce dose to wean), and drugs with anticholinergic effects.

Recognize and Manage Pain

Pain is considered a contributing factor for DHRRIs.[78] Many elder residents with middle- to late-stage dementia may fail to interpret physical sensations as painful, are often unable to recall their pain, or may not be able to verbally communicate it to their direct care partners.[395] Due to memory or other cognitive impairments, misperceptions, or language difficulties, the resident may not be able to describe or localize the pain.[396] As such, elders with more advanced dementia are often undertreated for pain.[395] They are left to suffer physically and emotionally, sometimes without the ability to convey it in words.

A large-scale study[397] examined the relationship between pain and "aggression" as a function of residents' communicative status (ability to self-report pain). The study, which used a sample of 71,227 nursing home residents age 65 years or older with dementia from the Minimum Data Set 3.0 (the largest federally mandated clinical dataset in U.S. nursing homes), found that in residents who could not communicate, pain was associated with verbal and physical aggression, whereas in residents who could communicate, pain was only associated with verbal aggression.

Another study has shown that the relationship between pain and engagement in DHRRIs may be a complex one—not as linear and straightforward as commonly believed. Forty residents in six nursing homes were involved as initiators in 123 resident-to-resident incidents over a 21-month period. Data related to these incidents were obtained through care professionals' referral, incident reports, and chart review, and resident data were obtained from the MDS 3.0. The study found that close to one-fifth of the residents involved had experienced pain during the same 7-day assessment period when they engaged in these incidents. A higher number of incidents was found among initiators without pain than among those initiated by residents with pain. However, incidents initiated by residents with pain were found to be more severe. A surprising finding was that as pain intensity increased, the number of incidents declined. In addition, the cognitive function of initiating residents was found to predict incident severity. Specifically, as cognitive functions were more intact, incidents tended to be more severe and offset the influence of pain intensity (Robin P. Bonifas, e-mail communication, June 14, 2021). Given the small sample used in the study, large-scale research is needed to improve our understanding of what appears to be a complex relationship between residents' experience of pain and their engagement in DHRRIs.

It is also important to recognize that myths about pain in this population may limit recognition, treatment, and relief from physical and emotional suffering caused by it. These myths include but are not limited to the beliefs that pain is a normal and expected part of aging, perception and sensitivity to pain decrease with age, and people who do not complain of pain do not experience it.[396]

The first thing that needs to be done in all efforts to address pain among elders with dementia in LTC homes is to recognize it as the "fifth vital sign" along with temperature, blood pressure, heart rate, and respiratory rate.[396] In Charles Wasserman's words, "The ethical and compassionate standard of medical and nursing care must include a strong commitment to pain relief for all of our patients." James Campbell of the American Pain Society states,[398]

> Vital signs are taken seriously. If pain were assessed with the same zeal as other vital signs are, it would have a much better chance of being treated properly. We need to train doctors and nurses to treat pain as a vital sign. Quality care means that pain is measured and treated.

The assessment of pain in people with dementia is essential and should be used to inform development of an individualized intervention plan to alleviate it. The approach for assessment of pain in this population as advocated by Wasserman[396] includes the following suggestions:

- Be proactive: Ask about it, look for it, listen to it, and smell for it.

- Know your resident's medical history and conditions that could cause pain. Examples of such conditions include arthritis, headache, angina, constipation, pressure sores, heartburn, urine infection, ill-fitting dentures, falls, and fractures.

- Know the common pain sites in elders—back, bone, chest, mouth, headache, hip, joints, incision site, soft tissue, and stomach.

- Have a high index of suspicion that any change in personality, affect, behavioral expressions, or patterns of eating, sleeping, and eliminating may reflect underlying pain.

- Check for changes in the other four vital signs (noted above).

- Use a system of charting pain, as it can be useful in the context of DHRRIs.

To begin the assessment of pain, it is important to first ask the person whether she or he is experiencing any pain or discomfort.[396] Although many people with early- and middle-stage dementia can report on their experience of pain, others may not be able to communicate it verbally. To detect signs of pain in people with advanced dementia, consider using the Pain Assessment in Noncommunicative Elderly (PAINE) scale.[399] The signs of pain in this population can include the following:

- Moaning

- Rigidity

- Facial grimaces

- Restlessness or repetitive movement

- Rubbing oneself

- Gasping or sighing

- Crying, whimpering, or whining

- Screaming or yelling

- Pulling others toward self

- Guarding or abnormal stiffness

- Bracing or leaning on wall or chair

- Moodiness, irritation, or depressed mood

- Apathetic or low energy

- Strange posture

- Decreased participation in meaningful activities (less than once a week)

Physical signs can include

- Falls

- Trembling or shaking

- Swollen joints

- Tight or swollen belly

- Bloodstains

- Changes in vital signs

- Broken bones or dislocated limbs

To fully characterize pain, Wasserman[396] suggests using the PQRST Assessment Protocol, which consists of the following parameters:

- Provocative or palliative (what aggravates or relieves it)

- Quality (such as burning, stabbing, throbbing, dull)

- Region (location and where it radiates)

- Severity (can be evaluated in three ways:

  o Verbal—mild, moderate, severe, worst

  o Numerical—0–10 (0 = no pain, 5 = moderate pain; 10 = worst pain)

  o Picture: Wong-Baker FACES® Pain Rating Scale—the person points to the face that best depicts the pain being experienced

- Timing (when, how long, constant, or intermittent)

Wasserman[396] describes the three aspects of the treatment plan,

> This information along with a physical examination and other diagnostic tests is used to implement a treatment plan that addresses the physical (unpleasant sensation), cognitive (thoughts about the sensation), and emotional (fear, anxiety, depression, hopelessness, anger, and guilt) aspects of the pain experience. If only the physical component is treated, the patient may still complain because the cognitive and emotional components are not addressed.

For review and guidelines of pain assessment tools (self-report and observational) in elders with dementia in LTC homes, see the article by Hadjistavropoulos and colleagues.[400]

In addition to observation and assessment, the importance of listening to the resident's description of his or her experience cannot be underestimated. Previous research has shown that, when dementia-supportive and dementia-friendly interviewing conditions are created, many people with early- and middle-stage dementia are capable of reporting meaningfully and reliably on their quality of life.[369] In addition, many can still communicate their needs verbally, so it is important for direct care partners to make every possible effort to continue to communicate with them in general, including about their medical needs, when appropriate. As explained by Judy Berry, "The person with dementia is still in there . . . still has the same feelings, thoughts, and needs that we do right through the end of their lives. It's so important that you continue to communicate with them."[401] In accordance, Peter Whitehouse shares,[402]

> As a medical student at Johns Hopkins, I remember some of the wiser senior clinicians telling me that the most important aspect of medical diagnosis, as well as ensuring care, was listening carefully to the patient's story, to the stories they bring to the clinic. The axiom went that 85% of diagnosis was reliant on listening to the patient's story, 10% on physical examination, and 5% on technology. In other words, the most important aspects of healing were bound up with the human relationship between the healer and patient.

Proactively Meet the Emotional and Psychological Needs of Residents with Dementia

There is a critical but all-too-often overlooked need to assess, document, anticipate, and proactively meet the varied emotional and psychological needs of residents with dementia. Lack of timely fulfillment of the psychological needs of these individuals often contributes to residents' frustrations and DHRRIs.

Based on years of observations, the late professor Tom Kitwood,[64] founder, Dementia Bradford Group, UK, identified the main psychological needs of people with dementia. These include the following needs:[64]

- Comfort

- Identity

- Occupation

- Inclusion

- Attachment

- To love and be loved (all-encompassing)

"The prime task of dementia care is to maintain personhood in the face of failing of mental powers," asserts Kitwood.[64] Meeting these psychological needs on a regular basis can enable direct care partners to help preserve residents' personhood and sense of self-worth, helping them to feel more secure and less frustrated and anxious and to move out of fear, grief, and anger and into the domain of positive experience. When a resident's emotional and psychological needs are fulfilled in time, it is less likely that she or he will engage in distressing and harmful interactions with other residents.

The critical importance of meeting the psychological needs of people with dementia is advocated by Power in his strength-based Experiential Model and Well-Being Framework, which is introduced in his book *Dementia Beyond Disease: Enhancing Well-Being*.[65] These psychological needs, building on the groundbreaking work of pioneers in this field such as Kitwood and Feil as well as the model developed by Fox and colleagues),[403] are shown in Figure 8.1.[404,65] Although research is needed to evaluate the effectiveness of this model, it is likely that successful implementation of its underlying principles and practices could lead to a substantial reduction of DHRRIs in the context of individuals with dementia.

Kitwood and Power have provided us with a precious road map for enabling elders with dementia to experience the highest practicable psychological well-being. We would all be wise to learn it and implement it in all care homes where people with dementia reside. The outcomes are expected to have far-reaching positive consequences on various other aspects of the lived experience of this population and the people caring for them.

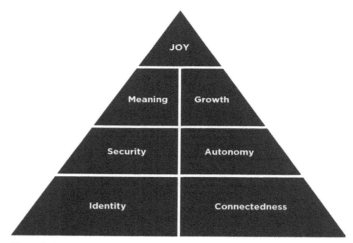

Figure 8.1   Well-being pyramid showing the hierarchy of domains to be addressed for restoring well-being. From Power,[65] based on Fox and colleagues.[403]

Regularly Move Around the Care Home

Direct care partners and other employees need to avoid the tendency to stay or congregate in one area of the care home (such as by the kitchen counter in the dining room). As noted earlier, DHRRIs may develop quickly at different areas of the care home or inside residents' bedrooms or bathrooms. Establishing the habit of regularly moving around the care home maximizes the likelihood that care employees will be in a position to identify frustrating interactions between residents at the early stages of their development.

It is helpful for all care employees and managers to remember the words of an excellent team leader with over 10 years of experience caring for residents with dementia:[34]

> CNAs always have to be alert . . . if you are not alert you could miss something . . . someone could fall or somebody can have a heart attack. Walking from point A to point B in the unit . . . the doors may be open and I am looking inside the room to see that there is no resident on the floor . . . always focused and always looking out because things can happen. They can happen fast.

Learn What Causes a Resident to Lose His or Her Temper

It is important to find out from the resident (cognitively able to convey it) and/or close family members what may trigger the resident to lose his or her temper or to become angry or upset with others.[83] Direct care partners could simply ask the person with early-stage dementia, and/ or when appropriate her or his close family members or friends, what specific situations tend to make the person become frustrated, upset, or angry; lose her or his temper; or react in a negative way toward others. It is important to take the advice of the interdisciplinary care team and/or the family as to whether these questions will cause the person to become distressed, and not ask the questions if so. Of course, it is preferable, easier, and potentially less stressful to the resident when these questions are being asked by a person who has already established a close trusting relationship with her or him. Psychologists Slone and Gleason[341] suggest asking residents with early-stage dementia,

> "What do you do when you get angry?" Next they suggest asking: "Do you ever get so angry you would [hit someone, swear, and so on]?" This question is often met with indignance. Then, reach out as if to grab an arm and ask, "What would you do if someone grabbed you like this?" An actual physical contact during this question is not recommended.

Below are some questions, recommended by the New York State Department of Health, that could be asked of family members of residents with advanced dementia, who are not cognitively able of answering on their own:[405]

- What does he or she dislike?

- What upsets him or her?

- What are the signs that show that he or she is becoming upset?

- What calms him or her?

- How does he or she currently show anger?

- How did he or she show anger in the past?

- Is there any history of episodes of explosive anger?

- Are there any usual triggers to his or her anger?

- What usually helped him or her to dispel anger at these times?

When the responses from either the resident or the family clearly suggest a potential for aggressive, violent, or abusive behavior, this information should be documented in the resident's clinical file, communicated to all care employees (not to label the person, of course, but to alert direct and non-direct care partners to information critical for prevention and de-escalation). The responses can inform the development of proactive individualized strategies aimed at avoiding these triggers and upsetting situations while focusing on those experiences that are known to enhance the person's emotional and psychological well-being. This background information should be collected during the preadmission behavioral assessment or, when not possible, during the admission process.

It is important to recognize that one of the risk factors for engagement in DHRRIs is being recently admitted to a LTC home.[367] This risk is at least partially due to the major personal adjustments and challenges a person with dementia faces during the first hours, days, weeks, and months after the move. In addition, in light of the progressive nature of dementia, direct care partners and the interdisciplinary care team need to continue to document information on personally upsetting situations and triggers for each resident throughout her or his residency and ensure that all employees in direct regular contact with the resident are informed about these promptly after each update. The same, of course, should be the case with documenting and sharing residents' individualized experiences that seem to calm and bring them joy.

Carefully Monitor and Eliminate Triggers in the Physical Environment

Examples of common environmental triggers of DHRRIs include excessive noise, crowdedness (too many people sharing a small public space), lack of adequate landmarks and signage exacerbating residents' wayfinding difficulties and unwanted entries into other residents' bedrooms, spending extensive periods of time confined indoors, upsetting or scary content on television, direct or indirect glare, and use of elevators. Being aware of these factors and working to proactively eliminate them or minimize their negative impact can help care teams reduce the incidence of DHRRIs. A detailed discussion of these and other factors in the physical environment that may contribute to the development of DHRRIs and suggestions for addressing them are presented in Chapter 5.

Eliminate Access to Objects that Can Be Used to Cause Injuries

It is fairly common for residents to use objects to injure others. One study that I conducted found that 27 out of 88 fatal resident-to-resident incidents (31%) in the context of dementia involved a resident using an object against another resident.[29] A more recent study in U.S. nursing homes found that 13 out of 101 fatal resident-to-residents (13%) involved a use of an object as a weapon.[30]

In light of these findings, a proactive anticipatory approach needs to be implemented by all employees in the care home. Specifically, it is important to rearrange, remove, or secure potentially dangerous objects and furniture to prevent their use as a weapon. An employee may need to secure a wheelchair's footrest to a wheelchair, footboard to a bed, hanger rod to a closet, or towel bar to a bathroom's wall so that residents will not be able to use them to harm other residents. In addition—depending on ongoing cognitive and risk assessment by the interdisciplinary care team—removing, locking, or limiting residents' access to knives, scissors, and heavy dishware might be necessary. Removing, securing, and limiting access to potentially harmful objects in a bedroom shared by residents who do not get along and/or engage in DHRRIs is essential. Selected examples of objects reportedly used by residents to harm their roommates include a plastic bag (used for suffocating), an electric cable (used for strangling), or objects that are heavy (such as a radio) or sharp (such as a glass lampshade).

Under the responsibility of a designated manager, direct care partners should survey all bedrooms and spaces regularly to remove or secure these and other objects that could be used by residents with dementia and serious mental illness as weapons. Residents have used all the aforementioned objects in the past during incidents, resulting in injuries and deaths. In addition, care employees will need to remove breakable objects that could have sharp pieces when broken (such as glass and ceramic figurines). Most importantly, direct care partners must think nontraditionally and creatively when it comes to the types of objects used by residents against other residents, and understand that residents—even those with significant cognitive impairments—clearly do.

Know and Use the Life History of Residents

A resident's life history may include, among other elements, her or his identity (who the person perceives herself or himself to be), premorbid personality characteristics (such as temperament or agreeableness), values, beliefs, prejudices, coping style, daily routine, likes and dislikes, fears, preferences, interests, passions, favorite activities, and cultural, spiritual, and religious background. It also includes a person's occupation, family life, close relationships and friendships, accomplishments and struggles in life, volunteering roles, military service, and traumas. When applicable, the life history must also include any history of behavioral expressions or acts reported as aggressive, abusive, or violent.

Collecting and using this information can assist direct care partners in building and maintaining a close trusting relationship with the resident with dementia (the single most important asset in supporting and caring for this population) and preserving her or his dignity and personhood (one of the primary goals of caring for elders with dementia). Carefully reviewing the resident's early life history is often useful in identifying the root causes and remote triggers for her or his engagement in various forms of behavioral expressions including DHRRIs.[406] Knowing the resident's lifelong preferences, likes and dislikes, and coping style often explains her or his frustrations and anger and thus they could inform individualized prevention efforts. Snellgrove,[407] who studied the phenomenon of DHRRIs, states that CNAs believe the more they know about particular residents, the more prepared they are to prevent and manage DHRRIs. According to Susan Desai and Ab McFadden,[156]

> Once a person with dementia moves into a LTC residence, vigorous effort needs to be made to help staff to get to know the new resident as much as possible. By getting to know the individual strengths and quirks of persons with dementia, the staff is able to better meet a key psychological need: recognition of their personhood.

The template/leaflet *This Is Me*, developed by the Alzheimer's Society and the Royal College of Nursing in the United Kingdom,[408] could be used as a good starting point. In addition, the 24-item "Whole Person Dementia Assessment Interview Form" developed by psychologist Benjamin Mast[409] could be used directly with residents who are cognitively intact and those with mild cognitive impairment or early-stage dementia to assist social workers, psychologists, nurses, and direct care partners in learning about their life history. The questions in the form could be modified for use with close family members when the resident has more advanced dementia and is unable to understand and/or respond to the questions due to cognitive impairment. However, it is important to recognize that getting to know a new resident takes time, and every interaction between a direct care partner and a resident with dementia or her or his close family members should be considered as an opportunity to get to know the life history of the resident a little better.

Ethelle Lord developed an excellent resource called *Knowing You At Glance*™. It contains the "essence" of a person with dementia and includes descriptions by close family members of their relative's important traits and recommendations for direct care partners for individualizing the care and meeting the person's unique needs. Using this tool could optimize residents' emotional well-being, prevent them from engaging in various forms of distressing and harmful behavioral expressions, and enable them to live their lives to the fullest despite having substantial cognitive disabilities.

To be of practical value, no matter which tool is used to collect life history information, it will need to be transformed into a short, clear, and easy-to-use "bio-sketch," one that is readily accessible and used by all direct and non-direct care employees who come in regular contact with the residents. At minimum, one recommendation is,[410]

> Prepare a 3×5 index card for all your residents. On each card write a brief introduction to that resident, including what things are important to her or him and good conversation topics so that any staff member that works on the unit can quickly pull the card out—it takes 5 minutes—and have a little bit of understanding about what might work well with the resident. Include in the card brief descriptions of strategies known to calm her or him down when she becomes upset, angry, or aggressive.

For example, the son of an older woman with advanced Alzheimer's disease who frequently engaged in DHRRIs in a secured care home for people with dementia, explained, "She is an animal lover. She loves animals more than anything else. When she is in a bad mood, if you bring her a dog or a cat, her mood will change."[34] All care employees and managers should be familiar with the early life history of the residents in their care who have dementia. For a detailed explanation, see my article, "Twenty Reasons Why We Need to Know the Early Life History of People Living with Dementia."[62]

Remote Triggers

It is important to remember that some residents with dementia may associate other residents with people they knew in their life before the onset of dementia or before they moved to the care home. That association can cause them to perceive the others as people they did not like or who had done them wrong earlier in their lives.[83] For example, one resident repeatedly told a CNA that she hits and pushes another resident because she "stole my husband." Misperceptions like this can cause some residents with dementia to experience anxiety and/or fear, which may lead them to avoid the individual or try to defend themselves by trying to harm them.

In other situations, a traumatic event from the person's distant past may trigger a reaction that could result in a DHRRI. As described by Flannery,[411] people with dementia "who have been able to hold past painful memories in check by cognitive distractions may find that painful memories of many decades past return in distressingly vivid detail as sense experiences and general health fail." Kitwood[412] explains,

> In many cases the psychological defenses which gave stability and protection against that
> which might overwhelm the psyche are breaking or have broken down; thus they are liable
> to be "invaded" by grief, rage, fear, a sense of terrible menace or desolation.

For example, during a spring horticulture session in a VA Medical Center,[116] residents were
transplanting blooming tulips. At one point, one of the men became pale, tremulous, and
anxious; he began to hyperventilate, and then he pushed another resident. He was restrained
and returned to the locked care home. While speaking with direct care partners, he recalled
becoming distressed on seeing the tulips and recounted an incident during World War II when
several of his platoon mates were killed after having been cornered in a tulip field. After learning this and capturing the information in the resident's care plan, the care partners were able
to avoid exposing the resident to this remote trigger from his past.

In another care home,[413] a resident was described by the care partners as "sexually aggressive" after incidents in which he was found in women's bedrooms early in the morning,
apparently disrobing them. In a review of his life history, care partners learned that this man
had been a physician who routinely did his rounds early in the morning during his years in
practice. The "behavior" made sense as a physical assessment and did not appear to be sexual.
The intervention was to encourage him to follow the nurse administering the 6:00 a.m. medications and to make his "chart notes" in a blank medical record. This approach promoted continuity of his lifelong practice and helped preserve his occupational identity, while protecting
other residents from his physical examinations. Knowing and using his life history enabled the
care team to develop this creative approach, avoid labeling him inappropriately, preserve his
dignity, and keep all residents involved safe.

In yet another care home,[307] a resident repeatedly grabbed, pulled, and shook other residents, direct care partners, and visitors—but only when they were wearing green clothes. A
review of his life history revealed that he had belonged to a fishing community where the color
green was perceived as unlucky because of its association with death in nature. The resident's
behavioral expressions were reframed as his efforts to protect others from the harmful effects
of the color green. Direct care partners conducted a 20-month experimental intervention in
which the resident would not see anyone wearing green clothes. When the policy was followed,
the resident's attacks no longer occurred; only one episode was observed during this long time
period when a new direct care partner did not redirect the resident quickly enough away from a
visitor who was wearing green clothes. This story demonstrates that identifying remote triggers
from a resident's distant past can involve a highly subtle process of inquiry of residents' life
backgrounds.

As these stories illustrate, it is important to understand key aspects of the early life history of residents with dementia—and to take the time to learn more—as an integral part of
direct care partners' efforts to help residents preserve their identity and personhood, prevent
DHRRIs, and keep them and others around them safe.

Build Close Trusting Relationships with Residents
During Routine Time Periods

As has been mentioned, direct care partners report that building a close trusting relationship
with residents with dementia is critical to their ability to prevent behavioral expressions such as
those considered as aggressive.[319] The way in which direct care partners relate to residents with
dementia during routine care when DHRRIs do not occur is as important as what they do or
say during these episodes. One CNA shared the approach she uses with residents,

> I don't walk down the hall without speaking, touching, hugging, or kissing someone. I . . .
> hardly ever walk by a resident without letting them know that I know they are there. I just
> don't. If you can make them feel good, they won't hit or kick anybody, at least for a while.

Regularly engaging in acts that build and nurture residents' trust during routine daily care, structured and unstructured activities, and downtime can make it easier to gain their cooperation when they are upset, angry, and engaged in DHRRIs.

According to Kane and West,[414] "The relationship between the caregivers and the resident proves to be the most important element of care." Echoing this view, Daniella Greenwood, former Strategy and Innovation Manager, Arcare Helensvale, Australia, states, "It's very easy to say, 'We believe that relationships are important and we really value them,' but this company says, 'It's the *most* important thing we do." Greenwood adds that the goal of building and nurturing close trusting relationships is not just with residents, "but with anyone involved in care." That is, to be successful in providing person-directed care practices, close trusting relationships must be built and maintained with all care employees and *between* all care employees. Building on Greenwood's inspiring statements, close trusting relationships with residents and care employees should be the first item on the mission statement of all LTC homes.

Snellgrove[407] has identified a theme across interviews with CNAs about DHRRIs by which they believed that residents are often "violent" because they are not receiving the attention that they need or desire. They reported that if one-on-one time is spent with them, "violence" directed toward CNAs and other residents can be avoided.

At the core of the trusting relationship is residents' expectation that direct care partners will protect them from the potential harmful effects of DHRRIs. In interviews with residents about DHRRIs, Lapuk[152] noted "their trust and confidence in the staff to step in, as needed, to protect their safety." In the words of one resident with middle-stage Alzheimer's disease,[27] "I want to know that someone will be there for me if something will happen to me."

Finally, beyond low and dangerous staffing levels that often limit care employees' ability to build and nurture close trusting relationships with residents with dementia, it is important to address another persistent barrier: the practice that most care homes have of rotating and rescheduling direct care partners, as Power[65] says, "such that a person sees a parade of different faces providing care and support from month to month. . . . The effect is devastating on people who are forgetful and need to build familiarity and trust with those who provide hands-on support."[65]

Care homes and their residents with dementia would benefit tremendously from implementation of consistent (dedicated, primary, or permanent) assignment that would enable direct care partners to strengthen their familiarity, relationship, and trust with the residents. Consistent assignment is defined as "the same caregivers consistently caring for the same residents almost (80% of their shifts) every time they are on duty."[415] This critically important practice could also apply, when possible, to housekeeping, dietary, and other staff members.

Knowing each resident as a whole person and her or his unique needs often leads to improvement in the quality of care. For example, a large-scale study by Nicholas Castle[416] examined the effects of consistent assignment of nurse aides on the quality of life provided to residents in 3,941 nursing homes. The study found that the numbers of survey agencies' deficiency citations for poor quality of life and quality of care were lower in nursing homes with the highest levels of consistent nurse aide assignment. Another study[415] among 3,550 nursing homes found that staff turnover was lower and family satisfaction with quality of care was higher in nursing homes with the highest levels of nurse aides' consistent assignments. Various quality measures examined in the study were better in the latter nursing homes.

In addition to the residents' perception of better care, direct care partners on consistent assignment are more likely to detect subtle changes from baseline in a resident's emotional and psychological states as well as to recognize and quickly respond to various forms of distressing behavioral expressions as they arise. Also important is that, especially when thoughtful assignment is implemented, direct care partners who take care of the same resident are likely to have higher job satisfaction, have less absences from work, and stay in their jobs longer.

Engage Residents in Personally Meaningful Activities

Several experts highlight the importance of engagement of residents with dementia in personally meaningful activities as an effective strategy for promoting positive emotions and preventing distressing behavioral expressions, including DHRRIs. Raia asserts,[128] "Activities are the main weapon against behavior difficulties and violent behavior." Soreff[78] states, "Having residents engaged in activities can remove the residents from a situation where an assault might have occurred." Stephen Long argues,[295] "The more often a person is involved in doing positive things, the less likely it is that he or she will behave in challenging ways."

Preliminary findings from a small study suggest that higher levels of DHRRIs occur during times when residents are not engaged in organized activities than when they are.[13] Raia[128] warns that, after an incident in which a resident has been injured, "A wise lawyer will first approach the activity director and ask: 'How did you engage the resident in a way that would have prevented the violence and injury against my client?'"

Although personally meaningful engagement is highly recommended in this population, it is important to acknowledge that residents with dementia *may* develop behavioral expressions, including DHRRIs, during activities. This can happen if, during an organized activity, a resident experiences unmet medical needs, pain, tiredness, situational frustration, or something negative in the physical environment such as crowdedness, overstimulation, excessive noise, and glare. If the activity is not planned or delivered effectively—for instance, when skillful guidance, cueing, and encouragement are lacking, or when the activity is perceived by residents as childish or devoid of personal meaning—residents with dementia may become frustrated and angry. Robert Davis, author of the book *My Journey into Alzheimer's Disease*, reflected on his reaction to being invited to perform childish exercises to rock music:[417]

> I would try to get back to my room and if stopped in this attempt I would become churlish and belligerent. If the insensitive [activity] director began to push or become condescending and began to pat my arm, I would probably explode with all the violence pent up in my six-foot-seven frame.

To summarize the above, it is important to regularly encourage and engage interested residents in all stages of dementia in activities that are personally meaningful, enriching, purposeful, appropriate, culturally specific, and age-appropriate throughout the day, evening, and, as needed, during the night. As Camp[418] observes, "If a person with dementia is engaged in a meaningful activity, the person cannot simultaneously be exhibiting problematic behavior."

In addition, meaningful engagement can also be used proactively to prevent DHRRIs. For instance, an activity could begin shortly before known times in which a resident's restlessness and engagement in DHRRIs tend to occur. In one care home for people with dementia,[176] residents would frequently walk around the public spaces during the early evening hours and invade the personal space of other residents, which resulted in resident-to-resident incidents. When care employees noticed this tendency, they began an intervention. Immediately after dinner, trained volunteers would lead a 30-minute walking group for 3 consecutive days. The effects were compared to the 4 days when walking groups were not offered. They found a reduction of 30% in episodes considered aggressive during the 24 hours after the walks.

It is important to recognize that, despite common beliefs, many elders with advanced Alzheimer's disease are capable of engaging in personally meaningful, well-planned, and skillfully delivered group and one-on-one activities. In my early study in two secured dementia care homes operated within an assisted living residence, I observed an older woman with advanced Alzheimer's disease (MMSE score 0) participating in a pet therapy group activity. The following transcript of my observation is presented here to illustrate the positive effects this activity had on this woman (the name of the resident used is a pseudonym):[161]

The group activity led by two pet therapists starts in the main activity room with trained pets such as puppies, kittens, rabbits, a chicken, a goat, and a piglet. 2:06 p.m. Mrs. Kendall notices a puppy and says: "Oh, look at the baby." [laughs] Mrs. Kendall looks at the black puppies and says: "They are so beautiful." One of the pet therapists gives Mrs. Kendall a rabbit wrapped with a soft fabric. Mrs. Kendall says to the rabbit: "Mommy is gonna give you some green . . ." When she holds the rabbit she says: "I like to be close to her." Mrs. Kendall calls a goat that is walking around the room: "Come on baby." 2:15 p.m. The director of recreation therapies brings a chicken to Mrs. Kendall and says: "Mrs. Kendall, it's a chicken," and adds: "Mrs. Kendall loves chickens." Mrs. Kendall hugs the chicken. Mrs. Kendall puts her finger in the mouth of a baby goat, looks at it, and says: "I love you." Then she sings: "La la la la la . . ." and tells the chicken: "I love you" and adds "Mommy wants you." [laughs] Mrs. Kendall says to a baby goat: "Oh my baby . . . mommy loves you." Director of recreation therapies: "Mrs. Kendall, he loves you," and adds: "You know, his mother abandoned him." CNA: "Mrs. Kendall, look at the pig." Mrs. Kendall: "Oh my God . . . where did you get that?" Mrs. Kendall is singing to the baby goat: "La la la la . . ." and tells the baby goat: "I love you" and adds "Be a good girl." Mrs. Kendall sings to the baby goat: "La la la . . . I love you and you like me . . . forever . . . poom poom poom," and adds: "I won't hurt you honey. If I could, I would take you to my house for a whole week." The baby goat gently sucks Mrs. Kendall's finger, who responds [in a playful tone of voice]: "You're a [missed word] bastard." A CNA hears what Mrs. Kendall said and tells her: "Mrs. Kendall." Mrs. Kendall immediately corrects herself and says: "Basket." CNA: "Yeah." When the baby goat is taken from Mrs. Kendall, she says: "She is trying to say: I am happy. Leave me alone."

Mrs. Kendall frequently engaged in DHRRIs throughout the study period but she was less likely to engage in these episodes when she was meaningfully engaged in an activity she enjoyed.

Finally, it is important to emphasize that there is a need to offer residents with dementia adequate periods of rest between organized activities based on their individual needs, preferences, cognitive and physical abilities and disabilities, and tiredness levels. However, it is also important to avoid excessive daytime napping, as this could have negative effects on their ability to sleep well at night. The goal is to use an ongoing individualized assessment to identify and strike an optimal balance between understimulation and overstimulation throughout the day and evening for each resident. The individualized meaningful engagement plan needs to be re-evaluated and adapted frequently in general and as the person's physical and cognitive abilities change over time.

Monitor and Avoid Distressing Content Shown on Television

As mentioned in Chapter 4, problematic television programs and content such as wars, car accidents, injuries, fires, airplane crashes, bridge collapses, the September 11 attacks, school shootings, and violence are commonly shown on televisions in LTC homes. Viewing this content may trigger anxiety or fear among some residents with dementia, and it can also lead to DHRRIs. My 10-month direct observation study in two care homes for residents with dementia showed that television viewing was generally a source of enrichment and enjoyment to residents, but it also identified a number of situations in which the use of television was a source of restlessness, anxiety, and resident-to-resident incidents.[34]

Residents often have differing preferences regarding television channels, programs, and volume (the latter may reflect variation in residents' hearing abilities). In addition, it is not uncommon for residents to argue about who should hold and use the remote control. Another explanation has to do with the fact that a substantial portion of people with advanced dementia people may have difficulty distinguishing the content shown on the television from what happens to them in the room.[186,250] Finally, the use of television in care homes often creates excess noise that is distracting and frustrating to certain residents (either those in the

TV lounge or those outside the area where the TV is located). And, as discussed earlier in this book, disagreements surrounding television use is also a common source of conflicts between roommates with dementia.

Direct care partners and all other employees need to carefully monitor any television programming containing violent, scary, and disturbing content and pay special attention to, assess, document, and monitor residents with a history of being negatively affected by these distressing programs (these triggers should be documented in their care plans, and all care employees need to be informed of them). When it is not possible to change the television channel or turn off the television altogether, direct care partners should encourage residents who are sensitive to such programming to move away from the television room and assist them in engaging in a different meaningful activity.

The television in LTC homes where a significant number of residents with dementia live should be used mostly as an enriching, therapeutic, enjoyable, and calming resource. Recreation therapists need to routinely work with direct care partners to make sure that the television is used for these purposes. In addition, it is important to remember that the LTC home is the residents' home, and television programs should be selected based on residents' interests, not those of direct care partners. As mentioned previously, it is helpful to remember that direct care partners work in the residents' *home*.

To the extent that it is practicable, TV programs and films should be chosen based on resident's preferences and cognitive abilities and disabilities; this is a complex daily challenge in care homes with a large number of residents who have varied interests and cognitive function levels. The recreation therapy department should have readily available a large collection of enjoyable old and new films that are suitable for the age cohort and preferences of residents. Other suggestions and considerations, identified in a guide to optimal use of television in LTC homes,[252] include the following:

- Ensure appropriate content for residents given their age and interests and their ability to follow, comprehend, and enjoy; content shown on the television needs to be adapted to residents with dementia who have limited attention span and decreased ability to sequence (such as follow a plot in a film). Shorter programs or carefully selected segments from full feature films may work better for a subgroup of residents with dementia.

- Pay attention to residents with limited physical mobility who may not be able to remove themselves from the area or turn the television off when they are no longer interested in watching the program shown on the television as this may causes them to experience tremendous frustration.

- Invite audiologists or other specialized health professionals to assess sound quality and speaker placement so that the television is adapted as much as possible to the residents' hearing needs.

Organizational Culture

Encourage Creative Approaches

Owners, administrators, managers, nurses, and social workers will want to encourage and support direct care partners' development and implementation of creative approaches for prevention of DHRRIs. In one example, a resident with dementia was exhibiting behavioral expressions considered as aggressive. The team at the care home decided to buy him a $79 manual lawn mower (push reel mower) that operated without electric or gas power. Berry, founder and former CEO of the care home, reported at the time on the outcome of this intervention: "He is now using it all the time to mow the lawn outside, and it reduced his aggressive behaviors. This is the best $79 I've spent."

Often, direct care partners come up with innovative person-directed ideas for prevention of behavioral expressions only to have these ideas dismissed or rejected by their supervisors without adequate exploration of the ways in which they could be implemented. Bonifas[419] found in her study in 10 nursing homes that nursing assistants developed creative individualized interventions that were devalued by other team members, which posed a barrier to quality of care provision. For example, nurse aides developed creative approaches (e.g., singing and dancing) to distract residents in the dining room where DHRRIs commonly occurred; some innovative approaches they devised to keep residents entertained during meal times were perceived as "goofing off" by supervisors and resulted in disciplinary action, which discouraged them from engaging in further efforts to prevent these episodes.[420] As one participant in the study explained, "They feel like they're so low on the totem pole that they don't recognize what they bring to the table." Even in situations where direct care partners' creative suggestions for preventing DHRRIs prove to be ineffective, supervisors should make it clear to them that they appreciate the intent behind the suggestions and that they should not feel discouraged from suggesting and trying creative approaches in the future.

Establish a Consistent Daily Routine

It is important to remember that small changes that people who are cognitively intact take for granted can be tremendously challenging and frustrating for people with dementia. To decrease restlessness, anxiety, and behavioral expressions and to promote positive emotional states, many people with middle- to late-stage dementia need a daily routine that is structured, familiar, meaningful, consistent, fairly repetitive, and anticipated. Small and large changes in the resident's daily routine, especially without adequate preparation and gentle and frequent reminders, often cause significant distress, frustration, and anger in residents with dementia, who find it difficult to adapt to and cope with these changes. Lucero and colleagues[192] argue that increasing structured time for residents with dementia can decrease DHRRIs. At the same time, it is important to be flexible and ready to change the plan on an as-needed basis using good professional judgment, because what worked yesterday or an hour ago may not work in the present. For a more thorough discussion of the need for a consistent routine, see Chapter 4.

Promote Effective Teamwork

Effective teamwork is characterized by a deep sense of interdependence, reciprocity, sharing, sensitivity, reflection, thoughtfulness, caring, ongoing mutual support, and shared goals. It can be characterized by a deep sense that "We are all in the same boat." Interprofessional collaboration is a critical component in addressing DHRRIs, because no single person or discipline has all of the knowledge, expertise, skills, or ability necessary to address these episodes. Stephen Long,[295] author of the book *Caring for People with Challenging Behaviors*, states:

> Team building requires open communication (promoted by good listening skills), acknowledgment of the importance of roles and contributions of team members (promoted by praise and compliments), respect for each person's independent work (promoted by allowing choices), cooperative problem solving (based on understanding that problems have triggers and, if they continue, have reinforcers), and a sense of a shared mission (providing for the needs of residents).

In the words of a nurse aide in a study[334] examining perceptions of aggressive behaviors, "You need teamwork—do something for me if I am busy. You need to look at the whole unit, not 'my side' or 'my residents.' You must work together, especially in the special care unit."

Other qualities of professional and effective care teams that can help care partners create and maintain good working relationships with co-workers and foster good teamwork, as identified in a study by Anderson and colleagues,[327] include being approachable, pitching in, seeking assistance, reciprocating, showing appreciation, giving respect, saying thank you, and giving praise. Routine use of these approaches can lead to positive outcomes for the care environment itself (e.g., reciprocity, respect, teamwork, learning, and better care processes and decision making), for direct care partners (e.g., feeling good, confidence, and satisfaction), and for residents (e.g., better quality of care and enhanced safety).

Besides being generally helpful and courteous, Anderson and colleagues[327] identified two additional forms of positive interactions among direct care partners. First, interactions that promote new information exchange can be of great benefit to all involved. These interactions help direct care partners and other interdisciplinary care team members give and receive new information about residents to and from the right people in a way that ensures everyone understands. Second, "cognitive diversity" interactions, in which care partners talk freely with each other about the residents in their care (while maintaining confidentiality), can help them notice changes in residents' emotional and physical/medical conditions, encourage them to act in a timely manner on what they see, and discuss multiple opinions for making sense of a problem and ensure the shared meaning of events.

By contrast, unhelpful approaches identified in the aforementioned study included blaming others, avoiding collaboration, ignoring others, saying "it's not my job," scolding others, and "passing the buck." These interactions did not support good relationships among direct care partners, hampered the flow of information (reduced their willingness to report their concerns about residents), and limited the variety of perspectives in decision making. These approaches have led to negative outcomes for direct care partners, such as dissatisfaction, burnout and stress, exhaustion, frustration, and not feeling valued, as well as for residents, with poor quality outcomes and poor safety climate.

Beyond an intentional and persistent effort to avoid these negative approaches, there is a need to promote "good interdepartmental relationships that help minimize burnout through reduction in departmental rivalries. The issue should always be, 'Let's solve the problem,' not 'Whose fault it is that Mrs. J. was not in activities this morning?' Teamwork is a great stress reliever."[421] It is recommended that administrators and interdisciplinary care team members interested in evaluating the quality of teamwork within the five domains of the work environment and job performance use the Interdisciplinary Team Performance in Long-Term Care Instrument developed by Temkin-Greener and colleagues.[422] Each of the domains is evaluated on a five-point Likert scale from 1, strongly disagree, to 5, strongly agree; below are the five domains, followed by examples of statements:

- Leadership: "The leader is sensitive to the needs of the team."

- Communication: "There is effective communication between team members about resident care."

- Coordination: "Written plans and schedules within our team are very effective."

- Conflict management: "In team meetings, we talk about and resolve issues."

- Team cohesion: "I identify with the goals and objectives of the team."

The study evaluating the instrument found that leadership, communication, coordination, and conflict management are positive predictors of team cohesion and team effectiveness.

Ensure Presence of an Employee in Key Areas During Low-Supervision Periods

A significant number of DHRRIs occur at times when direct care partners are providing personal care to residents inside their bedrooms but with no one supervising the other residents with dementia out on the floor, in the public spaces of the care home. It is important to implement a policy by which there is *always* at least one person—direct care partner, manager, or trained volunteer—actively present and supervising residents on the floor at each key location in the public spaces of the care home where residents with dementia tend to congregate, such as the main activity room.

Adequate staffing levels at all times are required to ensure the feasibility of this recommendation. The minimum number of direct care partners assigned to the public spaces of the care home (i.e., outside bedrooms) should be determined based on a combination of local factors. These include, among others, the following:

- Number of the residents living at the care home

- Number of residents with dementia at different stages of the disease

- Number of residents with serious mental illness

- Residents' physical function and frailty levels—the extent to which they need assistance in ADLs, including risk of falls

- Medical, chronic, and complex health conditions

- Frequency and severity of risky behavioral expressions

- Level of direct care partners' experience and skill in supervising residents, preventing and de-escalating various forms of potentially harmful behavioral expressions, and addressing other safety risks

- Size and physical layout of the care home—the extent to which it limits or enhances care employees' supervision of residents

Determination of adequate staffing levels—on all shifts—should take this important but often inadequately addressed supervision challenge into account in order to make the implementation of this recommendation feasible.

Increase Active Presence of Managers During Vulnerability Time Periods

Importantly, increased active presence of managers is often needed during evening hours and weekends; these are both vulnerability time periods for development of DHRRIs. Managers on the floor can provide direct care partners with hands-on guidance, role modeling, practical assistance, supervision, and emotional support. These critical but often overlooked supports can go a long way in enabling direct care partners to be more effective in recognizing, preventing, and de-escalating DHRRIs and keeping residents and themselves safe.

Train Care Partners in Effective Dementia-Specific Communication Techniques

Using respectful, effective, and safe communication techniques specifically designed for people living with dementia is critical to direct care partners' efforts to prevent and de-escalate DHRRIs. A description of dozens of effective communication techniques specific to DHRRIs in dementia is provided throughout Chapter 9. Additionally, owners and administrators of LTC homes should consider having direct care partners, interdisciplinary care teams, and managers trained in the principles and communication techniques of the Validation Method.[63]

Facilitate Communication About Previous Episodes

It is not uncommon for communication lapses, problems, and breakdowns between care employees within and across departments and shifts (verbally and in writing) to limit their ability to become informed in a timely manner about previous DHRRIs and thus to be able to anticipate and proactively prevent future episodes. Effective communication mechanisms must be developed and supported by leadership at all times to ensure that all employees (including dietary, housekeeping, maintenance, float staff, and external agency staff) who come in direct regular contact with residents will be informed about previous DHRRIs among the residents in their care. This issue is addressed in more detail in the section "Inadequate Communication Among Care Employees" in Chapter 6.

Use Structured Mechanisms to Transfer Information Between Team Members

Essential information regarding DHRRIs must be reported in a timely manner during and across shifts within disciplines (such as among direct care partners) and across disciplines (such as between nurses, social workers, and physicians); however, this often does not happen in many care homes. When this type of peer-to-peer communication is not maintained, critical information about DHRRIs is not reported in time, in a complete manner, or even at all to the director of nursing or the administrator of the care home. Communication lapses and breakdowns like these create gaps for distressing and harmful interactions to develop between residents without employees' awareness, until it is too late.

It is therefore essential to institute and utilize clear, easy-to-use, and structured mechanisms and procedures to promote effective transmission of information related to residents' negative emotional states, distress, and various forms of behavioral expressions including DHRRIs during and across shifts and days.[34] One such mechanism is the communication log (different terms may be used for this tool across care homes), where direct care partners and all other interdisciplinary care team members are instructed to write notes on distressing and harmful behavioral expressions experienced by residents immediately or at the earliest possible time after they occur.

The policy of the care home should be that *all* employees who come in direct regular contact with residents are required to read the communication log *before* they start their work shift, a few times during the shift, and as needed. Administrators and directors of nursing should require that managers regularly and carefully monitor use of the log to ensure that the policy is adhered to by all employees. When planning and implementing a structured communication tool, it is important to accommodate and, as needed, assist direct care partners for whom English is not the first spoken language; some of these individuals may not be able to read and/or understand portions of written reports.

The common problem of inadequate transfer of essential information about residents between direct care partners and other interdisciplinary care team members is addressed in Chapter 6. Recommendations for addressing this common problem, like many others, will more likely be implemented effectively if adequate staffing levels of well-trained care employees are in place at all times.

Other Measures

Train Direct Care Partners in Nonviolent Self-Protection Techniques

The Bureau of Labor Statistics[423,424] has found that CNAs in nursing homes represent the occupation most at risk for workplace assault. In the words of one CNA,[352]

I've been punched in the face several times. I've been punched in the jaw several times. Getting hit. Having your wrists twisted. That's the big thing. They're constantly twisting your wrists. Pulling and shoving at you. I mean that's a day-to-day thing. I work on the locked unit. Violence is an everyday occurrence.

It is the responsibility of the administrator of the LTC home to implement serious and ongoing measures to protect direct care partners and all other employees from any psychological and physical harm while at the care home. "Nursing homes have both an ethical and legal responsibility and obligation to protect all residents in their care, as well as all employees," according to Lachs and colleagues.[178] Beyond implementing the suggestions, strategies, and communication techniques described in this book, administrators are strongly encouraged to provide specialized training to all direct care partners and interdisciplinary care team members in self-protection techniques.

These techniques can increase the likelihood that both direct care partners and residents will remain safe during DHRRIs. When attempting to de-escalate a physical resident-to-resident incident, care employees need to use skilled strategies and techniques that not only de-escalate the episode itself but also ensure that none of the residents involved in it experiences a fall or is otherwise harmed.

Owners and administrators should consider enrolling experienced care professionals with good leadership skills in training programs such as the 3-day Train the Trainer Certification Course: *Non-Violent Self-Protection for Healthcare Trainers*[425] (TJA Protect-Systems International), which is endorsed by the National Council of Certified Dementia Practitioners. After completion of the training, these individuals should take on the role of champions in training all direct care partners and other employees in techniques for protecting themselves and residents during DHRRIs and other potentially harmful situations.

Use Assistive Technology

Thoughtful use of assistive technology can strengthen direct care partners' limited supervision abilities and resources (such as due to insufficient staffing levels). For example, motion sensor technologies could be used to alert direct care partners to situations that may develop into DHRRIs. Kutzik and colleagues[426] and Bharucha and colleagues[427] present excellent reviews of existing and future assistive technologies in LTC homes, and Freedman and colleagues[428] review the barriers for implementation of assistive technologies in these care settings.

An example of assistive technology is used here for illustration. According to Troy Griffiths, CEO, Vigil Health Solutions, Inc., installing assistive technologies such as the Vigil® Dementia System[196] in residents' bedrooms can alert direct care partners in real time to the entering of a resident into another resident's bedroom or bathroom (for example, through a silent, vibrating page with an alphanumeric message). This could assist direct care partners in recognizing and preventing DHRRIs that commonly occur as a result of such unwanted and intrusive entries. If a resident is at high risk of engagement in these unwanted bedroom entries, the system can be set up to alert direct care partners on the individual's bedroom departure and then again on entry to other residents' bedrooms. In addition, a centralized computer can track these entries over time to identify important temporal and spatial patterns (e.g., bedrooms and times of day when a resident enters other residents' bedrooms), which could inform individualized anticipatory preventative interventions.

My study examining fatal resident-to-resident incidents in the context of dementia[29] found that half (26 out of 50) of fatal incidents occurring inside bedrooms took place inside the bedroom of the resident who died (19 incidents) or inside the exhibitor resident's bedroom (7 incidents). Another study[30] in U.S. nursing homes found that two-thirds (23 out of 34) of fatal incidents taking place inside bedrooms were reported to occur inside the bedroom of the resident who died as a result of the incident (11 incidents) or inside the exhibitor's bedroom (12 incidents).

Using assistive technologies such as the Vigil® Dementia System[196] could have alerted direct care partners in time to the bedroom entries and enabled them to prevent the injuries and deaths. Although this type of technology seems promising, studies are urgently needed to evaluate the effectiveness of these as well as other assistive technologies in recognizing, preventing, and de-escalating DHRRIs involving people with dementia and serious mental illness in care homes.

Install Emergency Call Buttons and Use Handheld Communication Devices

Installing emergency call buttons in areas and rooms of the care home where DHRRIs tend to occur[63] can assist direct care partners in quickly alerting co-workers and managers to a DHRRI in progress and seeking their assistance without having to leave the area where the episodes occurs. In addition, hand-held radios or other portable communication devices should be provided to key (preferably all) direct care partners for the same purpose and for improving communication among direct care partners and interdisciplinary care team members in general.

In one incident,[34] a recreation assistant struggled to defuse a distressing and potentially harmful interaction between two residents with dementia during a group activity. No other direct care partners were in the area. The assistant left the activity room and walked all the way to the direct care partners' room, where he used the phone to call for assistance from other direct care partners. Leaving residents with dementia in these situations without supervision can contribute to escalation of these episodes and put residents at risk of psychological harm and/or physical injury.

For example, SecurAlert™ mobile technology enables direct care partners to signal an emergency situation immediately and summon help from co-workers, supervisors, security personnel, and police. It requires only one push on a duress button to generate two simultaneous signals (a wireless signal and a radio frequency signal—a double layer of protection). The button has a location tracker in the wireless device, pinpointing where the incident occurs. The alarm can be sent by using different devices, including the cell phone, portable radio, display panel, pagers, or computer with audible tones. Each button has an employee ID and code attached to it, allowing individual tracking of employees in distress. The device is often used in healthcare settings to signal threats or actual assaults and violent attacks. Co-workers, supervisors, and first responders can show up faster because they know exactly where the incident occurred.

In this time, when simple and affordable technological solutions are readily available, there is really no excuse for not exploring and incorporating these kinds of essential, potentially life-saving, devices into routine daily care as an integral part of a robust resident-to-resident incidents' prevention program. The modest investment is likely to pay off in reduction of harmful incidents and increased overall safety of residents.

9

Immediate Strategies
During Episodes

Every encounter is an opportunity to strengthen the relationship.
If the caregiver takes control, stops the vicious cycle of reactivity,
and looks for a way to let the person feel well respected and supported,
even a potential altercation can be such an opportunity.

Jitka Zgola[59]

This chapter describes dozens of psychosocial strategies that direct care partners and other members of the interdisciplinary care team (IDT) can use during distressing and harmful resident-to-resident interactions (DHRRIs) in the context of dementia; that is, interactions in which one or both of the residents involved has dementia. This comprehensive set of strategies consists of dementia-specific approaches and communication techniques that can be used to prevent an imminent conflict between residents and/or de-escalate it once it is already in progress. Equipping direct care partners and IDTs with these strategies can expand and strengthen their existing knowledge and skills for addressing these episodes. Using these strategies can enable them to more effectively recognize resident-to-resident incidents in their early stages of development and de-escalate them promptly and safely.

To ensure that these strategies and skills are internalized and implemented by direct care partners as intended and in a consistent manner, these individuals and all other employees in direct regular contact with residents will need to receive ongoing and close hands-on guidance on all shifts by qualified, experienced team members who are well-trained in person-directed care approaches and the strategies described in this book. Simply reading the book or presenting the material in a classroom setting will not enable direct care partners to realize the full potential of these prevention and de-escalation strategies.

Routinely demonstrating to all employees who come in direct regular contact with residents with dementia how these hands-on strategies work "on the floor" in real-time experiential learning—is key for achieving substantial reductions in DHRRIs with lasting effects. In addition, it is important to recognize that there is no prescription for which strategies should be used in a given situation. Every resident with dementia involved in an incident is different, and most scenarios are unique. The actual way in which many of these strategies should be used immediately prior and during incidents will likely vary across situations. The best professional judgment by direct care partners, other IDT members, and managers is needed for choosing the most suitable strategy or set of strategies for each situation. Care teams are encouraged to build on, modify, and refine some of these strategies in ways they think would result in more effective prevention and de-escalation of these episodes and keeping their residents and care employees safe and free from psychological harm.

Approach and Affect

Approaching the Situation

Use a Swift, Focused, Decisive, Firm, and Coordinated Intervention

The strategy needs to be orchestrated at the earliest practicable time under the supervision and close and continuous guidance of a qualified, well trained, and experienced care professional such as a nurse, social worker, or manager. Stephen Soreff,[78] who together with David Siddle trained more than 1,000 direct care partners in more than 100 long-term care (LTC) homes on dealing with residents' behavioral expressions considered as "aggressive," suggests,

> Once a violent episode erupts, a swift, focused, decisive and firm intervention is required. This means immediately separating the two residents and moving all other residents from the area. Securing physical distance between the two residents is the top priority. Yet at the same time all other residents must be removed from the area. The intervention must be a well-orchestrated and coordinated team effort. Having many staff available and working in a directed, coordinated fashion can bring the combative behavior to a prompt conclusion. The assaulting resident must be removed from the area but also not be left alone.

In addition, during the implementation of the strategy, as much as possible, the care team needs to avoid overcrowding residents involved in the DHRRI with too many direct care partners or other residents, as this may cause them to feel threatened ("outnumbered" or "cornered") and strike out in defense. Furthermore, it is important to remember that being firm and direct does not mean expressing anger or irritation. Every effort should be made to respond to DHRRIs in a calm and respectful manner rather than in an angry or irritated way. The former approach always works much better than the latter.

Slow Down

Person-directed care means that direct care partners need to do their best to move at a pace that feels comfortable to each resident with dementia and to match the speed of everything they do and say to the person. Moving quickly may frighten the resident. "Rushing scares and confuses people with dementia," says Judy Berry.[429] As much as possible, direct care partners should avoid surprising residents with dementia or using sudden movements with or around them. Instead, they will want to use slow hand gestures. One direct care partner reported,[430] "When I'm under [time] pressure and want to press on, I note that rushing is of absolutely no use with a resident with dementia. I simply have to take more time; otherwise it becomes worse. And then it is impossible to go on." In the words of a care professional,[186] "the truth is that when folks who have dementia are rushed, they are more likely to resist, and to become upset and distressed. We've learned that faster is not faster. Slower is faster."

In most situations, direct care partners need to do their best to move slowly. They should generally avoid acting as if they are in a hurry[251] or "outpace" the person with dementia. People with dementia tend to process information in their social and physical environment at a significantly slower pace than people without cognitive impairment. In the words of Christine Bryden, author of the book, *Who Will I Be When I Die?* "I'm like a slow-motion version of my old self—not physically but mentally."

However, in situations of potential or immediate risk to one or more residents involved in a DHRRI or risk to a care employee, direct care partners will need to move quickly to the area and *then* slow their pace as they get closer to the area of residents involved in the episode and approach them to de-escalate it. Moving slowly from a long distance all the way to the residents may mean loss of precious time that should be dedicated to de-escalation of the episode. For example, in incidents that involve one resident pushing another, causing a fall, the direct care partner's moving quickly but calmly and arriving at the scene even a few seconds earlier could literally mean the difference between a resident's serious injury or death and safe de-escalation.

Approach the Resident from the Front

In general, direct care partners should avoid approaching residents with dementia from behind or from the side. This is especially the case in most DHRRIs. It is important to approach the residents involved from the front and slowly attract their attention by establishing eye contact. When a direct care partner approaches a resident from behind or from the side, the resident may be startled and reflexively strike the direct care partner instinctively in defense.

In one case, a resident with dementia was walking to the sink in the dining room to wash her hands. On her way, her pants gradually slipped down (showing her adult Depends). A well-meaning private aide noticed it, approached her from behind, and started pulling her pants up without alerting her first. The resident, who was clearly startled by the touch, tried to strike the aide with her elbow in a quick backward motion.[34] In another incident, a nurse approached a resident from behind, and the resident responded by striking her in the jaw.[431] As explained by a person with dementia[251] after hitting a direct care partner: "I did not mean to strike you. I was protecting myself against insensitivity: My self-defense."

Approaching the person from the front is a good preventive strategy in general, but it is especially important during DHRRIs, as it creates the conditions necessary for a skilled de-escalation. Approaching the resident from the front is important also because, as one gets older and hearing ability declines, about 70% of speech intelligibility—the ability of a listener to hear and correctly interpret verbal messages—comes from the visual aspects of speech, such as movement of the lips, facial expression, and so forth. Complicating the situation is the fact that many nursing home residents do not have correct hearing aids or do not use them for various reasons, including memory loss, annoying amplified background noise, or lack of working batteries. Lip reading is therefore absolutely important for these residents. When interacting with a resident, the direct care partner must always ask him- or herself, "Can the person see my face and my lips?" (Steve Orfield, oral communication, September 19, 2013). As one older woman explained,[260] "I need my glasses to hear you. I look at your face and your mouth when you speak, and then I can understand what you say to me."

In addition, direct care partners will also need to be aware that certain elders with Alzheimer's disease may have a narrow field of vision, whereas others who have had a stroke may not be able to see direct care partners or other residents if they approach them from their side, as that may be their "blind spot."

Exceptions

Despite the general advice to approach from the front whenever possible, it is helpful to keep a few exceptions in mind. After approaching the close area of a resident engaged in a DHRRI, a direct care partner may want to stand at a 45-degree angle rather than facing the resident directly.[79] The following exceptions are presented not as an exhaustive list but rather as examples meant to encourage direct care partners and other IDT members to explore what approach is most effective with *each* individual person with dementia.

- *Visual limitation.* An individualized visual evaluation should indicate from which angle direct care partners should approach the resident to enable her or him to see them approaching and to avoid a startled response. For instance, depending on the specific scope and severity of a visual limitation, elders such as those with dry macular degeneration[432] may only have peripheral vision. The deficits caused by this condition vary across individuals but can include blurriness or a blind spot in central vision. Central vision is essential for many tasks, such as reading and recognizing faces. An individualized approach based on a visual evaluation will enable direct care partners to slowly and gently get the resident's attention and thus maximize the likelihood that the interaction with her or him will start, and proceed, in a positive way.

- *Frontotemporal dementia (FTD).* When helping residents with FTD, "You never want to stand in front of a person with FTD because what you are saying visually is, 'I'm the boss,'" according to Teepa Snow. "You are also presenting yourself as a target."[198]

- *Coordinated strategies that call for a different approach.* Another important exception to the advice to approach from the front is during implementation of techniques that are used simultaneously in a well-coordinated way by a few direct care partners to de-escalate a dangerous resident-to-resident incident. In these cases, team members will discuss and plan as much as possible in advance, with close familiarity with the triggers and ways of calming the residents involved. Examples of such techniques include "planned containment" and "unplanned containment," which are described in detail and demonstrated by Carly Hellen and Peter Sternberg in their staff training program (DVD and companion workbook) entitled *Dealing with Physical Aggression in Caregiving: Physical and Non-Physical Interventions* (Terra Nova Films).

When Possible, Maintain a Safe Distance from the Resident

Unless a physical intervention is immediately necessary, direct care partners should maintain a safe distance from any resident engaged in a DHRRI. As Power[49] advises, "Keep your face and sensitive areas out of arm's length." Maintaining a safe distance can reduce the number of physical injuries sustained by direct care partners as they try to protect residents from other residents. This advice cannot always be followed, of course, such as when care partners must physically separate two residents with dementia who are about to hit each other.

Be Patient and Supportive

Residents with dementia are trying to do their best in the face of an avalanche of aging-related, relational, occupational, functional, cognitive, and other losses. It is easy for direct care partners to forget this fact; it is up to managers and others who provide training and guidance to care employees to regularly remind them.

It may be difficult for care employees to remain patient and supportive when they are assigned to caring for 12 or more residents with dementia during each work shift each and every day. It is very common to hear direct care partners expressing frustration over their inability to spend more time with residents (beyond provision of assistance during personal care tasks). Governments, regulatory agencies as well as owners and administrators of LTC homes expecting delivery of excellent person-directed care must be committed to allocating sufficient funding to ensure adequate staffing levels at all times to reduce the daily pressures and burnout of dedicated but overworked direct care partners. Such commitment will enable these care workers to build and maintain close trusting relationships with residents and be more patient, supportive, and attentive to their needs. It may also increase their job satisfaction and retention.

As noted earlier, the emotional and psychological needs of residents with dementia are often inadequately addressed during routine care, day-to-day interactions, and DHRRIs in many care homes. Being as present and centered as practically possible during routine care and during these episodes is essential for working collaboratively in the "authentic partnership" with residents with dementia that is a critical but often overlooked component of prevention efforts.

Always *Show Respect to the Resident*

Respect is defined as "high or special regard" or "the quality or state of being esteemed."[433] It is the human right of people living with dementia to always be treated with respect, no matter how cognitively disabled they are. Residents with dementia who feel appreciated and respected are less likely to act out their frustrations in ways that are perceived by others as inappropriate or aggressive. The trust of the resident with dementia is considered the single most important asset a direct care partner can have, but it can be easily lost when a resident is approached by care employees with disrespectful attitudes, expressions, gestures, and acts.

Common examples are pulling a resident's chair backward without first asking his or her permission, ignoring a resident's requests for assistance, and not validating their distressed emotions. Once the resident's sense of trust in a direct care partner is threatened or lost, it is much harder to gain his or her cooperation and optimize his or her emotional well-being. As Zgola[59] suggests, "Every caregiver should make a habit of asking, 'Would I trust someone who had just done or said this to me?'"

It is crucial to maintain respect for the person with dementia while trying to prevent an incident about to happen (a resident walking angrily toward another resident with a tight fist held up in a threatening manner) or when de-escalating it. Respect during DHRRIs can be shown in many ways, including, among others actively listening to the resident, affirming her or his concerns, frustrations, and fears, making the person feel safe and save face, providing adult-to-adult reassurance, asking for the person's preference or permission, asking for her or his advice, following through with promises made, and apologizing sincerely. Respect is integral to a collaborative approach, which is more likely to result in an effective and safe outcome for all involved.

Never Laugh at a Resident

Laughing at a resident with dementia in general and during DHRRIs is, of course, extremely disrespectful and must be avoided; it will likely aggravate the resident and escalate his or her distressing behavioral expressions. Contrary to common beliefs, many residents—certainly those with early-stage dementia but also a significant portion of those with more advanced disease—are capable of detecting disrespectful approaches, such as when they are being made fun of by others.

Even when the person is not present, it is also important to avoid laughing at a resident with dementia, for instance, with co-workers. The mockery of the person behind closed doors is not only disrespectful but it can also spill over into direct care partners' later interactions with her or him and their attempts to prevent and de-escalate DHRRIs. The same is true when the mockery of a resident is done in the presence of other residents (when the target resident is not present), as it could reinforce negative perceptions of the resident by these other residents with whom she or he comes in regular contact. For example, when a care employee—perhaps with the intention of acknowledging or validating the experience of one resident—laughs at or speaks disparagingly of another resident who is not present, this can further shape these residents' perceptions of this person and their treatment of him or her in future interactions.

Remember: It Is (Usually) Not Intentional

In the context of residents with middle- to late-stage dementia, direct care partners sometimes make the mistake of considering the involvement of a resident as an exhibitor in these episodes as intentional. They may attempt to reason with the resident instead of recognizing that a different approach has to be used.[434] A study by Åström and colleagues[40] found that the majority of "violent" incidents directed toward direct care partners by residents with dementia were perceived and interpreted by them as intentional. The authors noted that direct care partners reporting these acts as intentional may really experience them that way. Gold[435] suggests, "Training should focus on helping staff see unwanted behaviors as clues rather than as random or malicious actions."

As mentioned earlier, it is important to recognize that the majority of residents living with a serious brain disease such as Alzheimer's disease do not try to make others' lives miserable. In most situations, they try their best to cope with their remaining cognitive abilities in an environment that increasingly becomes unfamiliar and/or threatening to them. Berry[429] adds, "Remember that for those with dementia their world can be confusing and frightening." Lachs and colleagues[6] state, "'Victim,' 'perpetrator,' or both may be 'blameless' in many of these episodes, in that they are facilitated by brain disease and not volitional ill will."

In one study[152] among residents who witnessed or were harmed during DHRRIs in a care home, the meaning assigned by these residents to the "aggressive behaviors" was that "the aggressor is not himself, and this person is not himself because the dementia has taken over him or something else has burdened or stressed him (pain or sadness)." These residents understood what is easy to forget, even by trained direct care partners, in the heat of a DHRRI. Even experienced and trained care employees need to be reminded sometimes. As Karl Pillemer[436] observes,

> I think that sometimes one of the most difficult things for staff is that even though we all *know* that residents are with dementia and that residents with dementia aren't doing what they do on purpose, it requires continuously reminding ourselves of that fact and looking for other kinds of solutions than being punitive or trying to extensively reason with someone.

That said, there are many instances in which residents without cognitive impairment intentionally psychologically and physically harm other residents. It is also true, though it happens rarely, that a subgroup of residents with early-stage dementia intentionally harm or injure other residents. For example, some individuals with no cognitive impairment or only early-stage dementia had a lifelong tendency to physically harm other people (for instance, people with a criminal record for violent behavior). In a portion of these individuals, these lifelong tendencies may continue or exacerbate after moving into a LTC home where they are forced to live in close quarters with large number of other residents or share a bedroom with a stranger as roommates. In others, such tendencies may often decrease after the onset of dementia or as their dementia progresses, especially for those with advanced disease.

Be Consistent in Approach and Strategy

Whatever the plan or strategy chosen by direct care partners and the IDT to address DHRRIs, it is important for it to be applied in a consistent manner (across all direct regular contact employees, work shifts, and days), with a strong commitment and persistence.[59] It is not uncommon for a resident's engagement in DHRRIs to worsen as a result of inconsistent approaches used by different direct care partners, and it also is not uncommon for care employees to send mixed and conflicting messages to residents within short periods of time (within the same shift, hour, or even minutes apart).

For example, in one secured care home[34] for elders with dementia operated within an assisted living residence, a male resident with early-stage Alzheimer's disease frequently engaged in DHRRIs as an exhibitor. Given his occupational background as a successful lawyer in a reputable law firm, the care team developed what they described as the "VIP approach" to this individual. Since many of the incidents in which he was involved occurred in the dining room, the team decided to allow him to use a small dining room that was typically used by up to five residents. The idea was that it was less crowded than the main dining rooms and thus could reduce the likelihood of DHRRIs caused by his interactions with a large number of other residents with dementia. When encouraging and directing him to sit there for meals, the direct care partners frequently told the resident that this was a VIP room. He clearly appreciated the idea and it helped reduce the incidence of these episodes.

However, there was only one problem: Some of the care employees either were not aware of the VIP approach or did not follow it consistently. Sometimes they did not make sure that he sat in the small dining room during mealtimes, and—worse—sometimes they made light of it by laughing in his presence when calling it the VIP room. This inconsistent approach was noticed by the resident, who reacted in frustration, anger, and behavioral expressions that were labeled as aggressive. This story is not meant to suggest that certain residents should receive a more favorable treatment than others; obviously, when possible, all residents should be treated in an equal manner. It is presented here to illustrate the potential negative effects of an inconsistent approach used by different care employees.

In general, any preventive approach developed by the IDT needs be implemented in a consistent manner by all employees (including housekeeping, dietary, and maintenance staff) who come in direct regular contact with residents with dementia (including across shifts, days, weekends, and holidays). This, unless an imminent risk to a person's safety in a particular situation warrants using a different strategy to prevent serious harm.

Life is hard enough when living with a cognitive disability caused by Alzheimer's disease and other forms of dementia. Consistency and predictability in approach are key when working with and caring for this population. Direct care partners need to be aware of the negative impact of inconsistent approaches on these individuals. Many residents with Alzheimer's disease, including a subgroup of those with middle- to late-stage disease, are able to recognize these inconsistencies, which often causes them to become frustrated and upset. This is important to reinforce with all care partners. As Zgola[59] asserts,

> It is the responsibility of supervisory staff to give that training and feedback as part of their ongoing supervisory and teaching roles. If the practice is left to the good will and insight of individuals, application is inconsistent and residents get incongruous messages. This is when behavior problems most often emerge.

Avoid Stopping a Resident Who Is Trying to Walk Away

It is not uncommon for direct care partners to try and physically stop a resident with dementia who starts to walk away during a DHRRI, such as by grabbing his or her arm. Trying to physically stop a person while he or she is angry and starting to walk away from a direct care partner could trigger a reflexive physical response toward the care employee (such as with a quick backward motion or hitting with the elbow) or other residents. Berry[429] suggests, "If the person starts to walk away while you are talking, don't try to stop them right away. Move along with them and keep talking." Alternatively, if there is no imminent risk to anyone involved in the episode, direct care partners may want to remain within a reasonable, unobtrusive distance from the resident, observe him or her carefully, and then decide whether and how to approach him or her to validate and minimize his or her emotional distress, meet his or her needs, and gently and empathically assist in calming the resident down.

Emotional Affect: What You Bring to the Situation

Do Your Best to Remain Calm

Direct care partners need to try their best to remain calm, and it is critical that they try as much as possible to give the appearance of not being intimidated during DHRRIs. Many residents with Alzheimer's disease and other forms of dementia are likely to sense it and react accordingly. Power[65] observes, "Many people underestimate just how much can be done to help an anxious person feel secure, simply by sharing a calm presence. One's own sense of calm can act as a life raft for someone swimming in uncertainty."

One research study showed that people with Alzheimer's disease tend to have increased sensitivity to and "mirror" the emotions of other people around them.[437] The study found higher "emotional contagion" (that is, a basic affective mechanism by which emotions spread across individuals) among people with Alzheimer's disease than among those with mild cognitive impairment and healthy controls. "This means that if caregivers are anxious or angry, their patients will pick up and copy these emotions. On the other hand, if the caregiver is calm, patients will emulate these positive emotions." According to Mahoney and colleagues, [255] "[Some] people with dementia have lost their ability to process the meaning of another's frustration. If a caregiver exhibits frustration, people with dementia may easily become frustrated themselves." In fact, direct care partners reported in a focus-group study[430] that their own fear of the resident may trigger aggressive behaviors. In the words of a CNA with over 20 years of experience caring for residents with dementia, "Try not to show a resident that you are afraid of him when he engages in an aggressive behavior towards you, your co-workers, and other residents."[34] Harry Urban,[438] a leading national educator and advocate who has lived with dementia for many years, has this advice for caregivers:

> Look me in the eyes when you are talking to me. Make me feel like you want to talk to me. I can tell by your eyes if you really are comfortable talking to me or afraid to be around me. I sense your emotions and will copy them. If you are angry or frustrated, you will pass these emotions to me.

For additional advice from this inspiring leader, readers are suggested to visit his blog *My Thoughts On Dementia* and his website "Dementia Mentors"; the latter is an essential initiative with services aimed at supporting and educating people who are newly diagnosed with Alzheimer's disease and other forms of dementia in coping with the disease and living life to the fullest extent possible. The mentors are people living with dementia who know best what it actually means to live with a cognitive disability.

As mentioned elsewhere in this chapter, direct care partners will benefit from speaking calmly, respectfully, and in a nondemanding manner with residents in general and those living with dementia in particular. They should never yell at a resident or use harsh tone, especially during an DHRRI, as it is likely going to further upset the person and "fuel up" and escalate the behavioral expressions.

Be Sincere

In contrast to a common belief, many people with advanced dementia are very good at detecting insincerity in those around them.[49] As explained by Feil,[63]

> We know that very old people, no matter how disoriented, know what is the truth, who is honest, and who is lying. If we want to develop a trusting relationship with our client, we must be honest and not lie. If we lie, the old person may quiet down but will not trust us.

People living with Alzheimer's disease can form new emotional associations—memories related to how they are treated or by an experience. Then, sometime later, they may exhibit the associated emotion, although they may not be able to consciously recall the incident related to that emotion.[439] It should be emphasized, however, that there is an important but often overlooked distinction between lying to people with dementia and "tuning in" to their subjective reality. As stated by Feil and Altman,[440] "Acknowledging the older person's reality in order to enter their world with empathy is not lying."

Direct care partners who are not aware of this distinction frequently make the mistake of lying to residents with dementia; in doing so, they risk losing these individuals' trust. This in turn makes it less likely that the residents with dementia will cooperate with them in general and, importantly, during DHRRIs. A related misconception is often conveyed in words such as, "They won't remember it anyway, so why does it matter?" But the truth is that many do recall on some level, and they will react accordingly, even if they do not remember the name of the person who has been lying to them. I have seen this dynamic many times in LTC homes. Lying can be devastating to residents with dementia at any stage, and this practice needs to discontinue.

Feil and Altman[440] state, "We do not believe that any kind of lying can be therapeutic. What we practice is not 'therapeutic lying' nor diversion." The Validation Method's principle related to being truthful with people with dementia is that people experience several levels of awareness, often at the same time. These authors explain, "This means we do not lie to persons with dementia, because we know that on a deeper level they will recognize it as such." They add, "When we lie, we lose that trust." The temptation for short-term cooperation in the heat of the moment may often prove costly in the longer term as many residents with dementia retain the ability to know and remember that the approach used with them was not truthful.

It is important to emphasize that my recommendation here is not meant to suggest that care employees should confront residents with dementia with painful intolerable truths such as repeatedly reminding residents of a loss of a beloved spouse. For example, in her book, Feil describes several elders with Alzheimer's disease who inaccurately accused their roommates of stealing their personal belongings and a resident blaming a roommate for spilling water all over the floor, when the resident felt too ashamed to admit that he could no longer control his bladder. After several decades of working with and supporting elders living with dementia, Feil shares that she learned not to confront these individuals with painful facts—a reality these people may not be able to tolerate. She explains that they may not have insights into the reasons for their behavioral expressions, and they may find it hard to deal with those reasons if they did understand them. Instead, she learned to listen to them, assist them in expressing their feelings, and validate their internal reality and underlying emotional states (such as soul-crushing loneliness, longing to be with a deceased spouse, and feeling ashamed of one's own incontinence). She learned to validate *their* truth; it is the only truth that matters when interacting with elders with advanced dementia if our goal is to meet the person's emotional needs and enable her or him to experience the highest practicable psychological well-being.

Pay Attention to **Your** *Body Language*

When direct care partners pay close attention to their own body language during DHRRIs and make sure it is adequate—that is, when it reflects a calm, empathic, and respectful approach— they are often in a much better position to gain the residents' cooperation and safely de-escalate the episode. Research by Mehrabian[441] shows that,

> In conversations where emotions and attitudes play an important role, only about 7% of the meaning we glean is communicated through the words themselves. Another 38% is paralinguistic, meaning that it is the function of *how* the words are spoken—the tone and inflection of the voice. The remaining 55% comes from facial expressions and body language.

It is likely that, when interacting during DHRRIs with elders living with Alzheimer's disease, the latter two aspects of communication (together consisting of 93% of the communication exchange) play a larger role than with people who are cognitively intact. A daughter of a woman with Alzheimer's disease reported that she is able to communicate with her mother more effectively than is anyone else in her family and that she is more successful in gaining her cooperation in various day-to-day and care-related tasks. The interesting part of this story is that the daughter is deaf; her mother can hear, but she does not know sign language. Effective communication with people living with Alzheimer's disease is less about the words we use and more about the emotions conveyed through our body language.

In the simple but effective words of Truthful Loving Kindness, a woman living with mild cognitive impairment who is a leading educator and advocate for people living with dementia, "What my system recognizes is body language." Readers are encouraged to visit her website (search on "Truthful Loving Kindness") for the inspiring and helpful insights and resources she regularly shares publicly.

As much as possible, direct care partners will need to try and keep their body relaxed and be aware of their stance to avoid sending negative messages to residents with dementia (such as standing with hands on hips or in a clenched fist). "Be sure that your verbal and nonverbal communication matches," advises Berry.[429] When the resident with dementia is speaking, direct care partners should avoid frowning or shaking their head in general and during DHRRIs; people with Alzheimer's disease "can 'read' your gritted teeth, anger, and impatience, rolling of your eyes, shaking your head or pointing a finger at them."[429] You should expect them to "mirror" your emotional states and respond accordingly.

Keep a Calm and Peaceful Facial Expression

As hard as it is to do sometimes, try as much as possible to remember, especially during resident-to-resident incidents, that many people with dementia are experts in detecting your nonverbal emotional cues. A study by Bucks and Radford[442] showed that "while persons with mild to moderate Alzheimer's disease may be impaired on tasks of general cognitive ability, they retain much of their ability to recognize nonverbal emotional cues in faces and voices." In accordance, Power[49] suggests that direct care partners consider the following during behavioral expressions labeled as aggressive:

> Because nonverbal signals are so important, the facial expression and body language will often trump the words that are spoken. If a stern face looks like a challenge and a smile looks like a sneer, then the best expression is often one that is placid (i.e., calm, peaceful with little movement), but also as expressionless as possible.

Jan Garard[262] further highlights the critical importance of staying calm during distressing behavioral expressions and avoiding using body language and tone of voice that convey impatience, frustration, and anger,

> We have to remember that persons with dementia often lose the ability to understand our language and words but they don't lose the ability to understand body language and tone of voice. So you may be saying something absolutely appropriate to a person with dementia . . . but your body language or tone of voice may be saying "I disapprove of this" or "I don't have time for this right now" or "I am mad"—and that is what the person with dementia reacts to . . . so they get angry at you and you wonder why because you didn't say anything wrong. Well, you didn't but your body language and tone of voice did. They respond to the unspoken!

The findings from the aforementioned study and the implementation of these experts' recommendations, through ongoing training and hands-on guidance and role modeling by experienced and skilled care employees, will often make the difference between a successful and safe de-escalation strategy and an unsafe one.

Communication Strategies

Acknowledging the Person

Acknowledge Feelings of Anxiety and Fear

Often, what underlies behavioral expressions labeled as aggression among elders with Alzheimer's disease is fear. Power[49] states, "Residents who are angry and potentially violent generally feel helpless and powerless. They need help with their self-control." In accordance, Richard Cheston observes in the context of people living with dementia, "If we understand that some forms of challenging behaviour are actually attempts to create emotional security, then the clear implication is that care providers need to find ways of creating greater emotional security."[443] He adds, "Good dementia care recognizes that people living with dementia, like all of us, have an enduring need for emotional security."

To acknowledge a resident who might feel frightened during a DHRRI, direct care partners can say, for instance, "Mrs. Allen, this must have been scary for you . . . Are you okay?"

and, "I will stay with you and make sure you feel safe." You can simply say (clearly and in an even tone), "You are safe here, nobody is going to hurt you,"[410] or "I am not going to let anyone hurt you."[205] Due to the residents' short-term memory loss and difficulties in regulating their emotions, direct care partners may need to repeat these reassuring statements frequently.

Avoid Contradicting What the Person Is Saying, Even If It Is Incorrect

When direct care partners insist on facts—*their* perception of the truth—with a resident who is cognitively incapable of understanding, remembering, and/or accepting it, this usually causes the person to become more frustrated and angry. It is important to be genuine—avoid pretending—when acknowledging, affirming, and validating what the resident says, as many with dementia retain the ability to sense insincere approaches and attitudes. Otherwise, direct care partners will risk losing the person's trust, which (as mentioned earlier) is critical for their ability to support and care for the person and encourage her or his cooperation. Gentle orientation is okay as long as the person with dementia wants it, can tolerate it, and can cognitively process the information.

The following story is presented for illustration. A resident with advanced dementia may take a shirt from another person's bedroom, wear it, and walk around the care home with it. When it is pointed out to him by a direct care partner that he is wearing someone else's shirt, he insists that it belongs to him, and he refuses to take it off. Attempts to convince him that the shirt does not belong to him will likely upset the resident, who truly believes that it is his. Clearly, wearing the shirt is important to this resident, and it allows him to be content.

As long as it does not trigger an altercation with the resident to whom the shirt belongs, it might be wiser to let him wear it. When appropriate, depending on the cognitive function level of the person, her or his close family members may need to be notified, especially so that they will not be surprised to discover it during a visit. Depending on the personality and level of cognitive function of the person to whom the shirt belongs, it might be possible to ask this individual whether he would be so kind, flexible, and willing to accommodate the other resident by allowing him to wear it.

One of the main goals of care is to enable residents with dementia to experience the highest practicable emotional well-being. Insisting that the person who took the shirt accept the truth—that the shirt is not his—would likely compromise the ability to realize this important goal of care. At bedtime, the resident may take the shirt off and put on his pajamas. It may be better to try to take the shirt at this point when the resident is fast asleep and give it back to the resident to whom it belongs. Alternatively, if the resident does remember it in the morning or continues to ask or search for the shirt, perhaps in the other resident's bedroom, it might be worth considering purchasing an identical shirt, when available and affordable, and giving it to the resident—making sure to name label each of the shirts. Often, it is possible for care teams to identify and use creative solutions that allow them to avoid insisting on the facts with a resident with a serious brain disease who has clearly lost the ability to recognize or tolerate them.

Validate the Subjective Truth and Feelings of the Resident

According to Tom Kitwood,[64] "[T]o validate the experience of another is to accept the reality and power of that experience, and hence its subjective truth." It often does not matter how illogical, chaotic, or paranoid the feelings of a resident with advanced dementia may seem to you.[63] Direct care partners should avoid denying the reality of and the feelings of the person. It is necessary to remember, as discussed throughout this book, the reality as perceived by the person with dementia "constitutes the reality of the situation."[444] Steve Ponath, an educator and advocate who lives with early-onset Alzheimer's disease, explains, "People have to learn how to live in my world. I can't live in your world anymore."

Trying as much as possible to see the world from the perspective of the person with dementia is one of the most effective approaches when working with, supporting, and caring for this population.[444] One resident with advanced Alzheimer's disease had run restaurants for decades as part of the family business.[34] While at the secure care home for elders with dementia, she clearly considered her role to continue in the dining room; her son reported, "She thinks this is her restaurant." She sat in a location where she could oversee the work of the kitchen staff and direct care partners as they served food for residents. She directed residents to tables and seats ("You take the seat you like" and, pointing to an open seat and saying, "Right there"), and she gave instructions, guidance, praise ("Very good"), encouragement ("We're almost there"), and critique to kitchen staff ("You're going the other place, honey") as they served meals. Occasionally, while in the dining room, you would hear her say, "This is my business," or "We were so busy today," and telling a direct care partner who is serving food, "You work so hard. Let the other girls help you." She would also frequently check the dining room floor with her hand to see how clean it was after housekeeping staff cleaned it.

Serving in this role enabled her to preserve her former occupational identity. It brought her tremendous joy over a period of many months. Affirming her misperceived cherished role, validating it, and genuinely nurturing it made all the difference. Outside of mealtimes, this resident frequently engaged in DHRRIs. Taking away her cherished role during mealtimes—by not validating her subjective truth when she acted as the manager of the "restaurant"—would have likely caused her frustration and anger, which could have contributed to more altercations with other residents and direct care partners. In fact, when direct care partners (such as float staff and external agency staff) were not aware of her role and, for example, directed her to sit in a different seat and table in the dining room (not knowing how important it was for her to sit in the special seat of the "restaurant owner"), she would immediately become furious and start cursing and pushing them, which triggered angry reactions from other residents. Not validating her subjective truth and feelings at this point and preventing her from returning to "her" seat could have resulted in physical harm to other residents, herself, or direct care partners. Despite her advanced cognitive impairment, this woman was ambulatory, though somewhat unsteady while walking, and very physically strong; she was not afraid to fight with others when she felt threatened. In short, genuinely validating her internal reality as "the manager of the restaurant" made the difference between optimal emotional well-being and safety and tremendous frustration, with resulting distressing and harmful incidents.

That said, direct care partners will need to use their best professional judgment to guide their approach when the situation might be putting a resident or those around him or her at serious risk—for instance, allowing a resident with late-stage dementia to leave a secure care home unattended because she or he does not perceive the LTC home as home. In addition, direct care partners should be formally trained in effective communication techniques such as the Validation Method[4] when working with older residents with Alzheimer's disease, especially when trying to understand the emotional and psychological needs underlying various forms of distressing behavioral expressions including DHRRIs.

Identify and Proactively Meet Physiological and Medical Needs

As discussed previously, when residents' physiological and medical needs are not met in general or in a timely manner, they may contribute to their engagement in DHRRIs. These conditions may include, among others, physical discomforts, pain (such as due to arthritis or constipation), acute illness such as urinary tract infection, delirium, or delusions and hallucinations. It is critical to routinely and proactively assess and treat these and other conditions in order to prevent emotional and physical suffering for residents. Feeling physiologically distressed and emotionally frustrated due to these conditions can put these individuals at risk of engagement in DHRRIs—sometimes because they are less able to tolerate others' distressing verbal or behavioral expressions. Physical distress may also exacerbate an ongoing episode.

Residents with advanced dementia who are unable to recognize and/or verbalize their unmet physiological or medical needs might be particularly vulnerable in this context. This aspect of care and prevention is discussed in Chapter 8 with illustrative examples in the area of pain, constipation, and delirium. When a DHRRI occurs, direct care partners should consider whether there might be an immediate medical or physical need at the root of it, and address that need quickly if it is identified.

In one instance, two residents with dementia were sitting in the dining room. One asked the other why he was not eating the food on his plate. After asking these question and making frustrated remarks about it a few more times without receiving an answer, the interaction escalated into physical altercation. The resident who was not eating his food reached a breaking point, picked up his walker, and threatened to hit his tablemate with it. Direct care partners intervened in time and prevented an injury. After evaluating the resident who was not eating his food, it was discovered that the resident had pain in his mouth due to a dental abscess. This resident was nonverbal and thus unable to verbally report the pain to direct care partners, nor could he explain to his tablemate why he would not eat his food. Routine and proactive mouth and dental assessment and treatment as well as awareness to this resident's pain during mealtime—not to mention a change of diet to allow him to eat with minimal pain—could have enabled direct care partners to prevent this incident from occurring.

Offer Reassurance to Help the Resident Feel Safe

Living with Alzheimer's disease can cause the person to experience frequent feelings of uncertainty, self-doubt, anxiety, and fear of failure. Due to a decreased ability to regulate one's emotions as the disease progresses, these feelings may exacerbate during stressful situations such as resident-to-resident incidents. To alleviate these feelings, direct care partners may want to consider saying to a resident in distress one or more of the following words of reassurance, "I know it is hard," "You are safe here," "I am sorry that you are upset. Is there something I can do to make you feel better?," and "I will stay with you until you feel better. Okay?"

Lisa Gwyther[186] of the Alzheimer's Disease Research Center at Duke University explains,

> If I have one message about dementia-related behavior . . . it is: Assume people are scared. They live in a world that doesn't make sense to them. They don't know who to trust and they are looking for reassurance that they are in the right place, doing the right thing, and that someone knows how to find them. And that explains *a lot* of the dementia-related behaviors. And if you think about that each time you see someone who looks like they are behaving uncharacteristically or aggressively, you'll do fine.

Berry[429] advises, "Remember that residents with dementia are more cooperative and trusting when they feel valued, safe, competent, successful, and understood." Skilled and effective direct care partners proactively interact and communicate with these residents in ways that focus on, promote, and nurture these feelings. Such reassurance can be a lifeline to a resident with dementia who is fearful and in distress. Providing reassurance to these individuals could be done during and after a DHRRI, and it should not be limited to residents directly involved in the episode. Residents who have just witnessed an episode can be afraid for their own safety; therefore, attention and provision of timely reassurance to these individuals are critical.

Apologize Sincerely

When things go wrong, direct care partners may want to try and take the blame, even when the resident's cognitive impairment clearly contributed to the situation or behavioral expressions. As Raia[129] suggests, "An apology goes a long way in defusing potential agitation." For example, direct care partners can say, "I apologize for turning off the television before asking your permission. Would you like me to turn it back on?" or "I am sorry that you had to experience and see this. It must have been scary. I will do everything I can to make sure that it will not happen again."

The following story illustrates the importance of a sincere apology during direct care partners' attempts to de-escalate DHRRIs. During one episode, two residents with dementia were arguing about a seat in the dining room; each insisted that this was where they always sat (a contributing factor to this disagreement was that different seating arrangements were used by different direct care partners across shifts). The argument intensified, and the two residents started pulling on the chair to gain possession of it, which placed them both at risk of experiencing a fall. The team leader noticed it, approached the two, and said, "Gentlemen, I am so sorry that *I* created the confusion by not placing the name tag in time next to your seats." She added, "I apologize. You are both right since both of you sit here on different shifts. Mr. Smith, here (pointing to another seat in the dining room), my co-worker prepared a seat for you closer to the bathroom where you prefer to sit. Let's go this way." On the way to the seat, the team leader told him, "Thank you for being flexible. I really appreciate it."

Ask for Permission Before Doing Something for the Person

Asking permission from a resident with dementia communicates respect and instills in the person a sense of control over the situation. Zgola[59] asserts, "A sense of mastery is one of the most important things a caregiver can offer a cognitively impaired person." For residents with advanced dementia who are unable to speak, universally known gestures may work well in seeking out their permission. For instance, universally known facial and hand gestures can signal a resident with advanced dementia that a direct care partner is asking—without words— whether it is okay to collect her nearly empty bowl of soup at the end of a meal. Many elders with dementia who live in LTC homes have lost control over so many aspects of their lives. Direct care partners are in an excellent position to identify every possible opportunity to enable them to feel some measure of control over their daily lives and care.

The following incident[13] illustrates the importance of asking permission from a resident during an attempt to de-escalate a physically threatening situation. One morning during my early study, resident A became increasingly frustrated and angry at resident B, who was sneezing repeatedly in the TV lounge before the first group activity of the day. At some point resident A said angrily: "She is spreading cold." When resident C tried to protect resident B from resident A, resident A verbally threatened her: "One more word from you . . ." Resident C, who was in her 90s, was physically frail, and used a walker, continued to confront him. Resident A stood up and walked very anxiously towards resident C with a body language as if he were about to hit her. In response, resident C shouted: "Help, help!" The team leader arrived at the TV lounge and told resident A: "Mr. [Resident A's last name], would you like to watch TV in the privacy of your own room?" Resident A: "No." Team leader: "Because in 15 minutes there will be an activity and the TV will need to be turned off anyway. Would you like me to turn your TV on?" Resident A (reluctantly): "Ok, you can turn it on." Team leader: "Come please . . . because I know you don't want me to go into your room when you are not there." Resident A: "That's right." The two left the TV lounge, and the episode discontinued.

Help Residents "Save Face"

During distressing or frightening resident-to-resident incidents, individuals with dementia may be more likely to say or do something that could be perceived by others around them (other residents, direct care partners, and visitors) as embarrassing or humiliating. It is important to make every effort to help all residents directly and indirectly involved to "save face" in order to preserve their dignity. The inability of residents with dementia to save face in these situations may "fuel up" and escalate these episodes. Erving Goffman[445] describes the potential consequences of losing one's face:

He may feel bad because he had relied upon the encounter to support an image of self to which he has become emotionally attached and which he now finds threatened. Felt lack of judgmental support from the encounter may take him aback, confuse him, and momentarily incapacitate him as an interactant. His manner and bearings may falter, collapse, and crumble. He may become shamefaced and chagrined. The feeling, whether warranted or not, that he is perceived in a flustered state by others . . . may add further injuries to his feelings.

Goffman adds, "The person who can witness another's humiliation and unfeelingly retain a cool countenance himself is said in our society to be 'heartless.'"

Remind Others that a Resident's Behavioral Expression Is Not Intentional

Residents with dementia impacted directly and indirectly during DHRRIs can often believe that the resident exhibiting the behavioral expression is trying to cause intentional harm. As mentioned earlier, however, in most situations involving residents with middle- to late-stage dementia, this is not the case. Direct care partners may need to quietly explain to residents without cognitive impairment and those with early-stage dementia that the resident's cognitive impairments may be contributing to his or her difficulty coping with situational frustrations, which lead to interpersonal stressors and, then, these episodes. However, providing this type of explanation must be done thoughtfully and sensitively in a way that does not inadvertently further stigmatize the resident in the eyes of his or her fellow residents. Examples of stigmatizing and labeling words to avoid include, "She is a difficult person" and "He is out of it." Helpful words to consider include, "He experiences significant challenges in organizing his thoughts due to a brain disease. It is not his fault. Please try to understand; he is not doing it intentionally to upset you" and "She has a condition that limits her ability to locate her bedroom. Please understand, when she enters your bedroom and interrupts you, it is because she is unable to locate hers."

Share Favorable Life Background Information About the Resident

Sometimes, sharing with residents a positive and meaningful piece of information about the life background of a resident frequently engaged in DHRRIs may assist, even if temporarily, to shift residents' negative perceptions of the resident. For example, some residents may become a bit more tolerant of a resident when they learn that he or she served in the army, contributed to a medical breakthrough, received a volunteer award, or was a loving, caring, and dedicated parent and/or spouse. Special events recognizing this resident's life achievements and frequent reminders about them to other residents could assist in instilling a more positive image of the resident with dementia who tends to engage in these episodes. This approach could be used prior and after DHRRIs but occasionally, when appropriate, it could also be used during an ongoing episode (some episodes may span over 15 to 30 minutes or longer, which allow for opportunities to use it). I have seen this approach used thoughtfully and effectively by direct care partners in a secured dementia care home.

Speaking with the Person

Establish and Maintain Eye Contact

Direct care partners should make eye contact with residents with dementia unless they know or sense that it may cause the resident to feel uncomfortable or somehow threatened. This is especially true during DHRRIs. An experienced and insightful music therapist, Wendy Krueger,[34] made the following observation: "When you look into the resident's eyes . . . and you are really looking into them, it makes them feel more real or more present . . . even more appreciated . . ." In accordance, Raia[122] explains, "Make eye contact even if the person may be looking at your mouth. As persons with dementia lose the ability to understand language they become inadvertent lip readers."

That said, it is important to avoid staring at the resident, as this may cause him or her (or anyone else for that matter) to become upset. In addition, avoiding eye contact with a resident with dementia is necessary when it is culturally inappropriate.[446] For example, direct eye contact is generally considered to be disrespectful in the Hmong culture. People in this culture customarily look down toward the floor as an indication that they are listening intently to the person. In addition, recommended practices specific to certain American Indian populations include avoiding looking directly into the person's eyes. For example, direct care partners attempting to de-escalate an episode in which a Vietnamese elder is involved—while making direct eye contact with the person—should not be surprised if their efforts are unsuccessful, as respect to Vietnamese elders includes avoiding direct eye contact.[447] It is essential to find out the culturally specific expectations for each of the populations and cultures represented among residents at the LTC home and adjust the approach accordingly to each resident's preferences (since cultural norms may change over time, the approach may need to be adjusted based on factors such as birth cohort).

Speak at the Resident's Eye Level

Often, well-meaning and overworked direct care partners, stand above ("tower over") residents with dementia when interacting with them. It is important to avoid this practice in general, but especially during DHRRIs, because it can be perceived by residents as disrespectful and threatening. In general and when it is safe to do it, if the person is seated, you should be at the same level. If the person is standing, you should be standing. When you speak at the level of the resident's eyes, it sends her or him the message that you are equals. This small act of respect is critical in care environments that are so often characterized by a gross power imbalance between direct care partners and residents with dementia. It will give the resident a small measure of control that is often desperately needed during DHRRIs; many of the more serious and frightening incidents are experienced by residents with dementia as episodes over which they have limited control—emotionally, socially, and physically.

In one example, from Power,[65] a nursing assistant was standing above a resident with her hands on her hips waiting to take the resident to the dining room. The resident asked, "What's the matter with you over there, 'standing so high and mighty' like that?" In response, the aide relaxed her posture, apologized, and spoke kindly to the woman, inviting her to lunch. The woman's demeanor followed suit, softening once again."

Use the Resident's Preferred Name

Every resident with dementia has a preference for how he or she would like to be called (for example, first or last name, professional title such as Doctor or Rabbi, or nickname). Knowing and using the resident's preferred name, especially during tense situations such as DHRRIs, is an important way to show respect and build trust with her or him. "Always indicate your name and say the person's name every time you have an exchange, even if it is several times in the course of the day," advises Raia.[122] Teepa Snow suggests,[448] "With older people, use the last name . . . though some may prefer to be called with their first name. You need to find out what the person prefers to be called. Ask the person how he or she likes to be called." If the person is unable to tell you due to advanced cognitive impairment, ask her or his close family members or friends. Once the person's preferred name is known, it should be noted in a central location in the resident's clinical record so that all direct and indirect care partners as well as float and external agency staff will use it during routine care times and DHRRIs.

Be Aware of Your Tone of Voice

Speaking fairly slowly and distinctly and using a gentle, relaxed, and friendly (not bossy or critical) tone of voice can be very helpful for many residents with dementia in general and during DHRRIs. A lower and deep voice pitch is more calming[448] and conveys an easygoing, nondemanding attitude. However, Feil[63] warns,

> Using a warm, loving voice tone with someone who is angry will only create increased anger or withdrawal. Also, be aware of your feelings and attitude. They are often communicated, unintentionally, through tone of voice.

As noted earlier, many people with dementia are able to pick up on and "mirror" the emotional states conveyed in the tone of voice of others around them. Power[49] explains,

> Using your voice and demeanor to try and restore calm can be extremely difficult if you feel surprised, angered, or frightened by the episode. It is essential to try, however, because failure to do so often results in failure to defuse the aggression. A calm voice works best with aggression, but the voice should also have a firm, steady quality. Fear can underlie aggression, and even in the midst of an outburst directed at you, the person may find calm in your tone of quiet assuredness. This is very different from using an authoritative tone of voice. Feeling loss of control is a major component of aggression, and a voice that tries to dictate behavior will likely meet with further resistance. Finding the right tone takes practice and is not always easy to master in the heat of the moment. You should adjust your tone as you observe the response you are getting. Avoid the tender or "singsong" voice that can calm feelings of anxiety but may magnify an angry outburst. In the resident's world, there is a serious and imminent threat to his well-being, and such tone of voice is inconsistent with the mood he or she is experiencing. These instances of emotional mismatch intensify distress in an environment that already feels confusing and threatening.

Make Sure the Resident Can Hear You Well

As an executive director gave a tour to a new employee, she leaned down toward an old woman, and yelled in her ear: "How are you doing?" In response, the resident "pulled her arm back like a major league baseball pitcher and swung an opened hand to the director's face." The director learned that louder is not always better. She also learned that she should have learned about this person's history—such as her hearing abilities and history of hitting others—prior to approaching her.[247]

Although a substantial portion of nursing home residents experience hearing impairments, the optimum volume of speech will depend on each resident's ability to hear. In addition, some residents hear better in one ear than the other. Knowing this personal information is key for direct care partners' ability to communicate effectively with residents with dementia during routine care and DHRRIs.

In addition, regularly assessing residents' hearing abilities and deficits and conducting an audiometric evaluation should guide decisions about the need for a hearing aid, for residents with dementia who can tolerate these aides and use them in ways that improve their ability to hear others around them.

Speak with the Resident, Not at the Resident

Many residents with dementia are able to sense the difference between these two communication styles (the underlying intonation and message conveyed in them) and they are much more likely to react negatively when they feel that they are being talked down to.[449] Regularly instilling and nurturing a collaborative, authentic partnership approach with the residents with dementia will increase the likelihood that they will cooperate with direct care partners during DHRRIs.

Speak Slowly and Clearly

Many people with dementia need extra time to process the information communicated to them. Avoiding fast-paced speech during DHRRIs will assist them in understanding what you try to convey to them; this is not easy to do in the heat of the moment, but direct care partners need to do their best, as it will assist them in their efforts to de-escalate these episodes. That said, it is important to avoid overdoing it by speaking too slowly, as this is likely to be perceived by residents with dementia as demeaning. Care employees will want to match the pace of their speech with the individual's current ability to comprehend it. It is important to allow the resident with dementia enough time to process what you said. This is no doubt a delicate balancing act that should be implemented based on an individual resident unique cognitive abilities, disabilities, and preferences.

Language Techniques

Use Simple Sentences and One-Step Directions

Speaking in simple sentences enables the resident with dementia to better process and understand what you are saying, and it may contribute to improved communication and cooperation during DHRRIs. Using too many words may be beyond what certain residents with a substantial cognitive disability may be able to comprehend. For example, to help reduce his emotional outbursts when his wife is talking, Robert Bowels, Jr.[438] noted, "I would suggest that those without dementia consider having a better listening ear and decrease the number of words that are used in their communication with someone with dementia."

People with dementia tend to understand, respond, and cooperate better when they are asked to do only one thing at a time. Raia[122] suggests, "Always 'chunk' information into short, explicit communications." Examples include "Please come with me" (pause to allow the resident to begin to move); "Take the dish from the shelf" (pause to allow the resident to complete the task) and "Put the dish on the table."

This "chunking" technique could be applied during DHRRIs. For example, consider this incident. During a group activity, Mr. Johns, who has early-stage Alzheimer's disease, is seated next to a resident with advanced disease who has asked the same question ("When will lunch be served?) 15 times within 2 minutes. After acknowledging the frustration and anger Mr. Johns is experiencing from these repeated questions, a direct care partner could say, "Mr. Johns, I saved you a seat next to me" (pause a couple of seconds); "Over there" (while pointing to the open chair many feet away from where he currently sits); "Come through here, please" (pointing to a safe route between the two rows of chairs); and "Right here" (pointing to the seat of the chair). When Mr. Johns sits down, the care partner quietly says, "Thank you for your patience and flexibility."

Use Language that Matches the Person's Comprehension Ability

Previous research[450] has shown that using language beyond the comprehension ability of residents with dementia may result in restlessness and negativism. The reason for this may have to do with the frustration experienced by residents with dementia when they cannot register, process, and/or understand what others are trying to tell them.

For example, at a certain stage of the disease, many people with Alzheimer's disease have lost their ability to understand the meaning of abstract phrases, figures of speech, and slang expressions, and some may even take them literally.[122] It is important to remember to use literal, sensory-focused language—words that can be seen, felt, heard, smelled, or tasted[451]—as opposed to more abstract words or idiomatic phrases. For example, instead of saying, "Jump into bed," care partners could use direct statements such as, "I prepared the bed for you. Would you like to go to bed?" or "It's time to go to bed."[452] With certain individuals with dementia, you may need to avoid saying figuratively, "It's just around the corner," when you mean to tell the person that a special event will be held in a few days; the person with advanced dementia may take it literally and look for it around the corner in the physical space where he or she is located.

It is important to remember that tense incidents between residents and their accompanying distress often exacerbate the situation by further limiting the person's ability to understand others around him or her; residents' cognitive functions are often reduced in many individuals under stressful and frightening situations. This, in turn, may limit care partners' ability to gain a resident's cooperation and de-escalate the DHRRI, such as when trying to get the resident's attention and guide him or her out of the area where the distressing situation has occurred. Using words the person can comprehend, preferably in simple sentences consisting of one-step directions, will increase care employees' ability to safely de-escalate these episodes.

Refocus or Switch the Topic

Direct care partners may want to refocus the resident's attention away from the episode, such as by turning to his or her favorite conversation topic (such as a beloved daughter or son, a previous occupation, hobbies, an enjoyable role in a faith community) or simply by offering to share an interesting story from the daily newspaper on a topic of known interest to the resident.[13] However, direct care partners will need to be mindful of the possibility that, although this is a strategy that can assist in de-escalating DHRRIs, refocusing may not address the residents' unmet needs and frustrations contributing to the development of the episode. As discussed earlier, causes of situational distress and anxiety among individual residents with dementia tend to occur in recurring patterns, so direct care partners have to do their best to proactively identify and meet these needs as early as possible to avoid further distress and anxiety for the same reason in a similar circumstance in the near future—minutes, hours, or days after the current episode has been de-escalated. Proactively meeting these needs, and preventing these frustrations from being experienced by the resident, will often enable care employees to prevent the episodes to begin with.

Turn Negatives into Positives

Instead of raising one's voice or shouting at a resident with dementia, "Don't go there!" or "That's not your bedroom. Don't go in there!," when possible, direct care partners should approach the resident slowly and calmly, establish eye contact, point to where they want the resident to walk, and say, "Let's go here." Instead of saying, "Don't sit here!" they can say "Mrs. Cohen, I prepared you a seat next to me. Would you like to sit?"[34] In accordance, Berry suggests, "Never say to a resident with dementia, 'You can't.' Instead say, 'Let's see what we CAN do.'"[429] It is best to ask for what you want the resident to do, not what you don't want him or her to do, especially during a DHRRI.

In fact, it's usually best to avoid saying "No" and "Don't do . . . ," both in daily practice as well as during a DHRRI. Raia[122] explains, "If one says no, muscles tense up, tone of voice changes, and the resident sees the caregiver as limiting his or her independence." One direct care partner[223] reflected, "If you always say 'NO' and slam the door in the face and say 'No, you have to stay here,' I can understand fully well why he gets so aggressive. Instead of saying 'No' all the time, we should try to think of something else." Sanjay Gupta[453] of CNN asked an experienced social worker the following question: "Are there absolute no–nos . . . things that you should never do when you're dealing with someone with dementia?" Social worker: "Yes—correct them. Saying, 'Don't do this. Don't do that.' They won't remember . . . so why would you?"

Listening to the Person

Listen Carefully to What the Resident with Dementia Is Saying

Actively listening to residents with dementia is a core component of an individualized person-directed care approach. It should also be considered as an integral practice in most risk-prevention programs, including those aimed at understanding, preventing, and de-escalating DHRRIs. Research[454] has shown that one of the main fears expressed by people living with dementia is that other people will no longer listen to them. Listening to people with dementia during routine care periods and during DHRRIs also meets the expectations of these individuals for an "authentic partnership" with their direct care partners. This expectation can also be reflected in the phrase "Nothing about us without us." This principle is never more important than when a DHRRI is in progress because every interaction, especially tense and potentially harmful interactions, should be seen as an important opportunity to build and strengthen trust with the resident with dementia.

Therapeutic listening is defined[455] as "An interpersonal, confirmation process involving all the senses in which the care partner attends with empathy to the client's verbal and nonverbal messages to facilitate the understanding, synthesis, and interpretation of the client's situation." To facilitate active listening, "the listener needs to be 'present' for the speaker, paying close attention to both the words and the feelings or other nonverbal signals being expressed."[456] In the context of residents with Alzheimer's disease, Raia[122] suggests, "Listen not so much to the often misused words and muddled sentences, but to the driving emotion behind them."

One resident with early-stage Alzheimer's disease frequently engaged in DHRRIs with other residents with dementia, nearly always as the exhibitor. A closer look revealed that he was often deprived of the basic respect he had been accustomed to receiving from his co-workers as a successful attorney. He was also experiencing ongoing depression due to his move to the secure dementia care home and separation from his wife. In addition, due to his frequent engagement in DHRRIs, he was labeled aggressive and violent, he became socially isolated as former friends increasingly distanced themselves from him. Intentional listening to these underlying emotions—such as during weekly one-on-one psychotherapy sessions in a private room—could have addressed his unmet needs and affirmed and alleviated his emotional suffering. Once his deeply painful experiences, emotions, and psychological and social needs were recognized, supported, and met, it would have likely helped to reduce the number of incidents he was involved in with other residents. For a discussion and additional suggestions related to active listening, see the excellent chapter "Encouraging Positive Behavior" in the book *Caring for People with Challenging Behaviors*, by Stephen Long.[295]

Encourage Expression of Feelings

People with dementia have the right to be angry and to express their anger. Direct care partners will want to let the person be angry if he or she needs to be, but also to make sure that the individual is expressing it in a safe way and place and that it does not violate the rights of other residents. Direct care partners will want to avoid telling a resident who is angry not to be angry. Many have good reasons to be angry, whether these reasons have to do with losses related to their aging process, cognitive disability caused by dementia, an unwanted move to the care home, or other causes. For example, due to dementia and memory loss, many people living with dementia have lost their job and were forced to retire, lost their home, or lost their life-long dreams for retirement. They may also have lost part or all of their support system if their spouse and/or close friends have passed away. Many were moved involuntarily to a care home, where they may frequently lose their privacy, freedom, autonomy, function, independence, and dignity. They are also often being cared for by well-meaning and hard-working people who may not have received sufficient specialized training in caring for, emotionally supporting, and communicating with people with dementia, which can add to their daily frustrations and anger. In the words of a direct care partner,[223]

> I wouldn't like it myself if when I'm really angry and someone comes in and says, "It'll be all right, everything's fine," "It will pass," or "Don't be angry." Personally I would get even angrier because no one wants to listen to what I have to say.

At other times, a simple but genuine acknowledgement of a resident's frustration with another resident can go a long way in affirming their experience and minimizing their negative reaction toward that resident. Marsha Frankel and colleagues[457] suggest saying, for example, "Mr. Jones, if I understand correctly, Mr. Brown's banging on the wall is more than you can put up with anymore." Not acknowledging a resident's repeated frustrations and anger with another resident may eventually lead her or him to reach a breaking point.

As important as encouraging expression of feelings is to pay close attention to the feelings that are expressed by residents with dementia; never ignore the emotions of a person with dementia. Raia asserts,[122] "If emotions are ignored, they fester and can lead to violent behavior." As explained by Naomi Feil,[63] "Painful feelings, such as anger, sadness, fear, frustration, and hurt, that are expressed, acknowledged, and validated by a trusted listener will diminish. Painful feelings that are ignored or suppressed will gain in strength."

Taken together, enabling a resident with dementia to express his or her anger during a DHRRI in a safe way will, if listened to and genuinely affirmed, assist the person to feel heard and to see that his or her frustrations and fears matter to direct care partners. That affirmation is essential to building and maintaining trust with the person. It is key to using a collaborative approach. Both are essential to direct care partners' ability to gain the person's cooperation when episodes arise and need to be de-escalated effectively and safely.

Wait a Bit, and Then Gently Assist with Difficulties in Verbal Expression

In general, due to cognitive impairment and especially during distressing situations such as DHRRIs, residents with dementia may experience difficulty organizing, formulating, and/ or expressing their thoughts—for instance, finding the right word or completing a sentence, or saying words that do not have the intended meaning. During these situations, direct care partners should be ready to gently assist residents at *their* (i.e., residents') pace and based on *their* expressive and emotional needs at that particular moment. It requires being attentive to striking a delicate balance with each individual resident—a balance between a resident's preserved but somewhat delayed response and unnecessary frustration. As suggested by Baker and colleagues,[458]

> If a resident is becoming very frustrated with their verbal skills, you can help supply the word if they are struggling, you should allow them to complete their thought—don't put words in their mouth, but mirror back to them their statement so that you can be sure of what they are saying to you.

Although every resident and situation differs and there is no magic one-size-fits-all guidance here, it is generally a good idea to wait a few seconds before assisting a resident with dementia who is trying to formulate and express a thought. Some people with dementia suggest waiting 10 seconds before trying to assist the person with dementia to express their thoughts. The optimal time will vary across individuals with dementia as well as within individuals over time—like us, people with dementia have good and bad days, and dementia is progressive.

Focus on Feelings, Less on Facts

Direct care partners will want to respond to the resident's underlying emotions, not the behavioral expression itself. Joanne Koenig Coste[251] suggests,

> Always listen to the emotion behind the person's failing words. The emotion is still intact; at some elemental level, you can still reach it. The actual words are not important if you can understand the feeling behind the attempt to communicate.

As Berry explains, "It is critical to pay attention to the emotional needs of residents with dementia. That has to be the focus because that causes the behaviors" (Judy Berry, personal communication, March 1, 2013). For example, when a resident with middle- to late-stage dementia tells a direct care partner angrily, "No," he or she may actually mean: "I don't understand" or "I am afraid." Raia and colleagues[129] give the following example: When a resident is saying angrily (while slamming her fist on the table), "You took my pocketbook, and I want it right back now!" maybe what she is really saying is "I don't know who I am," "I don't know what I should be doing," or "I feel panic." Instead of saying, "I didn't take your pocketbook. You just don't remember where you put it," which will only make her angrier, direct care partners should validate the resident's frustrating experience (whether the accusation is true or not) and offer to assist in resolving it. They can say (genuinely), "You must feel awful. I am so sorry. Let's see if we can find it." It takes time and practice to develop and hone this communication skill but it is critical if we want care partners to be able to de-escalate DHRRIs effectively, fulfilling the resident's unmet emotional needs underlying his or her behavioral expressions.

Try to Identify the Reason Behind a Resident's Refusal to Cooperate

The key to working with a person with dementia who refuses services is building and maintaining a relationship of trust.[123] In accordance, a direct care partner[34] with 20 years' experience working with and caring for residents with dementia explained, "When a resident refuses something, he has a good will . . . a good reason to refuse."

The following story[34] illustrates this general principle. One resident with dementia refused to be assisted with taking a shower for several months; she would kick direct care partners out of her bedroom when they tried to encourage her to take a shower. On her birthday, she finally agreed to be assisted. When she took off her shirt, direct care partners discovered that she had gone through mastectomy (surgery to remove her entire breast). Direct care partners reinterpreted her refusals as a way to protect her dignity and personhood. Power[29] observes, "Although this is not always easy to do, if a care partner can step back from a resistant person and think, 'What is he teaching me right now about my approach?' she can often discover how better to interact and eliminate the distress."

Encourage a Compromise

It can sometimes be helpful to remind and explain to residents with earlier-stage dementia the nature of communal living, such as the need to share limited available resources. Direct care partners need to regularly acknowledge residents' frustrations related to living with a large number of other people—some or many of whom have dementia—in close quarters as well as to share a bedroom with one or more roommates. For instance, when two groups of residents with early-stage dementia engage in tense arguments over which program or film should be viewed in the main lounge in the early evening hours, a thoughtful plan consisting of a compromise could be developed with direct input from the residents. The remainder of the evening could be divided in a way that enables each group to view its preferred film during separate times while offering the group that has to wait a separate meaningful activity in a different location of the care home. When this is not possible, viewing of preferred programs or films could be divided across days. In addition, some residents with dementia may be willing to compromise and watch their preferred programs inside their bedrooms, if they have a TV there; some of these residents may need assistance in finding the program or film and/or operating the remote control during their viewing.

Communication Strategies to Avoid

Avoid Smiling During Episodes

Smiling during certain DHRRIs can be perceived as devaluing the residents' emotional distress, which may further frustrate and upset these individuals, "fuel up" the situational tension, and contribute to escalation of the episode. As explained by Power,[49] "In the experiential eyes of the person who is feeling threatened, a smile can look like a sneer and is often interpreted as mockery or making light of one's distress." I have witnessed numerous DHRRIs in care homes over the years and, although smiling is not common, it does happen. That said, there can be exceptions and in some unique situations a gentle, genuine, and respectful smile by a trusted care employee may not result in a negative reaction from a resident, and it may even assist in calming certain residents with dementia. I have seen this too.

Some direct care partners might smile as a habitual reaction to anxiety, or in a misguided attempt to calm the situation; they may not be aware of the negative impact of smiling during these episodes. Others who are clearly insensitive and disrespectful should have never been hired to work with, support, and care for elders with dementia. When some of these employees perceive vulnerable and frail elders as lacking any value, or worse, as objects, they are more likely to disregard the emotionally distressing experience of a resident engaged in a DHRRI. They may lack empathy toward the person and may take the incident lightly. These employees may find these serious and frightening episodes funny, and they may smile at or even mock the residents with dementia involved in them. An employee may smile in a demeaning way and tell a resident with advanced dementia, "How many times do I have to tell you that this is not your bedroom?" Needless to say, this undignified attitude can only make things worse during an episode because most residents with dementia, including many with advanced dementia, will sense it and respond to it.

Avoid Arguing, Reasoning, Correcting, or Criticizing a Resident with Dementia

As discussed previously, it is generally good advice, particularly with a resident involved in a DHRRI, to avoid correcting or arguing a point with a resident with middle- to late-stage dementia, especially when the person is unable to tolerate it and benefit from it. When direct care partners argue with a resident with dementia, they may not really hear what the person is saying—the deeper meaning and underlying emotional states beneath the words. As a result, they may be less likely to identify the unmet human needs and situational frustrations contributing to or causing the behavioral expressions, and therefore, inadvertently, they will be more likely to worsen the situation.

The following conversation[34] between a nurse and a resident with Alzheimer's disease illustrates the problem caused when care employees argue with residents with dementia. Nurse: "You broke your tooth last week." Resident: "I did not. I broke it this morning." Nurse: "You broke it when you ate popcorn last week." Resident: "Why do you have to argue with me?" Nurse: "I don't." Resident: "You do, you argue, and make my life miserable." The following helpful reflective question was asked by dementia expert Teepa Snow,[198] "You can't let go of your point of view, and I can't let go of mine. Which of us has dementia?"

The following story[34] illustrates this point in the context of DHRRIs. A resident with Alzheimer's disease became frustrated and angry when he thought his tablemate was kicking his leg intentionally with her foot underneath the dining room table. At some point, he shouted at her (while raising his fist in a threatening manner), "Stop it, you are hurting me!" The tablemate suffered from tremor, which frequently caused her legs to move uncontrollably. Attempts to explain to the resident who complained about it that her kicking was not intentional were unsuccessful. In fact, they only made him more upset. A simple solution was then implemented. The resident with the tremor was asked to sit at another table, where only two residents sat during meals (most tables were designed for and used by four residents). She agreed to the change. The added space underneath the newly assigned table prevented further incidents.

Avoid Talking About a Resident in Her or His Presence

It is disrespectful and can cause the resident to feel devalued and excluded to talk about the person as if she or he were not there. This common but unhelpful practice is likely to cause many residents with dementia to become more upset than they already are during DHRRIs.

As explained by a nurse with over 20 years of experience working with residents with dementia, "People who are extremely compromised; even when they can't speak, they can really understand. It is amazing sometimes." Leading advocate Kate Swaffer,[438] who lives with dementia, asks, "Don't talk about me to someone else, in front of me."

During a visit to the doctor,[251] a person with Alzheimer's disease responded in the following way after the doctor spoke about his diagnosis with his wife as if he wasn't in the room: "Damn it all. Am I invisible? This is *my* disease you are talking about—I'm still here. Talk to me. Me!" Another physician suggests using body language and gestures to include a person with more advanced dementia in the conversation.

During one tense incident between two residents with dementia in the dining room, a well-meaning but inexperienced direct care partner told her co-worker about one of the residents involved in the episode in his presence, referring to his frequent attempts to take a cup of water from his tablemate. She said, "He always does it. He can't keep his hands to himself." The resident heard it and responded, "I am sorry but you should have known that I have glaucoma and it causes loss of peripheral vision. I am unable to see my cup of water when it is placed on my right side. I mistakenly think that my tablemate's cup is mine." Then he added, "I also ask that you refrain from speaking about me in my presence as if I am not here. It is disrespectful."

Avoid Questions that Challenge the Resident's Short-Term Memory

Short-term memory is one of the first cognitive functions damaged in Alzheimer's disease. Asking challenging questions is likely to further frustrate an already upset or angry resident and can escalate a DHRRI. For example, under pressure or in the heat of the moment, a care employee may say: "Don't you remember that . . . ?" or "Didn't I tell you already not to . . . ?" Barbara Haight and Barrett Haight[459] advise, "Do not make the mistake of asking, 'Do you remember?' For someone with memory impairment, 'Do you remember?' is a threatening question." Berg[146] explains, "Knowledge about memory loss provides us with a basis for caution when asking questions of residents whose memory loss disables them from giving an answer."

Never Command or Demand; Instead, Ask for Their Help

Feil observes that the need to feel useful is one of the main universal needs experienced by people with Alzheimer's disease. A study by Acton and colleagues[444] showed that the desire to remain useful was expressed by the majority of people with Alzheimer's disease. Robert Simpson, who lives with early-onset Alzheimer's disease shares, "I still want to be needed in some way. I would like you to talk things over with me, even if I can't respond well. I still need to hear 'I need you.' Even when I can't believe you do."

Despite this deeply important need of many people with dementia to remain useful to others, Desai and McFadden[156] observe that these individuals in LTC homes "rarely have the opportunity to gain a sense of meaning from helping other people." Many residents with dementia want to assist others, and direct care partners need to enable and assist them in meeting this basic need during routine care and—when possible, appropriate, and safe—also during DHRRIs. One way in which this need could help direct care partners de-escalate a DHRRI is by seeking the resident's assistance as part of an effort to redirect her or him away from the area where the episode takes place. For example, the direct care partner can ask the resident for assistance in another part of the care home: "Mr. Smith, you always loved working in the garden. I *really* need *your* advice. Would you be willing to help me in the garden?"

Avoid Asking Why the Person Is Doing Something

Many people with advanced dementia are not interested in understanding why they engage in behavioral expressions. Many, especially those with middle- to late-stage Alzheimer's disease, may have already lost the ability to identify and/or retain in their short-term memory the reason for their behavioral expression or have insight into it. Asking a resident (with an irritated or angry tone of voice), "Why did you do it?" often puts her or him on the defensive. Instead, as suggested by Feil,[63] direct care partners will want to use the factual questions: When? Where? What? or Who?—as these can assist them to "tune into" the subjective experience of the person and explore her or his perception of the situation. For example, angrily asking a resident with advanced dementia, "Why are you opening and closing bedroom doors in the middle of the night? Can't you see that it upsets the residents living in these bedrooms?" will not be helpful in most situations. The elder who used to work night shifts as a security guard in commercial buildings may not be able to explain why he is doing it. The "Why?" question, especially when asked in a critical or accusatory tone of voice, may upset the person; in his mind, he is only doing his job.

A more helpful approach could be characterized as an exploratory–validating one. The direct care partner may want to acknowledge the resident's efforts, telling him, "You are working hard here" and then ask, in a genuine, calm, respectful, and nonjudgmental tone of voice, "*Where* are you right now?" Continuing to explore the resident's internal reality, the care employee may ask, "*Who* works here during the day?" and "*When* does your shift end?" These kinds of questions can enable the care partner to affirm and validate the resident's experience (fulfilling his duties at his perceived workplace) and learn from him about the job he worked in for many years. Then, gradually and gently, the care employee can encourage the dedicated security guard (for example) to assist the care employee in a special task intended to ensure that the building is secure, for instance, sitting in a recliner chair by the windows overlooking the parking lot to make sure that the employees' cars parked there are safe and that no one approaches the building at night. The resident, who is tired, may gradually close his eyes and fall asleep. The care employee covers him with a soft blanket, lowers the recliner to a nearly horizontal position, places a pillow under his head, and goes on to complete her night duties.

Actions to Address Dynamics Between Residents

Immediately Discontinue and Defuse Chain Reactions

One of the reasons for defusing a DHRRI as quickly as possible is the "billiard effect," a term used by Raia (personal communication, November 2006), in which an episode can spread from two residents involved in an episode to others. For example, two residents with dementia engage in a tense argument in the dining room and, if the interaction is not recognized and de-escalated promptly, other residents with dementia may quickly "pick up" the negative emotional states and become distressed, anxious, and upset themselves. These residents who initially were not directly involved in the argument are now, and the expanded and increasingly distressful episode is now more challenging to resolve.

Camp[193] shares the following story: Two men without dementia did not get along at an adult day health center. They would regularly shout and call each other names. When the two would begin to argue, a woman with advanced dementia picked up on their negative emotional states, became overstimulated, and would go over to them and try to strike them with her cane as hard as she could. She thought that the shouting and name calling were directed toward her. Another fairly common scenario occurs when two residents engage in an episode and then at some point another resident approaches them (such as to protect one from the other or to separate the two). The third resident's involvement triggers a reaction by one or both residents involved in the episode (verbally such as "Stay away, it is not your business" or physically trying to push the approaching resident away). The reaction can trigger a verbal and/or physical response form the third resident, who then may become directly involved in the episode. At this point, if direct care partners do not intervene, other residents in the area may take sides, such as by making comments from another part of the room where the episode takes place, and before long, a handful of residents with dementia engage in this evolving episode, which is now harder to de-escalate. Needless to say, intervention as early as possible—at the first signs of irritability, restlessness, frustration, distress, and anxiety—is critical for prevention of harm to residents.

Position, Reposition, or Change Seating Arrangement

Problems related to seating and seating arrangements, such as in the dining room and activity room, are common contributing factors to conflicts between residents with dementia (see "Problematic Seating Arrangements" in Chapter 4).

Changes in seating arrangements should be done in a way that results in a decrease in direct physical and eye contact between pairs of residents who have been involved in DHRRIs; for instance, they could be seated back to back, facing different directions, or in different dining rooms, when available).[13] Direct care partners in a study by Rosen and colleagues[332] suggest moving one of the residents to a different seat or offering to find her or him an equally good seat.

It is important to remain vigilant to an assigned seating arrangement so that you can see when it no longer works, as well as to other quickly evolving problems with seating, for instance, when two residents grab hold of a chair in the dining room, each insisting that it belongs to her or him. Attentive direct care partners may need to make prompt, thoughtful decisions to reposition chairs as needed. If necessary, changes in seating arrangement can often assist in de-escalating an episode and reducing the likelihood that it will reoccur between the two residents in the future.

Physically Separate Residents

In situations where a resident verbally threatens to harm another resident, when there is potential for two residents to physically harm each other, or when there is already physical contact between residents, direct care partners need to quickly but calmly and skillfully separate the residents before the situation escalates further. One CNA[34] reported the following separation strategy: "Two residents can have an argument . . . and you just come and sit down and you separate them . . . sit down in the middle between them. When you sit down between them, there is no argument." Susan Snellgrove[407] has found that CNAs rely heavily on separating residents during DHRRIs.

CNAs should be trained in physically separating residents in a way that is safe to all involved, including themselves. In their often-courageous attempts to keep residents safe, CNAs have reported that they frequently use their own body as a barrier between residents involved in an episode or allowed behavioral expressions they considered aggressive to be manifested toward themselves while attempting to calm the residents. These CNAs were more concerned with protecting vulnerable and frail residents than they were in protecting themselves from harm. As noted earlier in this chapter, owners and administrators of LTC homes should ensure that their care employees learn and practice the specialized de-escalation techniques demonstrated by Carly Hellen and Peter Sternberg in their staff training program[460] (DVD and companion workbook) entitled "Dealing with Physical Aggression in Caregiving: Physical and Non-Physical Interventions" (Terra Nova Films).

However, simply watching a video training program will likely not enable care teams to implement them effectively and safely in real-life situations. It is very important that a well-qualified professional who is adequately trained and experienced in using these and similar separation techniques will regularly provide hands-on training and practice in using them to all employees who come in direct regular contact with the residents with dementia at your care home. Classroom training must be complemented with hands-on guidance to care employees on the floor when these episodes occur.

The following episode[34] took place between two residents with late-stage dementia. It started when a resident, Mrs. Kendall, who was known to be very protective of her bedroom, noticed the other resident, Mrs. Lewis, walking toward it from the dining room one afternoon.

Mrs. Kendall noticed this and shouted loudly and angrily to her: "Hey, don't open this door. This is my home." Mrs. Lewis turned around and walked back toward her. In response, Mrs. Kendall immediately told her, angrily, "No, no, you do what you want.' Then the two residents walked toward each other with a hand gesture as if they were about to hit each other. When the two were close to each other, a CNA physically separated them. Mrs. Kendall told Mrs. Lewis: 'I'll kill you.' Another CNA skillfully directed Mrs. Kendall aside, sat with her at a dining room table, and offered her a pizza. Mrs. Lewis left the dining room. The near-hit episode was de-escalated. (The names of both residents are pseudonyms.)

In some situations, however, direct care partners may need to be aware of potential negative effects of *routine* separation of residents engaged in tense interactions with other residents without a deeper understanding of the context in which these interactions occur. For example, some separations may potentially limit the social network of pairs of residents with dementia who tend to quarrel but also give social support to each other in an environment where personally meaningful social interaction can be scarce. Clearly, these situations require responses that aim to strike a balance between residents' need for companionship and peer support and their safety. Success in managing these complex relationships over time depends on the following:

- Adequate staffing levels of well-trained direct care partners who know the residents well

- Careful supervision and assessment of the two residents' interactions and relationship during all shifts

- Use of effective communication and timely information transfer among direct care partners

- Adequate documentation of areas of concern in each resident's care plan, including awareness of temporal, spatial, and other patterns underlying these episodes

- Use of proactive "anticipatory" prevention and de-escalation strategies

- Provision of personally meaningful engagement of the residents throughout the day and evening

That said, it is important to be aware that even pairs of residents with dementia who are known to be good or even best friends may at some point (due to progression in cognitive impairments or other reasons) reach a "breaking point" and turn against each other. A resident with advanced dementia who repeatedly shadows (walks closely to) another resident to feel secure at her presence might at some point be pushed away by this resident, who simply could not stand it any longer. The separation of these two residents should be considered before a DHRRI occurs, such as when the shadowing of the resident triggers the initial signs of frustration in the resident being followed.

The following tragic incidents illustrate this scenario. A 98-year-old resident[461] with dementia strangled to death her 100-year-old roommate in a nursing home in Dartmouth, Massachusetts; a plastic shopping bag was found tied around her head. The nursing home stated that "except for some minor arguments, the roommates acted like sisters, walked and ate lunch together daily, and said 'Goodnight, I love you,' to each other every day." The two women "generally carried on a caring friendship," the lawyers representing the nursing home stated.

However, there was no shortage of warning signs to this tragic death. According to a person briefed by police investigators, the younger resident had repeatedly complained that her roommate had more visitors than she did and had threatened to kill her. In addition, care workers at the nursing home had months earlier described the younger roommate as being "at risk to harm herself or others." Furthermore, although the son of the deceased resident said that his mother never told him that she had been threatened by her roommate, he knew of the tension between them. His mother had apparently complained on multiple occasions to staff at the nursing home. The son also stated that in the hours leading up to his mother's death, the roommate had "several violent episodes." It began when the deceased resident asked a nursing assistant to move a table from the foot of her roommate's bed so that she could get to the bathroom. In response, the roommate got out of bed, screamed, "was verbally abusive and hit" the nursing assistant. It took two staff members to calm her down."[462] The son claimed that the staff left the roommate in the bedroom with his mother and never let him know there was a problem. He added, "The thing that wakes me up at night is thinking that if I had been called, I would have taken her home."[463] He said that he did ask a staff member whether his mother should be assigned a new roommate but "the staff member did not think there was a problem." He stated, "She should not have been living in that room with my mother." In addition, according to the lawyers representing the deceased resident, the roommate was moved to live with her because of an "argument with her previous roommate."[462]

Redirecting Residents While Meeting Their Needs

Redirect Residents with Impaired Judgment Related to Personal Safety

Many residents with middle- to late-stage dementia have lost their ability to recognize a safety hazard, evaluate their need for help, and/or call for help.[464] As suggested by Berry,[429] "Remember that the person may have lost the ability to judge between safe and unsafe conditions. Evaluate each situation and do not let the person be in a potentially dangerous position." Zillmann[465] explains that under conditions of high arousal, a person's cognitive abilities may diminish and as a result he or she may be less likely to perform higher-level cognitive processes, such as evaluating potential consequences of behavioral expressions labeled as aggressive. During these times, the person's ability to inhibit a physically aggressive response may be reduced, which increases the likelihood of an impulsive act such as pushing or hitting another person.

The following story[34] illustrates this challenge and how it can be prevented. A resident with dementia hit another resident who had schizophrenia and Alzheimer's disease. Four minutes after being hit, in the main activity room, the resident went to sit right next to the resident who had hit her. A recreation assistant noticed her in time and redirected her to a remote seat in the activity room, preventing another potentially harmful episode. This resident frequently did things (such as burping) that were very irritating for the resident, who on several occasions responded with verbal and physical threats toward her. Kathy Burns[25] describes certain residents as "provocative victims," people who may have dementia or a psychiatric condition and repeatedly exhibit irritating behavioral expressions. They may "egg on" the exhibitor, and their behavioral expressions may be intrusive and a trigger for a harmful physical response. Remaining as vigilant as possible, and promptly redirecting residents away from other residents with whom they have a history of incidents can be helpful in reducing these episodes.

Redirect a Resident from the Area

The goal of redirecting is to carefully, skillfully, and safely assist the resident to leave the area that causes her or his distress, anxiety, and behavioral expressions considered as aggressive. Direct care partners can say (while pointing to the direction they want the resident to walk with them), "Let's take a walk to see if that clears our heads a bit," or "Why don't we get a cup of tea to help us figure this out?"

The following story[34] illustrates one successful approach. A recreation assistant was leading a group activity. Ms. Harris was sitting next to Mrs. Kendall, who was talking continuously. At one point, Ms. Harris put her hand on Mrs. Kendall's mouth and said, "Would you shut up?" In response, Mrs. Kendall spat on the floor, threatened to stab her, and then grabbed and pushed her. The recreation assistant tried to convince Mrs. Kendall to come with him but she refused. An insightful private companion of a resident not directly involved in this episode asked Mrs. Kendall to come with him. She did. When asked how he managed to redirect her, he said that he told her quietly and calmly, "Just relax," and then he started talking with her about meals as he redirected her out of the room. He explained that he chose this topic as a way to calm her because he knew that her family owned a restaurant where she had worked for decades since she was a teenager and that she loved to talk about food. Knowing the resident's life history and using it skillfully and calmly proved to be very helpful in redirecting this resident away from the area and de-escalating this physical incident.

Divert to a More Pleasurable Activity or Change the Activity

Although various organized activities can have tremendous positive effects on residents with dementia, it is not uncommon to see that an activity clearly causes a resident or a group of residents to become distressed, angry, or engage in distressing behavioral expressions that are labeled as aggressive. The best recreation therapists[34] always have "plan B and C" activities ready with them (such as ideas, materials, or equipment) as part a proactive approach for these situations. When the recreation therapist senses that the activity does not work despite her or his efforts and that it leads to distress among residents, she or he can "switch gears" quickly and transition seamlessly into leading a different activity.

This anticipatory approach can be very effective in prevention of DHRRIs during activity periods. It can also help avoid the potential danger of having the therapist leave the residents unsupervised in order to go in search of alternative activity materials and equipment. In situations where, despite all efforts and activity changes, a resident with dementia continues to feel distressed or angry due the something irritating in the activity or otherwise, additional direct care partners will need to step in and assist the group leader by gently and quietly redirecting the resident away from the activity room. They could offer to spend some quiet time together with the resident, or they could offer headphones with his or her favorite music and songs which may assist in calming the resident down in a separate quiet location, such as her or his bedroom.[466]

Depending on the resident's ability to communicate verbally, after settling down a bit, direct care partners may want to try and understand from his or her perspective, or from others who were around when it happened, what may have caused him or her to become distressed. That said, as mentioned earlier, it is important to be sensitive and avoid questioning a resident with dementia who has already lost the ability to attribute meaning or have insight into his or her negative emotional states and behavioral expressions. Identifying the unmet needs, situational frustrations, and triggers underlying the resident's distress and anxiety can assist direct care partners in avoiding exposing the resident to similar situations during organized activity periods in the future. It is important to document these situational triggers in the resident's care plan and inform all other recreation therapists, direct care partners, and IDT members about them. At times, however, these approaches simply may not work. Berry[66] explains,

> When you are seeing someone who is getting visibly upset and they are crying and you as a caregiver are going up to that person and trying to distract them to do something else, you think you are helping by doing that but in the meantime you skip the step that is validating what you're seeing in that person . . . the emotion. Say, for instance, you are crying and I walk up to you and say, "Oh, come on, let's go over here and bake cookies," What does that make you feel like? I've just de-honored all of your emotions.

Invite the Resident to Take a Walk with You

A direct care partner could offer a resident involved in a DHRRI a quiet one-on-one activity that they could do together, such as having the resident's favorite drink or a cup of coffee away from the area where the distressing episode has occurred.[13] Without touching the distressed resident who is engaged in the episode, using a supportive, nonthreatening stance, direct care partners may want to keep their arm down slightly away from their body while holding their palm up (a universal sign of friendly invitation) and let the resident choose if he or she wants and is ready to accept the offer.[413] When appropriate and true, direct care partners could say: "Mrs. Allen, the flowers in our garden have started to bloom. I would *love* it if you could come with me to the backyard to see them together." When direct care partners are successful in encouraging a resident with dementia to come with them to another quiet and calm part of the care home or a secure garden, they enable the person to decompress the negative emotions and gradually regain their calmness.

Pay Attention to and Redirect Immobile Residents

Care employees need to pay special attention to residents whose mobility is impaired and may be unable to move quickly from the "line of fire" during DHRRIs. People in the area of the episode who cannot walk should be assisted to be moved to a safe location. It is important to recognize that even if these residents are not directly involved in the episode, they may feel threatened and even terrified, but they may not have the physical ability to leave the area for a safe place without assistance from direct care partners. Many residents are ambulatory, but they may have cognitive impairments and they may experience overwhelming fear and feel "paralyzed" and therefore be unable to remove themselves from the area. They will need reassurance, guidance, and/or assistance from direct care partners to leave the area safely and go to another part of the care home.

Protect the Unintended Target

There is a need to proactively redirect away residents with dementia who may unintentionally walk into the path of a resident engaged in the episode or stand too close to him or her in a way that may be perceived by that resident as intrusive and/or threatening.[78] In other situations, residents may try to assist in resolving the situation, get close to the residents involved in the episode, and in the heat of the moment may be pushed or struck in return by one of them. For example, a man with dementia tried to help a woman open the door to her apartment. The woman resident refused his assistance, and he pushed her down. Her fall resulted in a significant injury, and she died a couple of weeks later. Her family filed a lawsuit and reportedly won a $1.2 million settlement (Mark Anderson, personal communication, April 6, 2018).

Adapting and Adjusting

Use the "Take a Step Back" Technique

At times, when efforts to de-escalate a DHRRI simply do not work, direct care partners may need to stop what they are doing and take a deep breath, count to 5 or 10 slowly, and encourage themselves with reminders and affirmations that can help strengthen their awareness and confidence. For example, a care partner can say, "I have the power to cope with anything that happens right now." They can say a prayer in their hearts, "God, give me the patience to deal with this situation calmly." Then, they will want to observe the situation carefully and try their best to see it from the point of view of the resident with a serious brain disease who is doing her or his best to cope with a distressing, frustrating, or frightening situation.

If a Strategy Is Not Working, Try Something Else

Paul Raia, developer of Habilitation Therapy for people with dementia, asserts, "the person's behavior cannot be changed directly, only indirectly by changing either our approach technique or the person's physical environment."[261] Consistent with this observation is Teepa Snow's suggestion,[448] "If what you are doing is not working, STOP! Back off. Give the person some space and time. Decide on what to do differently. Try again!" That said, it is important not to leave residents with dementia alone without supervision during and shortly after their engagement in a DHRRI; frequent gentle check-ins and monitoring will often be required in the minutes and hours following the episode. If the resident prefers to be alone to decompress and calm down in his or her bedroom after an episode, that should be allowed, but only with close monitoring of roommates when the person shares the bedroom with another person and prevention of unwanted entry of other residents with dementia—particularly those who were engaged in the most recent or previous episodes in general and with the individual as well as those who tend to walk into other residents' bedrooms.

Consider Taking a Time Out and Trying Again Later

Allowing a cooling-down period can prove helpful, unless there is an immediate danger to residents, direct care partners, or others around that must be immediately addressed. That said, an adequate number of well-trained direct care partners will need to continue and carefully supervise the residents involved in the episode during the cooling-down period and be ready to promptly respond to any signs of distress or escalation. Many injurious and fatal resident-to-resident incidents have taken place minutes or an hour or even a few hours after an earlier episode with one or both residents. Often, there were clear warning signs that were not adequately addressed.

During the cooling-down period, direct care partners may want to consider using the breathing technique called centering.[63] This important but underutilized technique can enable them to regain a sense of composure and calm during stressful situations. It can assist them to clear themselves from any negative emotions, such as feelings of hurt, anger, frustration, or fear. Feil[63] explains, "It is crucial to release one's own emotions in order to be able to listen empathetically to another person and tune into her/his world." The centering technique takes about 3 minutes. To center yourself:[63]

1. Focus on a spot about 2 inches below your waist.

2. Inhale deeply through your nose, filling your body with air. Exhale through your mouth.

3. Stop all inner dialogue and devote all of your attention to your breathing.

4. Repeat this procedure slowly, eight times.

Once centered and more relaxed, direct care partners are more likely to be in a better position to fully accept and validate the underlying emotions, such as frustrations and fear, experienced by a resident engaged in a DHRRI. They can now return to the area where the episode took place—or is still taking place—and try to act as if nothing has happened. A restless, anxious, or fearful resident with dementia who senses that her direct care partner is calm, centered, fully present, and attentive is more likely to respond in a calm and cooperative way. That said, the cooling-down approach may not be helpful to a care partner whom the resident does not trust, such as due to negative interactions with her or him in the past or due to other reasons.

Assistance and Support for Direct Care Partners

Seek Help from Co-workers and Supervisors

One of the most helpful strategies for solving distressing behavioral expressions in residents with dementia is to find out who works well with the resident and how he or she accomplishes this.[341] Direct care partners who struggle to prevent or de-escalate DHRRIs are encouraged to ask a co-worker who they know has a close, trusting relationship with the resident involved in the episode to approach the resident and try and calm her or him down. In accordance, Snow[467] suggests that care employees look for an authority figure whom the person respects (such as a nurse, social worker, psychologist, doctor, or clergy person). In addition, many employees who are not direct care partners (such as dietary, housekeeping, maintenance, or front desk staff) have a close, trusting relationship with residents involved in DHRRIs, and they can often be very effective in calming them down. In my early study[13,34] in an assisted living residence, beyond one outstanding direct care partner, the only other employee who was able to calm an older woman in advanced Alzheimer's disease when she was angry or engaged in DHRRIs was the receptionist. No matter how upset the resident was, the second the resident saw her, her emotional state changed, and she quickly calmed down. Clearly, the receptionist's presence during these episodes was a precious preventive asset for this care home, especially during times when the trusted direct care partner was not working.

Involve Skilled Bystanders

Often, other people in the area of the episode can be helpful in the response to it (such as volunteers, private companions, family members or friends of residents, and other visitors). Renee Garfinkel[468] explains in the context of bullying among seniors,

> If people see this, they should get involved. Go to the staff. Speak up the same way you would if you saw it at a bus stop. Sometimes people aren't sure what to do because the resident who engages in a bullying behavior might be impaired, not functioning on all cylinders. But you need to get somebody to come and help.

The aforementioned suggestion does not apply in most situations with the majority of residents who have middle- to late-stage dementia who are bystanders during these episodes. By contrast, many residents without cognitive impairment and those with mild cognitive impairment or early-stage dementia are capable of speaking up effectively during and after DHRRIs. For example,[13] after witnessing a potentially harmful incident, a resident said, "This is a matter of serious concern. It happens very often and will be fatal." After another serious episode, the same resident said, "The residents were trying to avert a huge disaster." It is also not uncommon for residents to be the first ones to witness these episodes and report them to direct care partners, both in the public spaces of the care home and inside residents' bedrooms and bathrooms. In a significant portion of the injurious and fatal resident-to-resident incidents I reviewed over the years it was a witnessing resident who alerted the care employees to the episode as it was unfolding out of their line of sight.

IDT members should regularly encourage and instill in the care community an atmosphere where all people—residents, direct and indirect care partners, family members, private companions, volunteers, visitors, and others—feel comfortable and safe speaking up and reporting to direct care partners, supervisors, and managers what they have witnessed and voicing their expectations for a safe and respectful care environment for all the people who live and work in the care setting.

Promptly Notify Your Supervisor and the IDT

A study[332] examining CNAs' responses to resident-to-resident incidents (classified in the study as aggression) in five nursing homes found that CNAs seldom notified nursing supervisors or colleagues in other disciplines about these episodes. Only 5 of 97 CNAs reported notifying their nursing supervisors, whereas only 2 notified social services. A different study,[420] in 10 nursing homes, found a barrier for collaboration between nursing staff and social workers. Specifically, social workers reported that sometimes they were not notified of DHRRIs, or were not notified about them in a timely manner.

Direct care partners must inform the nursing supervisor and social worker about DHR-RIs, and when they think that DHRRIs may take place if no intervention is taken. As reported by housekeeping staff, "We notify before something escalates."[14] Tony Rosen and colleagues[14] found in their study that one of the most common approaches used by direct care partners to manage these episodes was to contact social workers. Given the possible inconsistency in the findings between this study and the aforementioned one, additional research is needed to determine the extent to which CNAs report episodes to social workers and supervising nurses in care homes. For many reasons, it is likely that the use of this notification practice will vary significantly across LTC homes and even across care homes operated within the same care complex. In either case, the role of supervising nurses, psychologists, and social workers should be integral to every care home's effort to address these episodes.

Robin Bonifas[420] conducted a study in ten nursing homes to identify assessment and intervention strategies used by social workers to address DHRRIs and the ways they collaborate with nursing staff to manage these episodes. Social workers especially make unique contributions to addressing this phenomenon, but other care professionals, such as well-trained psychologists and nurses, can also assist in implementing some of these care practices. Examples of social workers' contributions are the following:[420]

- Providing assessment approaches that consist of gathering information and applying knowledge of causal factors, for instance, careful investigation of contributing factors, triggers, and unmet needs through a series of ad hoc interviews with eyewitnesses and other key individuals who seem to have insight into what may have caused the episode

- Determining the psychological impact of these episodes on residents, through conversations with cognitively able residents about their overall feelings of security and safety, as well as observation of emotional states of residents with advanced dementia through their body language and facial expressions; knowing a resident's baseline psychological state was reported as essential to their ability to detect significant changes in emotional states and mood

- Assisting in the decision process regarding appropriate prevention strategies, such as by communicating with different direct care partners and nurses regarding strategies that best fit the resident's cognitive abilities, disabilities, and needs.

- Helping to keep the focus on preserving each resident's dignity, identity, and personhood, seeing her or his value as an equal citizen with human rights and proactively address her or his psychosocial and other unmet needs instead of using a biomedical approach and perceiving incidents as "behavioral problems" that need to be controlled

- Helping to ensure thoughtful roommate assignments—a critical component of prevention—by matching up residents evaluated as likely to get along and supporting and monitoring residents' adjustment to life with a roommate

- Communicating resident needs and preferences to care employees

- Providing psychosocial interventions considered "social work-specific," such as negotiating behavioral contracts with cognitively able residents, facilitating bedroom changes, and providing one-on-one supportive counseling to assist residents in adjustment to placement or to help them process feelings of loss that may have contributed to development of the distressing and harmful behavioral expressions, such as depression or fear of being abandoned by one's family

- Working with family members of residents involved in DHRRIs by supporting them emotionally, as many may feel anxiety, fear or guilt; educating them about causes of behavioral expressions among people with dementia; gathering information from them about potential causes and triggers as well as what they think might work best with the person based on their lifelong and intimate knowledge of him or her; and discussing issues related to roommates and any needed changes in bedroom assignment

Inform, Involve, and Seek Advice from Physicians

A study[469] in five nursing homes has shown that physicians and psychiatrists are seldom called to assist in prevention and management of DHRRIs. Timely consultation with physicians well trained in person-directed care practices and treatment approaches for residents with dementia could yield invaluable insights regarding the root medical, physiological, and functional cause(s) of residents' engagement in these episodes. Physicians can also inform the development of individualized prevention strategies to address the medical needs underlying the identified causes, such as in the area of treatment for pain, which is often a contributing factor for these episodes.

In addition, timely psychiatric consultation should be considered,[14] such as for re-evaluation of unhelpful effects of psychotropic medications on a resident's behavioral expressions, including short-term and long-term adverse side effects. Psychiatric assessment can help determine whether a change in medication(s) is warranted—for instance, medical indication for use; appropriateness of type of medication; dose, frequency, time of day of administration, duration of use, and need for discontinuation—in accordance with the latest evidence-based gradual dose reduction protocols. As importantly, the appropriateness of as-needed (PRN) psychotropic medications should be carefully assessed by attending physicians and psychiatrists during and shortly after DHRRIs when the physicians are at the care home and, when not present, on the phone.

The need to more closely and frequently involve physicians and psychiatrists in psychotropic medication consultations and management in the context of DHRRIs is based on studies demonstrating that many may be insufficiently involved. For example, a U.S. General Accounting Office report[470] found that, in close to half of 116 community living centers (formerly called VA nursing homes), "staff administered psychotropic medications as a restraint and beyond the scope of the physician original order (e.g., using psychotropic medications to calm residents before trying other non-pharmacological interventions to manage behavior)."

The Role of Security Personnel

When direct care partners and other IDT members struggle to de-escalate potentially dangerous resident-to-resident incidents, they may need to seek assistance from the care home's security personnel. However, the response of security personnel will only be as effective as their experience working with people with dementia, their level of specialized training in dementia-specific approaches and communication techniques, and their skill set in using DHRRI-specific prevention and de-escalation strategies in a safe way for all involved. Security guards should be encouraged by managers to take the time during routine care to visit with residents with dementia, get to know them, and build trust with them. This proactive practice may assist them later on in gaining cooperation from these residents during DHRRIs.

As importantly, in care homes where in-house security cameras are used in the public spaces of the care setting, such as hallways, dining rooms, activity rooms, and living rooms, security personnel who are trained, attentive, and vigilant may detect on their monitors that a DHRRI is about to take place or that one is already in progress. This can help direct care partners who may be busy providing personal care to other residents in another part of the care home. Using direct communication devices, the security personnel can alert direct care partners, nurses, a social worker, and managers to the exact location of the episode and who is involved, and share in real time any other pertinent information about the incident. They could also alert direct care partners to situations in which a resident with dementia is about to enter or has already entered the bedroom or bathroom of another resident. In alerting direct care partners in real time to these potentially harmful situations, security personnel can assist them in their efforts to prevent and de-escalate these episodes, which otherwise may remain unwitnessed. Preventing and de-escalating DHRRIs must be viewed as a care community–wide effort, and every person in the care home can contribute to its success.

Consider Calling the Police

A study conducted by Lachs and colleagues[6] found that serious resident-to-resident incidents were the most common (89%) reason the police were called to nursing homes in Connecticut; other reasons included residents with dementia leaving the care home unattended, theft, and alleged abuse by staff. Police officers may be called to nursing homes to help de-escalate and investigate DHRRIs. It is important to ensure that law enforcement personnel are well trained in understanding Alzheimer's disease and other forms of dementia as well as the varied human needs and rights of this population. They need to be trained in the use of dementia-specific communication techniques and skills for safe prevention and de-escalation of resident-to-resident incidents, including those considered aggressive and violent. It is also important to recognize that a subgroup of residents with serious mental illness (such as schizophrenia and antisocial personality disorder) may be involved in these episodes. Therefore, care employees and police officers must be trained in specialized approaches for interacting with these individuals, including the safe use of de-escalation techniques during potentially dangerous resident-to-resident incidents.

In order to help prepare police officers to respond when called to LTC homes where people with dementia live, dementia expert Teepa Snow developed a training program[471] called "Improving Emergency Services for Dementia Patients." This excellent 105-minute DVD for first responders such as police officers and medical emergency services personnel enhances understanding regarding various issues with direct relevance to DHRRIs. These include, among others, signs and types of dementia; disease stages; brain changes; limitations caused by dementia; issues related to abuse, neglect, and safety; and behavioral expressions, such as unwanted touching, impulsive behaviors, intrusion into personal space, and verbal and physical aggression. Through engaging role-modeling and participants' practice, Snow demonstrates effective dementia-specific approaches (such as validating the person's internal reality), effective interaction and communication techniques (use of visual cues, gentle nonthreatening physical guidance, and distraction and separation techniques during resident-to-resident incidents), suggestions for helping the person during medical emergencies, how to get the person who has difficulty following instructions to cooperate, and strategies to protect the safety of the person with dementia and others around. As importantly, Snow demonstrates *ineffective* approaches commonly used with this population and provides descriptions of their negative consequences.

Another helpful practice for owners and administrators of LTC homes is to invite police officers for special events and visits with residents with dementia during routine times, such as during special intergenerational events and celebrations. Getting to know the residents with dementia and their direct care partners, nurses, and social workers could assist police officers in interacting and collaborating with them more effectively during emergency and crisis situations, such as when they are called to assist in de-escalating resident-to-resident incidents.

10

Post-episode Strategies

*The way the environment responds to the person in
her or his attempts to have her or his needs met is likely
to influence future patterns of behavior.*

Benjamin Mast[409]

A critical but commonly overlooked component of any effective prevention program
aimed at reducing distressing and harmful resident-to-resident interactions (DHRRIs)
in long-term care (LTC) homes is the aftermath. Below is a description of strategies
that direct care partners and managers should consider implementing immediately or shortly
after these episodes. The practical insights learned from using a "360–degree" debriefing procedure, as well as detailed and skilled documentation and reporting, should be used after every
single DHRRI. Routine implementation of this procedure can assist in identifying critical
patterns underlying episodes and thus inform and improve future individualized prevention
efforts. In response to what is learned, for example, direct care partners can change or refine
existing personalized psychosocial strategies, avoid ineffective approaches or reinforcers, or implement other protective measures, such as in the areas of seating arrangement and roommate
assignment.

Direct care partners' responses and events that take place immediately or shortly after a
DHRRI often influence the nature, frequency, complexity, and severity of future episodes in
similar circumstances. Below are general strategies for addressing the residents' unmet needs
after episodes, followed by recommended procedures for care team debriefing and skilled documentation as the basis for future prevention efforts.

General Strategies

Reassurance, Reassurance, Reassurance

Thomas DeBaggio,[472] who lived with Alzheimer's disease, wrote, "I live on the edge of fear and
insecurity and I am filled with insecurity." Direct care partners must routinely and promptly
offer reassurance and emotional support to residents with dementia, including those who were
directly involved in a DHRRI as well as those who were not. Witnesses to these incidents may
become restless, anxious, or frightened afterward. The focus should be on validating each resident's emotional states, experiences, and perceptions of the situation and her or his subjective
reality, even when what the person with dementia says may be factually incorrect.

It is important to remember that many residents with Alzheimer's disease, especially those
with middle- to late-stage disease, may have difficulty regulating their emotions and calming
themselves down on their own. Direct care partners will want to enable residents to express
their frustrations, anger, and fear while showing genuine concern and empathy.[63] Julie Ellis and
colleagues[199] suggest providing support to all residents involved in a DHRRI by "listening to

each resident's interpretation of the events without blame or condemnation." Dementia expert Carly Hellen[460] suggests,

> A really important piece that is very often overlooked is going back to the resident when he is settled down. Telling him that he is okay. "Everything is okay, [name of resident]." "I am going to be here this afternoon." "We'll share the afternoon together." And reminding him that he is safe . . . because there is a part of him that really knows that he raised a problem and his adrenalin has been up and he is feeling badly about it.

Direct care partners will want to send residents with dementia a clear and consistent message that their sense of security and safety are of the highest priority. This could be done, for example, by demonstrating to them in action that these episodes are being taken seriously, and that measures are being promptly put in place, and will be frequently evaluated and improved upon, as part of an effort to prevent similar episodes from occurring in the future. The care home is the residents' home. Residents must feel safe in these care settings exactly as all other people in the community expect to feel safe in their homes. It is their basic human right.

Direct care partners need to pay special attention to the body language and facial expressions of those quiet residents who might be negatively affected by a DHRRI but who may not be able to verbally articulate their fear due to cognitive impairment, for example, a frail resident in middle-stage Alzheimer's disease whose hands are shaking from fear at the corner of the activity room. It is important to remember that certain residents with dementia may not remember what happened during an episode but they may be left with negative emotional states (such as anxiety and fear) for which they may not be able to attribute a cause. "A couple of times I had the daylights scared out of me," a resident reported.

Providing timely reassurance and emotional support to a resident who is anxious or fearful after being involved in or witnessing a DHRRI may include holding her or his hand—if wanted and tolerated by the resident—gently stroking it, and saying, "It's okay. You are safe here with me." Slone and Gleason[341] highlight the need to emphasize that direct care partners are here to keep the residents safe by saying, "I do not want you to be scared or to have to fight to protect yourself." As importantly, direct care partners will need to routinely reassure residents with dementia that they and the managers of the care home will do everything they can to prevent similar episodes from occurring in the future. The reassurance must be done in a way (body language, facial expressions, and tone of voice) that reflects an adult-to-adult reassurance, as opposed to a demeaning and infantilizing adult-to-child reassurance, which is disrespectful to the elder living with dementia and is also ineffective.

Offer Psychological "Holding"

Immediately after a DHRRI, direct care partners could consider offering "psychological holding" to residents with dementia. Tom Kitwood[64] describes this important but underutilized emotional supportive strategy in this way:

> To hold, in a psychological sense, means to provide a safe psychological space, a 'container'; here, hidden trauma and conflict can be brought out; areas of extreme vulnerability exposed. When the holding is secure a person can know, in experience, that devastating emotions such as abject terror or overwhelming grief will pass, and not let the psyche disintegrate. Even violent anger or destructive rage, directed for a while at the person doing the "holding," will not drive that person away . . . Psychological holding in any context may involve physical holding too.

In one case,[34] an older woman with vascular dementia was known to have experienced sexual abuse during her teenage years. Whenever a male resident with dementia mistakenly entered her bedroom at night at the secured dementia care home, she became terrified for her safety.

One night, after a male resident entered her bedroom and was quickly redirected back to his bedroom by direct care partners, she experienced a panic attack. She looked very frightened and was sobbing. A direct care partner she trusted entered her bedroom, closed the door behind her, and sat on the edge of her bed. She held the resident's hand and simply listened to her expressing her fear that she would be sexually assaulted by male residents. Centered and fully present, the care partner acknowledged her experience and validated her fears. She promised her that she would stay with her until she went back to sleep. She also told her that first thing in the morning, the interdisciplinary care team (IDT) would meet to discuss, develop, and implement a new strategy to prevent male residents from entering her bedroom. While listening to her, the direct care partner gently stroked her back and massaged her shoulders, something she knew the resident enjoyed. The woman leaned toward the direct care partner and hugged her. Gradually, after fully expressing her fears for several minutes, her crying lessened; she seemed calmer, breathed a sigh of relief, and fell asleep.

Direct care partners could also use psychological holding during routine care as well as when the resident is experiencing any form of great distress or fear, such as the perception of having been abandoned by family members and existential fear that arises from that, or during scary times when a resident's trauma from childhood or young adulthood is reactivated and experienced vividly by the person in the present.

Avoid Arguing and Accusing

It is not respectful or helpful to try reasoning, arguing, scolding, lecturing, patronizing, confronting, or placing blame on a resident with dementia after a DHRRI. Instead, as mentioned above, direct care partners must reassure residents that they are safe and valued. It is important to remember that certain residents with dementia have lost their ability to have insight into the reasons for their behavioral expressions, explain them, or recall what made them engage in them in the first place. Therefore, care employees must remain sensitive and careful during their communications with residents after DHRRIs. Insisting on questioning a resident with advanced dementia and demanding an explanation for his or her behavioral expressions is cruel and is likely to worsen his or her anxiety, frustration, and anger. Importantly, this kind of interaction limits direct care partners' ability to identify the root causes, unmet needs, and situational frustrations that led to the behavioral expressions and thus decreases their ability to prevent similar episodes from occurring in the future. Although some residents with dementia, especially those with early-stage disease, are able to report reliably on episodes they observed or were involved in recently, including what they believe were the causes and triggers for these episodes, many others are limited in their ability to do so. It is important to recognize that there is great variation across individuals with dementia in this ability and even within individuals over time—different parts of the same day, or over a period of months and years as their dementia progresses.

Assist with Locating Missing Personal Belongings

It is common for certain residents with middle- to late-stage dementia to take personal items from others and place them in different locations in the care home (such as in their own bedrooms and bathrooms). At times, the items taken may be placed in locations that make it difficult to find them; for instance, a resident may take a piece of clothing from another and place it underneath his or her mattress and then forget that he or she put it there. The removal of personal items from residents' possession can be a trigger of DHRRIs. If there is a tense episode after one resident has accused another of stealing, a thorough search for the lost item must be conducted promptly, even if direct care partners have already managed to separate the residents. If the unmet need underlying the accusation of theft is not addressed, it is more likely than not that a similar incident will reoccur between the two residents in the near future (within minutes, hours, or days). In the words of Julie Ellis and colleagues,[199] "If personal items are missing, staff should inform the resident that a room-by-room search will be conducted to locate the items and then ensure that this search happens promptly." When appropriate, the family of the resident with dementia will need to be notified about the missing item, including the effort made to locate it.

Without a prompt search and a return of the missing item or replacement with a similar—preferably identical—item, when possible, the post-episode strategy may remain incomplete and thus likely ineffective in preventing similar episodes from occurring in the future. For a detailed discussion of this common problem and a series of suggestions for addressing it, see the section "Perceived Theft of Personal Belongings" in Chapter 4.

Gather Practically Useful Information and Document the Episode Fully

The minutes and the hour or two immediately after the episode should be considered a critical time period for learning and improvement through a thorough collection of detailed, accurate, and practically useful information about the episode—especially the situational circumstances and sequence of events leading to it. To be successful, the process must be a well-coordinated interdisciplinary collaborative effort that is orchestrated skillfully by a qualified manager. The care team and managers must make every effort to speak with *all* the people who were present and saw and/or heard the episode. As explained by a social worker[420] in the context of DHR-RIs, "People depict things in different ways . . . that's why we try to get a witness statement from everyone possible, to piece together as much [of the events] that seem the same." Those people who were present in the area of the episode and who should be interviewed typically include the following:

- Residents who are cognitively capable of reporting; many are able to report important pieces of information when they are well into the middle stage of Alzheimer's disease, some even with more advanced stages of disease

- Direct care partners

- Nurses

- Non-direct care partners, such as housekeeping staff, dietary aides, and maintenance staff

- Social workers and psychologists

- Recreation therapists

- Managers

- Physicians

- Visiting family members and friends

- Volunteers and other visitors

Speaking with private companions, volunteers, family members, and other visitors who may have observed the episode can often be very helpful, as they may be the only ones who have witnessed these episodes; sometimes a DHRRI takes place in a public space while direct care partners are busy providing personal care tasks inside bedrooms. As noted throughout this book, although speaking with the people who saw the episode is a high priority, it is also important to speak with employees and other people who were at the care home during the hours and minutes *before* the episode occurred, given that many DHRRIs are influenced by events, interpersonal stressors, and triggers that have taken place earlier.

Identification of recurring patterns of stressors, situational frustrations, and triggers for DHRRI is fundamental for development of individualized preventative strategies that work in the long-term. As explained by Ellis[199] in the context of DHRRIs,

> It is only through reporting and documenting incidents that a process of discussion of appropriate strategies and relevant issues can occur, and it is through such discussions that appropriate interventions can be implemented and documented in the nursing care plan.

Under the direction of a qualified manager, direct care partners should follow up with as many people as possible to gather information about the possible causes, unmet needs, circumstances, interpersonal stressors, and situational triggers that led up to the DHRRI. They must also gather and document information about the nature of the behavioral expression itself. However, documenting only or primarily the nature of the behavioral expressions without documenting the circumstances and situational context in which they occur is a common missed opportunity for prevention. Consider, for example:

> Mr. Cohen hit Mrs. Smith in the face this afternoon.

A more complete, and more helpful, description is the following:

> Mr. Cohen hit Mrs. Smith in the face this afternoon after Mrs. Smith unintentionally but repeatedly blocked Mr. Cohen's view of the TV when she was walking in small circles with her walker—trying to find a place to sit—while his favorite program was on.

The latter description not only tells what happened and how it could have been prevented (by helping Mrs. Smith to a seat) but also how it can be prevented in the future.

In addition, documenting what happened immediately *after* an episode occurs is just as important. The reactions of care employees and all residents directly and indirectly involved, which could reinforce the behavioral expression, making it harder to de-escalate or prevent in the future) should be included. Furthermore, gathering information about what in residents' and direct care partners' reactions seemed to have been helpful in restoring calm and safety to all people in the area of the episode is obviously key for future prevention efforts.

Routinely Use a Behavioral Expressions Log

The Behavioral Expressions Log is a way of systematically and consistently documenting the circumstances surrounding and the nature of DHRRIs. Each log entry should include detailed descriptions answering the following questions, which could be summarized using the acronym "5WSOS":

- *When* exactly did the episode take place?

- *Where* exactly did the episode take place?

- *Who* was involved in the episode?

- *What* happened? Describe the sequence of events occurring *prior* to the behavioral expression, the nature of the behavioral expression itself, and what happened immediately *after* it occurred (for example, reinforcers).

- *Why* did it happen? Provide your best explanation of the cause and/or situational trigger of, or frustration leading to, the behavioral expressions.

- Describe the *strategy* or *strategies* used to address the episode (if any).

- Describe the *outcome(s)* of the intervention.

- Provide your *suggestion(s)* for future preventive strategies.

Over time, persistent use of this 5WSOS approach can enable direct care partners to identify underlying patterns (for example, temporal, spatial, or environmental circumstances
or triggering events, persons, or objects), which are key for informing the development and
refinement of individualized prevention strategies. Once a pattern is identified, a hypoth-
esis about its origin and a plan for a personalized prevention strategy should be developed.
This approach, which is a central component of a behavioral risk management program,
directly builds on the behavioral log approaches developed by leading dementia experts
Raia,[122] Zgola,[59] and Cohen-Mansfield and Schindel Martin.[204] An example of a behavioral
expressions log, including rationale and detailed instructions for using it, is presented in
the downloadable files available with this book at https://healthpropress.com (see p. viii for
access information). The Behavioral Expressions Log is the basic tool on which the Evaluation of Urgency of DHRRI Form, the Interdisciplinary Screening Form, and the Behavioral Expressions Prevention Plan Form should build (these latter assessment tools are also
described and available in the downloadable files). The Behavioral Expressions Log is the
foundation. If it is not used skillfully and consistently, the rest of the assessment building
blocks are unlikely to work, and important opportunities for prevention and de-escalation
of DHRRIs will remain limited.

Use the Resident's Care Plan to Document Effective and Ineffective Approaches

Getting into the habit of routinely writing descriptions of effective, partially effective, and
ineffective prevention and de-escalation psychosocial strategies in the care plans of residents
involved in DHRRIs (both exhibitors and residents on the receiving end) is likely to prove
invaluable in the long term. When direct care partners, other IDT members, and managers
regularly revise and read residents' care plans, they are in a better position to be aware of, as
well as improve and refine, existing prevention and de-escalation strategies.

Direct care partners can learn from their own experiences and those of other care professionals when there is consistent, habitual documentation. Strategies that worked can help
all care employees learn and build on them in future interactions with residents. Carefully
documenting those strategies that did not work or worked only partially is an effective means
of making sure they are not repeated. However, this practice can only work well in care homes
where managers are successful in instilling a culture in which direct care partners and all other
employees are not afraid to report on approaches and strategies that did not bring about the
desired preventive effects. If care employees fear that they will be reprimanded or disciplined
for documenting failed approaches, the potential for prevention of DHRRIs will likely remain
limited. As mentioned earlier, a strong culture of learning is critical to any successful risk-management program.

Strategies contained in residents' care plans should inform discussions during care plan
meetings in general and those held with residents and/or their close family members (cognitively intact residents and those with early-stage dementia should be regularly invited to
participate in these meetings). A community-wide approach, one that values residents and
family input, has the greatest potential to result in care plans that actually help the care home
in reducing these incidents and keeping residents safe.

Find an Appropriate Time and Place to Vent

After a distressing or harmful episode, direct care partners should be encouraged by managers
to take some quiet time to speak with a trusted co-worker or supervisor to express their frustrations and emotions and to receive support. They should be encouraged to share with their
co-workers or supervisors how they *felt* when the DHRRI occurred (e.g., "It was scary" or "My
hands were shaking"), what they *thought* when it took place (e.g., "I thought that he was going

to kill someone"), and how they feel now (e.g., "I feel better now but I don't know how we can continue this way. It happens every day. I am afraid that if we don't do something about it, someone is going to get hurt").

When speaking with these supportive individuals, direct care partners could seek out acknowledgment of their experience during the episode, reassurance, and emotional support. It is critical that they find an outlet—a safe place where they can ventilate and process their negative emotions, particularly after being involved in or witnessing a serious DHRRI. This enables care employees to decompress their negative emotions and therefore minimize the likelihood that they will carry these negative emotional buildups into their future interactions with residents, co-workers, supervisors, and family members of residents. In the words of a direct care partner who reflected on the value she sees in this practice,[430] "It helps me a lot when I can talk it over afterwards. When I can tell others what happened to me. I think that also teaches me how to get over it. Then I suddenly realize that it not only happens to me."

Post-incident Debriefing Procedures

The 360–Degree Approach

Lanza and colleagues[473] suggest that after a DHRRI occurs, the IDT should implement a 360–degree approach to understanding the episode by interviewing all of the relevant participants and observers for their perspectives on contributing factors, as described earlier in this chapter. In this way, a collaborative, community approach to preventing DHRRIs is encouraged, as all are seen as contributing to understanding, and therefore prevention, of such incidents.

To this end, several typically brief meetings should be held after each potentially harmful or harmful resident-to-resident incident. It is important to recognize that "near-miss" incidents are as important for learning and prevention as harmful incidents; when a resident pushes a frail resident away, the difference in factors leading to the pushed resident falling and sustaining and injury versus regaining balance and remaining steady on his or her feet is often minimal.

A separate meeting should be held with each resident involved in the episode. Another meeting should be held with other residents, especially those who were in the area and witnessed or heard the episode. Whether or not to hold meetings with residents with dementia will depends on their cognitive ability to recall and report on these episodes, a determination that should be made by the IDT based on adequate cognitive assessment. As noted earlier, when the right elder-friendly and dementia-friendly interviewing conditions are thoughtfully created, many elders with early- to middle-stage Alzheimer's disease are able to provide invaluable input into the circumstances surrounding DHRRIs.

In addition, a meeting should be held with the families of the residents involved, both the exhibitor and the one on the receiving end to the extent that that is possible and known—as described earlier in the book, it is not always straightforward or even possible to know who is truly the exhibitor and who is the one on the receiving end. Furthermore, a meeting of direct care partners is needed; this should include, at the very least, CNAs, nurses, a nurse supervisor, a social worker or psychologist, and a manager. A nurse practitioner and the attending physician should make every effort to participate in the meeting—in fact, they should be required to attend when the meeting addresses a serious and injurious episode. The latter meeting should include review and open discussion of the episode, based on its documentation in the Behavioral Expressions Log and residents' care plan. Topics discussed should include, among others, possible causes, contributing factors, unmet needs (such as emotional/psychological and medical needs), interpersonal stressors, situational frustrations and triggers, prevention and de-escalation strategies used, and suggestions for improvement in future strategies and (when appropriate) pharmacological treatments. Finally, these meetings and the decisions taken in them must be summarized and documented in residents' clinical records and care plans, including clear and concise instructions regarding specific measures and prevention strategies planned.

Promptly Consult with the Nurse Supervisor and Physician

The nurse supervisor and physician should be consulted immediately after any serious episode to evaluate whether first aid or medical treatment is needed for one or more of the residents involved. In fact, whenever possible, they should be notified about the episode while it is still taking place; their presence could not only allow them to assist the care employees in resolving the episode but their experience with the situation could also inform their decision-making process regarding future prevention efforts and/or treatment.

Lachs[203] suggests that when an incident results in physical injury, it is important to monitor the residents not only right after the incident but several hours afterward, especially in the case of head injury, where serious symptoms can sometimes appear hours after what seemed like only a minor injury. For example, a blood clot can form in the brain some time after a person's head is hit. It is important to emphasize that, in a significant portion of serious incidents, a resident sustains a head or brain injury due to direct hitting, with or without an object, by another resident, or after being pushed, falling, and hitting his or her head on the floor.[26,29]

In addition, the nurse supervisor and physician will need to promptly assess whether an underlying medical condition may have contributed to the episode (such as pain, constipation, or a urinary tract infection) and whether there is a need for a change in a resident's medications. In one case,[199] a resident with dementia who used a wheelchair suffered physical pain from a wound on her back that caused her to scream, "Ow! Ow!" These expressions led to several incidents with other residents who told her to "shut up." At one point, she and another resident began to hit, push, and curse each other. The other resident picked up a fork and repeatedly stabbed the woman on her arm. A CNA moved her to a distant corner of the room, which temporarily discontinued these episodes. However, to address the root cause (back pain) of the triggering event (screaming), assessment of the resident's back wound was needed to inform physical intervention and pain management, in this case, using pain medications.

Communicate with the Resident's Family

Inform the Resident's Family or a Legally Authorized Representative

Any potentially harmful or harmful resident-to-resident incident—whether the harm is physical, psychological, or sexual (or any combination of these)—should be reported promptly to the resident's close family members or legally authorized representatives so they will know about it and how the resident is doing. It is important to provide a *complete* and *reliable* report on what actually happened, including a description of her or his physical or psychological/emotional state during the episode, immediately after it occurred, and in the present. Soreff[78] adds,

> It is important that staff inform the family *before* they hear it from other sources. All too often a family member coming on a regular visit could be shocked to hear for the first time that their loved one had been attacked. This also gives staff an opportunity to tell the family the steps taken to ensure their loved one's safety.

The following tragic story[57] about a Korean War veteran who lived with Alzheimer's disease illustrates the importance of this recommendation. One evening after 9:00 p.m., he walked into another resident's bedroom and climbed into the empty bed. Moments later, the person whose bed it was, who also had dementia, walked in and beat him repeatedly with his cane.

That night and over the next 4 days, direct care partners told his wife that the man had merely fallen and needed to go to the hospital for x-rays. During another phone conversation, the wife asked if everything was okay with him; the social worker reportedly said yes. The wife asked if she should drive the hour from her home to visit him, and a nurse reportedly said that he had no broken bones and was doing fine. A couple of days later, the wife went for a visit, and when she walked into his bedroom she was shocked to see his injuries. She reported, "I walked into the room and gasped. He was black and blue all over, swollen, and on oxygen. I ran out of the room and got a nurse." The nurse told her that her husband had fallen. She approached a direct care partner and said, "He couldn't have possibly gotten that from a fall." The direct care partner's reaction was: "No one told you? He was beaten." She then learned that direct care partners had found him in a fetal position on the floor, unconscious and bleeding, with the man still beating him. The wife watched her husband grow weaker by the day until he took his last breath several days later.

One has to wonder whether she could have done something to save her husband's life had she been informed during the first report to her—4 days prior to her visit—that his severe injuries were due to beating by the other resident. The deep and lasting psychological trauma experienced by his wife due this untruthful report should encourage owners, administrators, and all care employees in LTC homes to always tell the truth when communicating with family members in general, but especially right after serious resident-to-resident incidents.

Often, family members may feel embarrassment or guilt upon being told that a resident with dementia—their loved one—has engaged in behavioral expressions that are harmful or considered as "aggressive." It is important to be sensitive when communicating about this and reassure the family members that the cognitive disabilities of their relative, combined with distressing factors in the social and physical environment, often contribute to these episodes—unless of course the IDT determines that a physiological or medical condition caused it. That said, it needs to be recognized that some residents without cognitive impairment, and those with early-stage dementia, as well as individuals living with a serious mental illness, may have a lifelong propensity and/or the current ability to deliberately cause physical harm to another resident. Even with these individuals, caution and sensitivity should always be practiced before labeling a person as aggressive, violent, or abusive, especially when speaking with his or her family members. It can be deeply painful and extremely difficult for family members to hear such labels used to describe their relatives.

Being careful not to blame residents with dementia involved in DHRRIs is critical, as the majority are trying their best to cope with situational and interpersonal stressors with their remaining cognitive and physical abilities while living with a serious brain disease. This reassurance may also be helpful in gaining the family's cooperation and seeking out their invaluable insights into possible causes, unmet needs, or situational triggers that may have led to their relative's behavioral expressions, as well as suggestions for developing individualized strategies for preventing similar episodes from occurring in the future. By contrast, being quick to label a resident as aggressive during communications with family members may not only make them feel bad or guilty, but it may cause them to react defensively while trying to protect their loved one's identity, dignity, and personhood. This, in turn, may limit the family members' ability to share useful insights for prevention and de-escalation of future episodes.

Seek Input from Family Members

For a resident engaged in DHRRIs, direct care partners and managers should try and learn from those in close relationship with the person about possible causes or triggers of the behavioral expressions and explore with them ways to prevent similar episodes from occurring in the future. Family members often hold invaluable information about the person, such as personality traits, coping style, likes and dislikes, what tends to upset and calm the person, and remote triggers from the distant past, including traumatic experiences in early life (such as being physically or sexually abused or suffering a war trauma); some of this key information may be unknown to direct care partners.

Cindy L. Kincaid,[166] a regional LTC ombudsman for the Centralina Area Agency on Aging (Charlotte, NC), has this advice for direct care partners:

> Really recognize that family needs to be included as a full partner in care. Families have dealt with these residents for an extended period of time before they ever came to the tough decision to place them in the special care unit. Allow families the opportunity to really have the input into what works well for their family member and what doesn't. Make sure they have the opportunity to be included in all the components [of care planning]. This often can reduce difficult behaviors and staff getting frustrated with residents when the care they provide is counterproductive to what the family has known works and doesn't work.

The value that input from family members can have in resolving one resident's fear of another can be surprising. Lisa Gwyther[186] shares a situation in which the family was able to identify that the janitor at the care home looked like a man who had been very aggressive toward their relative. Every time he would appear with a mop, the relative, who had vision deficits, feared the janitor was going to attack him with it. Being sure that the janitor cleaned the area when the resident was in another part of the building reduced his anxiety, fear, and yelling.

Consider a Change in Seating Arrangement

Problems with seating arrangements, such as in the dining room of the care home, are a frequent contributing factor to engagement of residents with dementia in DHRRIs, such as due to personality clashes, tense arguments, a resident mistakenly thinking that a chair and/or table belongs to him- or herself, residents taking food from tablemates, or residents with early-stage dementia not tolerating verbal or behavioral expressions exhibited by residents with more advanced disease. This common problem is discussed in detail in Chapters 4 and 9.

A change in the seating arrangement might be needed in the dining room, activity room, or other locations where DHRRIs repeatedly occur.[13] The task of changing a seating arrangement, however, is not always straightforward. In a "domino effect," designating a new seat and/or table for a particular resident frequently requires a change in seating for one or more other residents; this will depend on a number of factors, such as dining room size, number of dining rooms, number of tables available, and number of residents using each table.

For instance, resident B may need to give up his or her seat for resident A, and a different table and seat now must be assigned for resident B (meaning that another resident may need to move). After a rearrangement, the IDT should conduct a careful and ongoing evaluation of the new seating to avoid the possibility that, in the effort to prevent DHRRIs involving resident A, resident B ends up sitting with residents with whom he or she does not get along or that they are incompatible in some other way, which may negatively impact resident B's and/or his new tablemates' mealtime experience. Even when no resident has to move from the table to which resident A moves (as when there is an open seat at that table), direct care partners will need to be aware of the possibility that the social dynamic between the new tablemates may change in a negative way, which could result in new DHRRIs.

In one case, a CNA reported[34] about a woman with late-stage dementia, "She is picky about her place in the dining room, and if you change her place it will be a disaster. . . . She starts cursing or takes her plate and goes to another table." She added that the woman also would get upset when the people with whom she usually sits are moved. This woman, who was a participant in my early study, had a long history of engaging in verbal and physical incidents with other residents, often as the exhibitor. The CNA's concern for potential harm was real. Many residents with dementia may be very sensitive to any changes made in their seating arrangement.

Whatever the new seating assignment is, there is a need to make sure that all employees in direct regular contact with residents (including float staff and external agency staff) on different shifts, days, and weekends are aware of the change and implement it *consistently*. An experienced CNA[34] at a care home for people with dementia reflected on the problem caused by inconsistency in the seating arrangement in the dining rooms across breakfast, lunch, and dinner, as well as across days, shifts, weekdays versus weekends, and across different team leaders. She said that this inconsistency creates confusion for the residents and causes them to become upset, as it makes it harder for them to locate their pre-designated seats (a significant portion of residents with middle- to late-stage dementia experience visuospatial disorientation and wayfinding difficulties). She added that the inconsistent seating arrangement is confusing also for her and her co-workers and makes their job harder. In general, consistency in seating arrangements often helps in reducing tense arguments and DHRRIs that can occur, for example, when two residents with dementia insist that a particular seat in the dining room belongs to them (a common trigger of DHRRIs). When changes are needed, it is important to carefully consider each person who may be affected by them, and then to apply the changes consistently and with careful monitoring and adequate documentation.

Consider Changing a Resident's Bedroom

When incidents reoccur between roommates, or even when there is a single serious incident between them, the IDT should consider the possibility of a change in the roommates' assignment. It is important to inform and consult with the residents about their preferences, when cognitively capable, and with their close family members a sufficient time prior to the intended change. In addition, nursing homes must adhere to the following requirements in the federal nursing home regulations (effective November 28, 2017):

> Residents have the right to receive written notice, including the reason for the change, before the resident's room or roommate in the facility is changed. Moving to a new room or changing roommates is challenging for residents. A resident's preferences should be taken into account when considering such changes. When a resident is being moved at the request of facility staff, the resident, family, and/or resident representative must receive an explanation in writing of why the move is required. The resident should be provided the opportunity to see the new location, meet the new roommate, and ask questions about the move. A resident receiving a new roommate should be given as much advance notice as possible.

In addition, under federal regulations,[32] the resident also has a right to refuse to transfer to another room in the facility, if, among other reasons, the purpose of the transfer is solely for the convenience of staff. Readers are strongly encouraged to consult and adhere to other requirements pertaining to this right.

That said, if the IDT and administrator determine, based on careful assessment, that there's imminent risk of serious harm (serious bodily injury or death) to one or both roommates if they were to continue and share the same bedroom, the bedroom change will need to be implemented urgently, and one of the residents will need to be reassigned a new bedroom and/or roommate. However, every effort must still be made to consult and notify the resident about it (if cognitively able) and her or his family—prior to the change, if possible—especially when the resident is cognitively unable to be consulted and informed about the bedroom change.

Careful attention needs to be given to the selection of a new bedroom and the thoughtful matching of a new roommate for the resident who is moved out of the shared bedroom where the DHRRIs have taken place. This is often a complex task given the limited space available in other bedrooms, especially in care homes with high occupancy rates, combined with the fact that one bedroom change could lead to a need for a new bedroom change due to incompatibility of certain pairs of residents. Needless to say, the task often becomes even more challenging when the need for the roommate reassignment and bedroom change is urgent to protect residents' safety.

In certain emergency circumstances, a temporary bedroom assignment may need to be considered, to separate the roommates *before* harm is caused, but then after a short period of time of careful IDT assessment, a permanent bedroom assignment could be determined. This should be done in close consultation with the resident when cognitively capable and/or her or his family when appropriate. Enhanced emotional support, guidance, cueing, reassurance, and monitoring are needed during the temporary period, even if it spans only minutes or hours instead of days, especially with residents with middle- to late-stage dementia for whom any bedroom change can be very distressing, disorienting, and challenging to cope with and adjust to.

When at all possible, the assignment of a new bedroom to a resident due to conflicts within a shared bedroom should take into consideration the physical distance of the new bedroom from the old one. A farther away bedroom, as opposed to one located only two or three doors down the hallway, can sometimes decrease the likelihood that the two residents with dementia will interact with each other in general or enter each other's bedroom after the bedroom change. The routine walking routes each of these residents tends to follow and the frequency at which these routes tend to intersect spatially and temporally will also have an impact.

When a temporary or permanent bedroom change has been implemented, it is important for all care employees to stay aware of the fact that certain residents with dementia will try to return to their old bedroom after being assigned to the new one; this may occur in the minutes, hours, days or even weeks after the bedroom change. While living in his first nursing home, a resident with Alzheimer's disease, whose story[57] was told earlier in this chapter, was moved to another bedroom to allow a prisoner to use his bedroom. Shortly after the change, the resident returned to his previous bedroom, where he was attacked and beaten by the new resident.

Private Bedrooms

As recommended in Chapter 4, a substantial portion of DHRRIs would likely be reduced if more LTC homes would shift toward constructing the vast majority of the bedrooms and bathrooms as private living spaces. Legislation at the state and federal level, such as the one implemented in British Columbia,[141] could go a long way toward not only keeping a higher number of residents with dementia safe but also realizing their human right for privacy and dignity; residents' bedrooms and bathrooms are their last frontier of privacy in nursing homes and assisted living residences, and these settings are their homes.

Empirical evidence from research studies on the deadly effects of COVID-19 transmission between roommates could lend further support for the need to commit to this paradigm shift in nursing homes and in assisted living residences that have not yet made this sorely needed transformation. The deeply scary and traumatic experiences of residents who had to face the possibility of sharing a bedroom with a roommate with COVID-19 have been described in media reports.[474,475] One simulation study of COVID-19 outbreaks in LTC homes in Ontario, Canada,[270] found that 31% of infections and 31% of deaths "could have been prevented if all Ontario LTC residents had single rooms."

Carefully Consider Using Temporary Seclusion as a Last Resort

An extreme protective measure is a temporary involuntary confinement of a resident alone in a safe room or area from which he or she is physically prevented from leaving. The room needs to be one that is designed in a way that enables direct care partners to closely supervise the resident for the entire duration of the seclusion, such as through a secured window or small observation window within a door. Before the resident arrives, the predesignated room must be cleared of all objects that could be used to harm him- or herself or others.

Seclusion in the context of resident-to-resident incidents may only be used for the containment of dangerous and violent behavioral expressions that cannot be discontinued using other psychosocial and pharmacological measures. It could be used in those rare emergency situations to ensure the immediate safety of the resident, other residents, care employees, visitors, or others, and it must be discontinued at the earliest possible time when the IDT, in close consultation with the administrator, director of nursing, and attending physician, determines that it is safe to do so. This measure should be used as a last resort and only for the shortest period necessary to protect the safety of the resident and others around him or her; direct care partners and managers need to be aware that residents with dementia have the right to be free from seclusion, of any form, imposed as a means of coercion, discipline, or retaliation by care employees.[476]

Residents with dementia, serious mental illness (such as schizophrenia), or medical or physical conditions requiring close medical supervision *must be constantly supervised* while in seclusion to ensure the protection of their own health and safety as well as that of all others around the secluded area. As importantly, the emotional and psychological well-being of residents in seclusion must be constantly monitored; seclusion can cause these individuals serious emotional distress, fear, suffering, trauma, and harm. An explanation, ongoing reassurance, emotional support, and frequent reminders must be offered to the resident in seclusion to minimize the emotional distress as much as possible while in temporary seclusion.

Close family members of the resident in seclusion must be immediately notified about the decision to place the individual in temporary seclusion, including a detailed report regarding the reasons leading to the last resort decision. The IDT should also discuss and consult with the family about psychosocial approaches and strategies that could be used to prevent the person's engagement in similar incidents in the future. They should be invited to the care home to emotionally support their relative and work closely with the care team on developing a revised care plan that will enable him or her to experience the highest practicable well-being and safety for all involved.

For important details about the requirements for implementing this extreme procedure, readers are strongly advised to consult with the latest guidelines from the Centers for Medicare & Medicaid Services. Federal and state regulations and guidelines related to seclusion may change over time, so the owner, administrator, director of nursing, and IDT members will need to consult the latest guidance and best practices, as well as the relevant state regulations governing the care home. Adherence to the latest regulations and guidelines will increase the likelihood that the safest and least restrictive seclusion strategy is implemented and that the care home is in full compliance with federal and state regulations.

Comply with External Reporting and Investigation Requirements

It is the responsibility of the administrator or her or his designee to ensure that a timely, detailed, complete, and truthful written report on any serious resident-to-resident incident and its thorough internal investigation is submitted to the relevant state survey agency and, when applicable, to law enforcement, as required in the state and federal regulations governing the care home. Unfortunately, it is not uncommon for some care homes to ignore these requirements. For example, in the tragic death of one resident with Alzheimer's disease,[57] an investigator from the state Department of Health found the nursing home had not properly notified the agency about his injurious beating.

Not reporting on serious incidents (such as those that put residents at risk of physical harm), incomplete reports, and delays in submission of such reports to the state survey agency often compromises its ability, and local law enforcement's ability, to promptly and effectively investigate these episodes. This, in turn, limits important opportunities to gain insights into the causes and triggers of the episode and ensure that appropriate preventive measures and corrective actions are taken as soon as possible to protect residents with dementia from harm during future incidents in similar circumstances.

Lack of reporting, delayed reporting, incomplete reporting, and unreliable reporting may also limit the ability of residents and their family members to hold accountable those responsible for these injurious and deadly incidents. For example, a delay in external reporting often compromises regulatory and law enforcement agencies' ability to substantiate allegations, such as of neglect of supervision contributing to injurious incidents; obtain necessary evidence; and build a case for prosecution against the care home (e.g., when it has neglected to protect one resident from another who has a history of behavioral expressions considered as aggressive) or against a resident without cognitive impairment who may have intentionally harmed another resident.

For residents whose physical and/or cognitive functions are already in significant decline, allowing too much time to pass without reporting it to the state survey agency after an incident makes it harder to establish an accurate account of what happened and the factors that led to it. In addition, these residents' ability to communicate verbally may have deteriorated, physical injuries may have changed and/or healed since the incident occurred, threats of retaliation against a resident could have been made, and evidence from the scene may have been tampered or removed. For these and other reasons, a timely written report and thorough internal investigation of serious incidents submitted to the state survey agency must be considered the standard of care.

Federal and state survey agencies must use strong enforcement measures to ensure that the LTC home is in compliance with the applicable reporting requirements. In the words of the commissioner of health of the state of Minnesota, "Our protections in law are only as good as the enforcement capabilities."[477] Without adequate reporting and enforcement, the state survey agencies' ability to realize its mission to protect vulnerable and frail residents' right to live in safe LTC environments will remain limited.

Acute Treatment Options

In extreme circumstances in which immediate physical harm to residents or others could result (or may already have), and when all other psychosocial approaches and appropriate pharmacological treatments have been tried and have failed, the administrator and director of nursing may need to consider transferring the resident exhibiting the dangerous behavioral expressions to a psychiatric hospital or neurobehavioral unit for evaluation and acute treatment. Power[49] observes and warns, however, that in many cases,

> An acute care hospital is not a "transformed" environment. The person's aggressiveness will be rapidly "controlled" through a combination of restraint and sedation. This means that even though the individual's aggression is halted, little else will be done to identify the underlying cause or help him or her to reintegrate successfully back into his living environment. Therefore, this approach is for true emergencies only and will not help you to provide a long-term solution.

Well before the person with dementia returns to the care home, the administrator, director of nursing, and key members of the IDT should carefully review and evaluate the discharge summary and recommendations provided by the interdisciplinary care team of the psychiatric hospital or neurobehavioral unit where the person has been evaluated and treated. A conference call should be held with the care team of the discharging care setting prior to the person's discharge to ensure that the observations and recommendations are fully understood by the administrator and IDT of the LTC home.

This review and the preventive and treatment insights gleaned from the discharge summary should inform the development of a revised individualized care plan, and the IDT should consider all or part of the recommendations contained in the discharge summary as potentially useful in enhancing the emotional well-being and safety of the resident, other residents, and care employees. It is important to work closely with the resident when cognitively capable and not distressed by the process, and/or his or her close family members when appropriate, on development of the new or revised care plan during the readmission process to the LTC home, as they may have insights and suggestions that could make the new prevention plan more effective.

Once the new or revised care plan is developed, the administrator or director of nursing needs to make sure that all direct care partners and all other employees, such as housekeeping, kitchen staff, and maintenance staff are informed about it in a timely manner, or at least by the time of readmission. Each care employee needs to know what her or his specific role and tasks are and how they fit into and support the overall individualized prevention strategy. In the days, weeks, and months after the readmission, the administrator and director of nursing must continuously verify that everyone in direct regular contact with the resident—including any float staff or external agency staff—the resident (when cognitively capable), and/or his or her family member are fully informed and on the same page regarding the revised care plan and what their roles are in implementing it. The same must apply to any further modifications and revisions made in the care plan going forward.

It should also be the responsibility of the administrator or the director of nursing to require and verify that all direct and non-direct care partners and managers read the discharge summary and the revised care plan, including any further modified versions, and initial them to indicate that they have done so *before* their first work shift after the resident's return to the LTC home. A subgroup of residents returning from psychiatric hospitals and neurobehavioral units to LTC homes may experience substantial emotional distress as they try to cope with the adjustments to life at the care home. Some of these people will engage in DHRRIs within the first few minutes, hours, days, and weeks after readmission. That is why having a new and well-thought-out preventive care plan in place by the end of the readmission process—one that all involved are informed about—is critical to the safety of everyone.

Successful implementation of this process can assist the IDT in improving the support and care provided to the resident, meeting his or her psychological and medical needs, decreasing his or her frustrations, and ultimately reducing his or her engagement in DHRRIs and keeping everyone safe.

Alternatively, if after reviewing the discharge summary and recommendations, the administrator and director of nursing determine that the LTC home does not have the ability to care for the resident in a safe way, for all involved, they may need to consider the possibility of recommending the person and/or his or her close family a more suitable LTC setting. However, given that the care setting is going to be the person's home, such a high-stakes decision about this major life event must be done in good faith, only after thorough, well-documented assessment by the IDT, and in compliance with the requirements in the care home's state and federal regulations pertaining to transfers, discharges, and discharge planning. Eric Carlson, directing attorney, Justice in Aging, adds (in the context of CMS–certified nursing homes),[478]

> In planning for discharge, residents and their advocates should be vigilant to ensure that necessary services are in place when the resident moves from the facility. The facility shares responsibility for identifying and securing the assistance that the resident will need.

Avoid Wrongful Evictions and Implement Adequate Discharge Plans

According to federal nursing home regulations, a "resident has the right to reside and receive services in the facility with reasonable accommodation of resident needs and preferences except when to do so would endanger the health or safety of the resident or other residents" (Resident Rights, 42 C.F.R. 483.10[e][3]). Although certain transfers and discharges are warranted, it is not uncommon for LTC homes to improperly evict residents such as those with dementia because the IDT considers them to be "difficult" in general or due to their engagement in resident-to-resident incidents. According to the National Consumer Voice for Quality Long-Term Care,[479]

> The threat of transfer or discharge from a nursing home can be both frightening and stressful for residents and their families. Too often, a facility may respond to resident's difficulties or increasing need for care or repeated questions or complaints from family members by attempting to transfer or discharge a resident.

Robyn Grant, public policy director of this advocacy organization, explains,

> A lot of individuals, residents, and families, if they're told, "You have to find another home," just accept what the people in authority tell them and don't think they have any choices. They may not know that they have rights to challenge that eviction.

Under the new federal nursing home regulations, there are only six legitimate reasons for transfer and discharge of a resident from a CMS–certified nursing home.[478] These include the following:

1. The resident's needs cannot be met (this reason applies only if the resident's needs cannot be met in a nursing home generally, for example, if the resident needs placement in a subacute unit or locked psychiatric ward); a nursing home cannot use its own inadequate care as a justification for eviction under this reason.

2. The resident no longer needs the nursing home services.

3. The safety of other residents is endangered due to the clinical or behavioral status of the resident.

4. The health of others is endangered.

5. Resident's nonpayment but only if the resident does not submit the necessary paperwork for third-party reimbursement (such as Medicaid).

6. The nursing home closes.

The federal nursing home regulations require, in part, that before a nursing home transfers or discharges a resident, it must notify the resident and the resident's representative(s) of transfer or discharge and the reasons for the move in writing in a language and manner they understand. Most discharge notices must be given at least 30 days prior to the discharge date. Residents and their families have the right to appeal the decision and must do so before the date of discharge. The nursing home must also send a copy of the notice to the state office of ombudsman for long-term care.[478,479] When residents receive a discharge notice, they can contact the state office of ombudsman for LTC to receive information about their rights and the ways in which these rights could be protected.

According to the National Consumer Voice for Quality Long-Term Care and Justice in Aging,[478] for evictions based on a nursing home's supposed inability to meet a resident's needs, the nursing home must document the "specific resident need(s) that cannot be met, the facility attempts to meet the resident's needs, and services available at the receiving facility to meet the need(s)."

According to the aforementioned national advocacy organizations, it is important to limit the nursing home's ability to "dump" a resident at a hospital. In this form of mistreatment, in an effort to evade eviction safeguards, some nursing homes effectively evict residents by refusing to readmit them from hospitalizations. Now, with the new federal nursing home regulations, a nursing home must comply with transfer and discharge procedures and give a hospitalized resident an opportunity to appeal, when the nursing home claims that the resident cannot return. When the nursing home has decided to discharge the resident while the resident is still hospitalized (a "facility-initiated" discharge), the nursing home must send a notice of discharge to the resident and her or his representative, and must also send a copy to the office of ombudsman for LTC. For any other types of facility-initiated discharges, the nursing home must provide notice of discharge to these three parties at least 30 days prior to the discharge or as soon as possible. Additional requirements (such as those pertaining to emergency transfers and resident-initiated transfers) can be found in the CMS Survey and Certification Letter/ Guidance (May 12, 2017) *and* in the most updated guidance related to transfer and discharge released by CMS (such as CMS waivers during COVID-19 emergency period).[480]

Under certain circumstances, nursing home residents have a right to have their bed saved for them when they are hospitalized (also called bed-hold rights). These rights are established in the federal nursing home regulations. A useful description of bed-hold rights and current federal requirements pertaining to nursing homes (including, among others, types and timing of notices, "therapeutic leave" with family and friends, and right to appeal) can be found in the Issue Brief entitled *Return to Facility After Hospitalization* (developed by the National Consumer Voice for Quality Long-Term Care, the Center for Medicare Advocacy, and Justice in Aging). However, CMS requirements and guidance regarding bed-hold rights may differ, for example, during pandemics and other emergency conditions, and thus it needs to be consulted until these periods and emergency declarations discontinue.

In general, the nursing home must give the resident a notice of its bed-hold policy, and it must allow the resident to return to the next available shared ("semi-private") bedroom; it must be the resident's previous bedroom, if available. Transfer and discharge are not permitted while appeal is pending, without documented endangerment to health or safety of resident or others.

It is important to point out that owners and administrators of nursing homes are responsible for consulting with and adhering to the new federal regulations for nursing homes (which are more detailed than described above) and the relevant CMS Interpretive Guidelines related to transfer and discharge of residents.

How does a resident challenge the assertion that their condition or behavioral expressions presented danger to others as we think about the reasons for transfer and discharge? Eric Carlson, directing attorney, Justice in Aging, suggests,[481]

> You put evidence that the person is not a danger or demand that the facility present [its] evidence that supposedly shows that the person is a danger. In my experience, a lot of these cases are overblown. You've got a resident who is physically frail with Alzheimer's that lashes or swings his or her arms . . . that sort of thing. The point is to put the onus back on the facility to back up the allegations, to emphasize that facilities are set up or should be set up to care for people with dementia. Also, look back on the care planning process . . . oftentimes there is a deficit there (such as the nursing home's failure to address the underlying problem). The first response in these situations should be care planning . . . to try to figure out and find solutions instead of a facility moving to involuntarily transfer or discharge first. That's getting things backwards.

Nursing homes and assisted living residences are the homes of people living with dementia. It is of utmost importance that we cherish and protect their human right to live in these care homes as required by federal and state regulations. The practice of wrongful involuntary discharges of these individuals is a violation of this right. Moving vulnerable and frail elders with dementia from the care home to another care setting can often be traumatic for them and their families. We must use our best clinical judgment when making this high-stakes decision—a decision that often results in far-reaching psychological, functional, and medical consequences for these people. As described earlier, there are unique circumstances when well-planned discharges and transfers are appropriate, but we should always try to imagine how we would feel if someone were to try and evict us from our own homes.

In Closing

If there are three words I want you to remember from reading this book, they are:

> *Fighting for Dignity*

If there are three things I hope you'll take away from reading this book, they are the following.

1. In the vast majority of distressing and harmful resident-to-resident interactions, people living with dementia "fight" with each other in an effort to preserve their dignity. In the words of Joanne Koenig Coste, "Alzheimer's disease doesn't take the person's dignity away. We do." Next time you notice a resident with dementia engaged in an episode with another resident, observe it carefully, and try to look at it through the lens of *dignity*. That is, do your best to discover the ways in which the situation threatens this person's dignity and the ways in which he or she is trying to preserve it.

I guarantee you that if you are able to be centered, attentive, and fully present, and if you dedicate enough time to this effort, in most situations the insights you will gain from direct observation will open up new and exciting opportunities for proactively meeting residents' needs and thus more effective prevention of these episodes, while preserving these individuals' dignity.

2. Only a very small subgroup of elders living with dementia engage in behavioral expressions that are truly aggressive. The vast majority of these individuals are not aggressive. This biomedical term is often unhelpful because it is not only inaccurate in most situations but it is also labeling, and deeply stigmatizing. It prevents us from seeing the whole person behind the dementia. It limits our ability to see that people living with dementia have the same human needs we all share. They live with a cognitive disability caused by a serious brain disease. They are trying their best to use their remaining cognitive and physical abilities to cope with factors in their social and physical environments they often experience as distressing, frustrating, and frightening. For far too long, we have been inadvertently dehumanizing people with dementia when we commonly but mistakenly labeled them as "aggressive." I am afraid that this and the other biomedical and harmful terms "violent" and "abusive" reflect more on us than on people living with dementia. The time for a paradigm shift is long overdue.

I would like to ask you: How would you feel if you had a serious brain disease, could not express yourself verbally, and were forced to share close quarters in a care home with 30 other residents with dementia 24 hours a day, 7 days a week, 365 days a year? How would you feel if other residents with dementia repeatedly invaded your personal space or entered your bedroom or bathroom? How would you feel if you have not gotten along with your roommate for months and your desire for a bedroom change is not happening? Then, when you can no longer stand it, reach a breaking point, and express your deep frustration and anger, you learn that one of the care employees described you as an "aggressive" or "violent" person. How would that make you feel? I encourage you to think a lot before using these terms in the future.

3. Care homes can be successful in assessing, identifying, and proactively meeting the emotional, psychological, social, medical, and other basic human needs of residents living with dementia. With the *full commitment* of owners and administrators of care homes to this effort, direct care partners can prevent and de-escalate the majority of these episodes. This commitment can go a long way in restoring residents, families, and the public's trust in nursing homes and assisted living residences as safe care environments for residents with dementia and a safe work environment for direct care partners.

Hopes, Dreams, and Not Giving Up

The song "Hopes and Dreams" was written in 2007 by 11 residents with early-stage dementia in a songwriting group facilitated by music therapist Wendy Krueger:[34]

> Hopes and dreams will carry us through.
> In work in play and all that we do.
> Friends will help us on our way.
> Lest we should fall or go astray.
> In times of trouble, in times of woe,
> When we have nowhere else to go . . .
> We stand together, hand in hand,
> to make this world a better land.
> Now take heart, do not despair,
> hopes and dreams are always there.

Never give up on your dreams, and drive forward until the end. You can still make a difference. Try to advocate for the ones who cannot, because we will be them one day.

Michael Ellenbogen,[143] a leading educator
and advocate living with dementia

References

1. Woolford MH, Stacpoole SJ, Clinnick L. Resident-to-resident elder mistreatment in residential aged care services: a systematic review of event frequency, type, resident characteristics, and history. *Journal of the American Medical Directors Association*. Published online March 13, 2021.

2. Tutton M. N.S. woman shocked by lack of probe into mother's nursing home death. *The Canadian Press*. https://atlantic.ctvnews.ca/n-s-woman-shocked-by-lack-of-probe-into-mother-s-nursing-home-death-1.2927742. Published June 2, 2016. Accessed May 11, 2021.

3. CBC News. Probe Winnipeg care home death: family. https://www.cbc.ca/news/canada/manitoba/probe-winnipeg-care-home-death-family-1.1056782. Published March 31, 2011. Accessed May 11, 2021.

4. McLaughlin A. Family of elderly man attacked at nursing home demand changes to Alzheimer's care. CBC News. https://www.cbc.ca/news/canada/hamilton/hamilton-man-assaulted-nursing-home-1.3965905. Published February 3, 2017. Accessed April 19, 2021.

5. Surr C. The task of cultural transformation. In: Kitwood T. *Dementia Reconsidered, Revisited: The Person Still Comes First*. 2nd ed (edited by Dawn Brooker). London, UK: Open University Press; 2019:170-177.

6. Lachs M, Bachman R, Williams CS, O'Leary JR. Resident-to-resident elder mistreatment and police contact in nursing homes: findings from a population-based cohort. *Journal of the American Geriatrics Society*. 2007;55(6):840-845.

7. Oved MC, Consiglio A, Green J. Woman killed, another injured, in attack at seniors residence in Scarborough. *The Toronto Star*. https://www.thestar.com/news/gta/2013/03/15/woman_killed_another_injured_in_attack_at_seniors_residence_in_scarborough.html. Published March 15, 2013.

8. Lock M. *The Alzheimer's Conundrum: Entanglements of Dementia and Aging*. Princeton, NJ: Princeton University Press; 2013.

9. U.S. House of Representatives Special Investigation Division. *Abuse of Residents Is a Major Problem in U.S. Nursing Homes*. 2001. https://www.cbsnews.com/htdocs/pdf/waxman_nursing.pdf

10. Government Accountability Office. *Nursing Homes: Improved Oversight Needed to Better Protect Residents from Abuse*. 2019. Accessed April 19, 2021. https://www.gao.gov/products/gao-19-433

11. Caspi E. A federal survey deficiency citation is needed for resident-to-resident aggression in U.S. nursing homes. *Journal of Elder Abuse & Neglect*. 2017;29(4):193-212.

12. Caspi E. MDS 3.0: a giant step forward, but what about items on resident-to-resident aggression? *Journal of the American Medical Directors Association*. 2013;14(8):624-625.

13. Caspi E. Aggressive behaviors between residents with dementia in an assisted living residence. *Dementia*. 2015;14(4):528-546.

14. Rosen T, Lachs MS, Bharucha AJ, et al. Resident-to-resident aggression in long-term care facilities: Insights from focus groups of nursing home residents and staff. *Journal of the American Geriatrics Society*. 2008;56(8):1398-1408.

15. Lachs M. Resident to resident elder mistreatment (RREM) in long term care. In: 1-Day Meeting for Development of Research Agenda on Resident-to-Resident Aggression in Canada. Hosted by the Institute for Life Course & Aging, University of Toronto. Funded by the Canadian Institutes for Health Research Institute of Aging; 2014.

16. Lachs MS, Teresi AT, Ramirez M, et al. The prevalence of resident-to-resident elder mistreatment in nursing homes. *Annals of Internal Medicine*. 2016;165(4):229-236.

17. Teresi JA, Ocepek-Welikson K, Ramirez M, et al. Development of an instrument to measure staff-reported resident-to-resident elder mistreatment (R-REM) using item response theory and other latent variable models. *The Gerontologist*. 2014;54(3):460-472.

18. Creno C. Chandler woman, 76, experiences bullying at retirement community. *Deseret News*. December 29, 2010. https://www.deseret.com/2010/12/29/20163411/chandler-woman-76-bullied-by-other-seniors

19. Bonifas RP. Insights for understanding and preventing senior bullying. In: *The 38th Annual Fall Aging Conference, Senior Workers Association, Minneapolis and St. Paul, MN*. 2012.

20. Trompetter H, Scholte R, Westerhof G. Resident-to-resident relational aggression and subjective well-being in assisted living facilities. *Aging & Mental Health*. 2011;15(1):59-67.

21. Hawker DS, Boulton MJ. Twenty years' research on peer victimization and psychosocial maladjustment: a meta-analytic review of cross-sectional studies. *Journal of Child Psychology and Psychiatry, and Allied Disciplines*. 2000;41(4):441-455.

22. Walker S, Richardson DR. Aggression strategies among older adults: delivered but not seen. *Aggression and Violent Behavior*. 1998;3(3):287-294.

23. Bonifas RP. Identifying, preventing, and responding to bullying in long-term care facilities. Webinar. The National Long-Term Care Ombudsman Resource Center; 2015. https://ltcombudsman.org/library/identifying-preventing-and-responding-to-bullying-in-long-term-care-facilit.

24. Pillemer K, Chen EK, Van Haitsma KS, et al. Resident-to-resident aggression in nursing homes: results from a qualitative event reconstruction study. *The Gerontologist*. 2012;52(1):24-33.

25. Alcon A, Burns K, Frankel M. Social bullying: training older adults to make a difference. Workshop delivered at the American Society on Aging Annual Conference, San Diego, CA, March 14, 2014.

26. Shinoda-Tagawa T, Leonard R, Pontikas J, et al. Resident-to-resident violent incidents in nursing homes. *Journal of the American Medical Association*. 2004;291(5):591-598.

27. Caspi E. Deaths as a result of resident-to-resident altercations in dementia in long-term care homes: a need for research, policy, and prevention. *Journal of the American Medical Directors Association*. 2016;17(1):7-11.

28. Murphy B, Bugeja, L, Pilgrim, J, Ibrahim, JE. Deaths from resident-to-resident aggression in Australian nursing homes. *Journal of the American Geriatrics Society*. 2017;65(12):2603-2609.

29. Caspi E. The circumstances surrounding the death of 105 elders as a result of resident-to-resident incidents in dementia in long-term care homes. *Journal of Elder Abuse and Neglect*. 2018;30(4):284-308.

30. DeBois KA, Evans SD, Chatfield SL. Resident-to-resident aggression in long-term care: analysis of structured and unstructured data from the National Violent Death Reporting System, 2003-2016. 39(10):1069-1077.

31. Bettinger G. *Moving on by Standing Still: A Different View of "Problem Behavior."* Victoria, BC, Canada: FriesenPress; 2017.

32. Centers for Medicare & Medicaid Services. *State Operations Manual. Appendix PP. Guidance to Surveyors for Long-Term Care Facilities*. Centers for Medicare & Medicaid Services; 2017. https://www.cms.gov/medicare/provider-enrollment-and-certification/guidanceforlawsandregulations/downloads/appendix-pp-state-operations-manual.pdf

33. Centers for Medicare & Medicaid Services. *Reporting Reasonable Suspicion of a Crime in a Long-Term Care Facility: Section 1150B of the Social Security Act. Memorandum from Director, Survey and Certification Group, CMS, to State Survey Agency Directors*. 2012. https://www.cms.gov/Medicare/Provider-Enrollment-and-Certification/SurveyCertificationGenInfo/downloads/scletter11_30.pdf

34. Caspi E. Preventing agitated behaviors and encouraging positive emotions among elders with memory-loss in an assisted living residence. Unpublished doctoral dissertation. Published online 2010.

35. Frankel M. Is it bullying? Strategies for assessing and intervening with older adults. *Meeting of the Minds Dementia Conference*. March 1 2014. St. Paul, MN.

36. Castle NG. Resident-to-resident abuse in nursing homes as reported by nurse aides. *Journal of Elder Abuse & Neglect*. 2012;24(4):340-356.

37. Kutner NG, Brown PJ, Stavisky RC, et al. "Friendship" interactions and expression of agitation among residents of dementia care unit. *Research on Aging*. 2000;22(2):188-205.

38. Rosen T, Pillemer K, Lachs M. Resident-to-resident aggression in long-term care facilities: an understudied problem. *Aggression and Violent Behavior*. 2008;13(2):77-87.

39. Herbert B, Bradshaw YS. Aggressive behaviors and injuries among nursing home residents. *Journal of the American Medical Association*. 2004;291(17):2074-2075; author reply 2075.

40. Aström S, Karlsson S, Sandvide A, et al. Staff's experience of and the management of violent incidents in elderly care. *Scandinavian Journal of Caring Sciences*. 2004;18(4):410-416.

41. Fitzwater EL, Gates DM. Testing an intervention to reduce assaults on nursing assistants in nursing homes: a pilot study. *Geriatric Nursing*. 2002;23(1):18-23.

42. Cohen-Mansfield J, Jensen B. Nursing home physicians' knowledge of and attitudes toward non-pharmacological interventions for treatment of behavioral disturbances associated with dementia. *Journal of the American Medical Directors Association*. 2008;9(7):491-498.

43. Ballard C, Lana MM, Theodoulou M, et al. A randomised, blinded, placebo-controlled trial in dementia patients continuing or stopping neuroleptics (the DART-AD trial). *PLOS Medicine*. 2008;5(4):e76.

44. Schneider LS, Dagerman K, Insel PS. Efficacy and adverse effects of atypical antipsychotics for dementia: meta-analysis of randomized, placebo-controlled trials. *The American Journal of Geriatric Psychiatry*. 2006;14(3):191-210.

45. Malone ML, Thompson L, Goodwin JS. Aggressive behaviors among the institutionalized elderly. *Journal of the American Geriatrics Society*. 1993;41(8):853-836.

46. Jalbert JJ, Eaton CB, Miller SC, Lapane KL. Antipsychotic use and the risk of hip fracture among older adults afflicted with dementia. *Journal of the American Medical Directors Association*. 2010;11(2):120-127.

47. Morley JE. Antipsychotics and dementia: a time for restraint? *Journal of the American Medical Directors Association*. 2012;13(9):761-763.

48. Taylor R, Power AG. *Living with Dementia: To Change Your Minds About People Whose Minds Have Changed*. Brilliant Image Productions; 2011. https://terranova.org/film-catalog/living-with-dementia-to-change-your-minds-about-people-whose-minds-have-changed/

49. Power AG. *Dementia Beyond Drugs: Changing the Culture of Care*. Baltimore, MD: Health Professions Press; 2010.

50. Jackson-Siegal JM, Schneider LS, Baskys A, Haupt DW. Recognizing and responding to atypical antipsychotic side effects. *Journal of the American Medical Directors Association*. 2004;5(4 Suppl):H7-H10.

51. Cohen-Mansfield J, Thein K, Marx MS, Dakheel-Ali M. What are the barriers to performing nonpharmacological interventions for behavioral symptoms in the nursing home? *Journal of the American Medical Directors Association*. 2012;13(4):400-405.

52. Mayers KS. Combativeness in the demented patient. *American Journal of Alzheimer's Care and Related Disorders and Research*. 1995;10(1):6-9.

53. Souder E, O'Sullivan P. Disruptive behaviors of older adults in an institutional setting: staff time required to manage disruptions. *Journal of Gerontological Nursing*. 2003;29(8):31-36.

54. Florida Agency for Health Care Administration. *Long Term Care Review: Florida Nursing Homes Regulation, Quality, Ownership, and Reimbursement*. Tallahassee, FL: Florida AHCA; 2007.

55. Gruszecki AC, Edwards J, Powers RE, Davis GG. Investigation of elderly deaths in nursing homes by the medical examiner over a year. *The American Journal of Forensic Medicine and Pathology*. 2004;25(3):209-212.

56. Stevenson DG, Studdert DM. The rise of nursing home litigation: findings from a national survey of attorneys. *Health Affairs (Project Hope)*. 2003;22(2):219-229.

57. Bartelme T. Alzheimer's and violence: state fails to take care of combative patients. *The Post and Courier* (Charleston, SC). 2009.

58. Menio DA. Advocating for the rights of vulnerable nursing home residents: creative strategies. *Journal of Elder Abuse & Neglect*. 1996;8(3):59-72.

59. Zgola JM. *Care That Works: A Relationship Approach to Persons with Dementia*. The Johns Hopkins University Press; 1999.

60. Karasik R, Berry J. Reimagining care for persons with severe dementia-related behavioral challenges: The Lakeview Ranch Model of Specialized Dementia Care™. *The Journal of Dementia Care*. 2013;21(3):28-31.

61. Brooker DJ, Woolley RJ. Enriching opportunities for people living with dementia: the development of a blueprint for a sustainable activity-based model. *Aging & Mental Health*. 2007;11(4):371-383.

62. Caspi E. Twenty reasons why we need to know the early life history of people living with dementia. ChangingAging. Published April 16, 2019. https://changingaging.org/dementia/20-reasons-why-we-need-to-know-the-early-life-history-of-people-living-with-dementia/

63. Feil N, de Klerk-Rubin V. *The Validation Breakthrough: Simple Techniques for Communicating with People with Alzheimer's-Type Dementia*. 3rd ed. Baltimore, MD: Health Professions Press; 2012.

64. Kitwood T. *Dementia Reconsidered: The Person Comes First*. London, UK: Open University; 1997.

65. Power GA. *Dementia Beyond Disease: Enhancing Well-Being*. Revised edition. Baltimore, MD: Health Professions Press; 2017.

66. Dignity. In: *Merriam-Webster.Com Dictionary*. Accessed January 23, 2021. https://www.merriam-webster.com/dictionary/dignity

67.   Alzheimer's Association. Activity-based Alzheimer's care: building a therapeutic program. In: *Training Presentation.* 1998.

68.   Harrington C Schnelle, JF, McGregor, M, Simmons, SF. The need for higher minimum staffing standards in U.S. nursing homes. *Health Services Insights.* 2016;9:13-19.

69.   Woods B. The Caring Organization. In: Kitwood T. *Dementia Reconsidered, Revisited: The Person Still Comes First.* 2nd ed (edited by Dawn Brooker). London, UK: Open University Press; 2019:137-142.

70.   Cohen-Mansfield J, Mintzer JE. Time for change: the role of nonpharmacological interventions in treating behavior problems in nursing home residents with dementia. *Alzheimer Disease and Associated Disorders.* 2005;19(1):37-40.

71.   Rasin J, Kautz DD. Knowing the resident with dementia: perspectives of assisted living facility caregivers. *Journal of Gerontological Nursing.* 2007;33(9):30-36.

72.   Negley EN, Manley JT. Environmental interventions in assaultive behavior. *Journal of Gerontological Nursing.* 1990;16(3):29-33.

73.   Almvik R, Woods P, Rasmussen K. Assessing risk for imminent violence in the elderly: the Brøset Violence Checklist. *International Journal of Geriatric Psychiatry.* 2007;22(9):862-867.

74.   Bharucha AJ, Vasilescu M, Dew MA, et al. Prevalence of behavioral symptoms: comparison of the minimum data set assessments with research instruments. *Journal of the American Medical Directors Association.* 2008;9(4):244-250.

75.   Shah A, Chiu E, Ames D, et al. Characteristics of aggressive subjects in Australian (Melbourne) nursing homes. *International Psychogeriatrics.* 2000;12(2):145-161.

76.   Voyer P, Verreault R, Azizah GM, et al. Prevalence of physical and verbal aggressive behaviours and associated factors among older adults in long-term care facilities. *BMC Geriatrics.* 2005;5:13.

77.   Marx MS, Cohen-Mansfield J, Werner P. A profile of the aggressive nursing home resident. *Behavior, Health, and Aging.* 1990;1:65-73.

78.   Soreff S. Violence in the nursing homes: understandings, management, documentation, and impact of resident to resident aggression. In: Olisah V, ed. *Essential Notes in Psychiatry.* IntechOpen; 2012:221-241.

79.   Frankel M. Combating social bullying among older adults. Webinar for Jewish Family & Children Services of Greater Boston; 2012.

80.   Freed G, Silverlieb C. Supporting cognitively impaired residents in independent senior housing. Presentation at the American Society on Aging Annual Conference, San Diego, CA; 2014.

81.   Hamel M, Gold DP, Andres D, et al. Predictors and consequences of aggressive behavior by community-based dementia patients. *The Gerontologist.* 1990;30(2):206-211.

82.   Archer N, Brown RG, Reeves SJ, et al. Premorbid personality and behavioral and psychological symptoms in probable Alzheimer disease. *The American Journal of Geriatric Psychiatry.* 2007;15(3):202-213.

83.   Sifford-Snellgrove KS, Beck C, Green A, McSweeney JC. Victim or initiator? Certified nursing assistants' perceptions of resident characteristics that contribute to resident-to-resident violence in nursing homes. *Research in Gerontological Nursing.* 2012;5(1):55-63.

84.   Brush JA, Fleder HA, Calkins MP. *Using the Environment to Support Communication and Foster Independence in People with Dementia: A Review of Case Studies in Long-Term Care Settings.* Kirtland, OH: I.D.E.A.S., Inc. 2012. Available at https://brushdevelopment.com/articles/

85.   Schumacher J, Zedlick D, Frenzel G. Depressive mood and cognitive impairment in results of old age nursing homes. *Zeitschrift für Gerontologie und Geriatrie.* 30(1):46-53.

86.   Menon AS, Gruber-Baldini AL, Hebel JR, et al. Relationship between aggressive behaviors and depression among nursing home residents with dementia. *International Journal of Geriatric Psychiatry.* 2001;16(2):139-146.

87.   Pillemer K, Teresi JA, Chen EK, Lachs MS. Correlates of resident-to-resident mistreatment in nursing homes. Symposium at the 67th Gerontological Society of America Annual Scientific Meeting, Washington, DC; 2014.

88.   Alexopoulos GS, Abrams RC, Young RC, Shamoian CA. Cornell Scale for Depression in Dementia. *Biological Psychiatry.* 1988;23(3):271-284.

89.   Yale R. *Counseling People with Early-Stage Alzheimer's Disease: A Powerful Process of Transformation.* Baltimore, MD: Health Professions Press; 2013.

90.   Cheston R, Jones K, Gilliard J. Group psychotherapy and people with dementia. *Aging & Mental Health.* 2003;7(6):452-461.

91.   Borson S. Posttraumatic stress disorder and dementia: a lifetime cost of war? *Journal of the American Geriatrics Society.* 2010;58:1797-1798.

92. Breslau N, Kessler RC, Chilcoat HD, et al. Trauma and posttraumatic stress disorder in the commu-nity: the 1996 Detroit Area Survey of Trauma. *Archives of General Psychiatry.* 1998;55(7):626-632.

93. Qureshi SU, Kimbrell T, Pyne JM, et al. Greater prevalence and incidence of dementia in older veterans with posttraumatic stress disorder. *Journal of the American Geriatrics Society.* 2010;58(9):1627-1633.

94. Yaffe K, Vittinghoff E, Lindquist K, et al. Posttraumatic stress disorder and risk of dementia among US veterans. *Archives of General Psychiatry.* 2010;67(6):608-613.

95. Mittal D, Torres R, Abashidze A, Jimerson N. Worsening of post-traumatic stress disorder symptoms with cognitive decline: case series. *Journal of Geriatric Psychiatry and Neurology.* 2001;14(1):17-20.

96. Hamilton JD, Workman RH. Persistence of combat-related posttraumatic stress symptoms for 75 years. *Journal of Traumatic Stress.* 1998;11(4):763-768.

97. Weintraub D, Ruskin PE. Posttraumatic stress disorder in the elderly: a review. *Harvard Review of Psychiatry.* 1999;7(3):144-152.

98. Macleod AD. The reactivation of post-traumatic stress disorder in later life. *The Australian and New Zealand Journal of Psychiatry.* 1994;28(4):625-634.

99. van Zelst WH, de Beurs E, Beekman ATF, Deeg DJH, van Dyck R. Prevalence and risk factors of posttraumatic stress disorder in older adults. *Psychotherapy and Psychosomatics.* 2003;72(6):333-342.

100. Flannery RB. Restraint procedures and dementia sufferers with psychological trauma. *American Journal of Alzheimer's Disease and Other Dementias.* 2003;18(4):227-230.

101. Bernsten D, Rubin DC. Flashbulb memories and posttraumatic stress reactions across the life span: age-related effects of the German occupation of Denmark during World War II. *Psychology and Aging.* 2006;21(1):127-139.

102. Messner SE. Levels of aggression and alcohol use in populations with dementia. *American Journal of Alzheimer's Disease & Other Dementias.* 2000;15(2):109-120.

103. Klein WC, Jess C. One last pleasure? Alcohol use among elderly people in nursing homes. *Health & Social Work.* 2002;27(3):193-203.

104. Joseph CL, Ganzini L, Atkinson RM. Screening for alcohol use disorders in the nursing home. *Journal of the American Geriatrics Society.* 1995;43(4):368-373.

105. Leurs P, Huvent-Grelle D, Lelievre-Leroy S, Roche J, Puisieux F. La consommation d'alcool en établissement d'hébergement pour personnes âgées dépendantes est excessive. *La Presse Médicale.* 2010;39(12):e280-e288.

106. Castle NG, Wagner LM, Ferguson-Rome SML, Handler SM. Alcohol misuse and abuse reported by nurse aides in assisted living. *Research on Aging.* 2012;34(3):321-336.

107. Moss BH, Tarter RE. Substance abuse, aggression, and violence: What are the connections? *The American Journal of Addictions.* 1993;2(2):149-160.

108. Kuerbis A, Sacco P, Blazer DG, Moore AA. Substance abuse among older adults. *Clinical Geriatric Medicine.* 2014;30(3):629-654.

109. Brennan PL, Greenbaum MA. Functioning, problem behavior and health services use among nurs-ing home residents with alcohol-use disorders: Nationwide data from the VA minimum data set. *Journal of Studies on Alcohol.* 2005;66(3):395-400.

110. Moore AA, Karno MP, Grella CE, et al. Alcohol, tobacco, and nonmedical drug use in older U.S. adults: Data from the 2001/2 National Epidemiological Survey of Alcohol and Related Condi-tions. *Journal of the American Geriatrics Society.* 2009;57(12):2275-2281.

111. Hughes JR. Genetics of smoking: A brief review. *Behavior Therapy.* 1986;17:335-345.

112. McGrew KB. Residents with severe mental illness: How nursing homes respond. *Journal of Geron-tological Social Work.* 1999;31:149-168.

113. Bell K. St. Charles nursing home patient dies after catching fire while smoking in her wheelchair. *St. Louis Dispatch.* Published May 18, 2017.

114. Forde E. Assaults between care home residents reported daily. *BBC News.* https://www.bbc.com/news/uk-39962700. Published May 23, 2017.

115. Ryden MB. Aggressive behavior in persons with dementia who live in the community. *Alzheimer Disease and Associated Disorders.* 1988;2(4):342-355.

116. Johnston D. A series of cases of dementia presenting with PTSD symptoms in World War II com-bat veterans. *Journal of the American Geriatrics Society.* 2000;48(1):70-72.

117. Office of the Chief Coroner of Ontario. *Report on the Inquest into the Deaths of Ezzeldine El Roubi and Pedro Lopez. Jury Verdict and Recommendations.*; 2005.

118. U.S. General Accounting Office. *Long Term Care Facilities: Information on Residents Who Are Regis-tered Sex Offenders or Are Paroled for Other Crimes.* GAO Publication No. GAO-06-326. 2006.

119. Appleby J. Lawmakers look at sex offenders in nursing homes. *USA Today.* July 25, 2008.

120. Mulder JT. CNY nursing home didn't call cops after sex offender abused resident 3 separate times. *Syracuse.com—The Post-Standard*. February 16, 2021.

121. McNeal MH, Warth P. Barred forever: seniors, housing and sex offense registration. *Kansas Journal of Law and Public Policy*. 2013;22(2):317-378.

122. Raia P. Habilitation therapy: a new starscape. In: Volicer L, Bloom-Charlette L, eds. *Enhancing the Quality of Life in Advanced Dementia*. New York: Brunner/Mazel; 1999:21-37.

123. Marshall M, Tibbs MA. *Social Work and People with Dementia: Partnerships, Practice, and Persistence*. 2nd ed. Bristol, UK: Bristol University Press. 2006.

124. Junaid O, Hegde S. Supportive psychotherapy in dementia. *Advances in Psychiatric Treatment*. 2007;13:17-23.

125. National Institute on Aging. *Caring for a Person with Alzheimer's Disease: Your Easy-to-Use Guide from the National Institute on Aging*. Bethesda, MD: National Institute on Aging. 2012.

126. Sabat SR. Excess disability and malignant social psychology: a case study of Alzheimer's disease. *Journal of Community and Applied Social Psychology*. 1994;4(3):157-166.

127. Bowlby C. *Therapeutic Activities with Persons Disabled by Alzheimer's Disease and Related Disorders*. New York: Aspen Publishers; 1993.

128. Raia P. If you do it well there is no resident to resident violence: standards of Alzheimer's care in nursing homes. Meeting of the MA Alzheimer's Association Annual Conference—Map Through The Maze. 2006.

129. Raia P, Reiter W, Katt-Lloyd. *Caring for People with Alzheimer's Disease: A Habilitation Training Curriculum*. Alzheimer's Association, MA/NH Chapter; 2011.

130. McShane R, Keene J, Fairburn C, Jacoby R, Hope T. Psychiatric symptoms in patients with dementia predict the later development of behavioural abnormalities. *Psychological Medicine*. 1998;28(5):1119-1127.

131. Doll GA. *Sexuality in Long-Term Care: Understanding and Supporting the Needs of Older Adults*. Baltimore, MD: Health Professions Press; 2012.

132. Merriam-Webster.com dictionary. Intimate. In: Merriam-Webster. Accessed February 20, 2021. https://www.merriam-webster.com/dictionary/dignity

133. Bitzan JE. Emotional bondedness and subjective well-being between nursing home roommates. *Journal of Gerontological Nursing*. 1998;24(9):8-15.

134. Everard K, Rowles GD, High DM. Nursing home room changes: toward a decision-making model. *The Gerontologist*. 1994;34(4):520-527.

135. Kane RA, Baker MO, Salmon J, Veazie W. *Consumer Perspectives on Private versus Shared Accommodation in Assisted Living Settings*. American Association of Retired Persons; 1998. https://assets.aarp.org/rgcenter/consume/9807_living.pdf

136. Wiltzius F, Gambert SR, Duthie EH. Importance of resident placement within a skilled nursing facility. *Journal of the American Geriatrics Society*. 1981;29(9):418-421.

137. Hartman S. Even in dementia, Korean War medic cares for his men. *CBS News*. https://www.cbsnews.com/news/even-in-dementia-korean-war-medic-cares-for-his-men/. Published August 31, 2012. Accessed April 20, 2021.

138. Miles SH, Sachs GH. Intimate strangers: roommates in nursing homes. In: Kane RA, Caplan AL, eds. *Everyday Ethics: Resolving Dilemmas in Nursing Home Life*. New York: Springer Publishing Company. 1990:90-91.

139. Snow R. Middle-aged persons' perceptions of their intergenerational relations. 1981. https://elibrary.ru/item.asp?id=7290135

140. Snow R, Crapo L. Emotional bondedness, subjective well-being, and health in elderly medical patients. *Journal of Gerontology*. 1982;37(5):609-615.

141. Pemberton K. Sharing of nursing home rooms saves dollars in B.C., but at what cost? *The Vancouver Sun*. https://vancouversun.com/news/metro/sharing-of-nursing-home-rooms-saves-dollars-in-bc-but-at-what-cost. Published February 11, 2016. Accessed April 20, 2021.

142. Hubbard G, Tester S, Downs MG. Meaningful social interactions between older people in institutional care settings. *Ageing & Society*. 2003;23:99-114.

143. Ellenbogen M. *From the Corner's Office to Alzheimer's*. Self-published book. 2014.

144. Teresi JA, Holmes D, Monaco C. An evaluation of the effects of commingling cognitively and noncognitively impaired individuals in long-term care facilities. *The Gerontologist*. 1993;33(3):350-358.

145. Lillesveen B, Berg G, Skjerven L. *Fra Huggu Tel Nava'n. Tonsberg/Oslo: Nasjonalt Kompetansesenter for Aldersdemens*. 1999.

146. Berg G. *The Importance of Food and Mealtime in Dementia Care: The Table Is Set*. London, UK: Jessica Kingsley Publishers; 2006.

147. Zeisel J. The physical environment's impact: using effective design to reduce the behavioral symptoms of dementia and improve care. Webinar. *American Society on Aging.* 2014.

148. Murtaugh CM, Kemper P, Spillman BC. The risk of nursing home use in later life. *Medical Care.* 1990;28(10):952-962.

149. Spillman BC, Lubitz J. New estimates of lifetime nursing home use: have patterns of use changed? *Medical Care.* 2002;40(10):965-975.

150. Thein NW, D'Souza G, Sheehan B. Expectations and experience of moving to a care home: Perceptions of older people with dementia. *Dementia.* 2011;10(1):7-18.

151. Snellgrove S, Beck C, Green A, McSweeney JC. Resident-to-resident violence triggers in nursing homes. *Clinical Nursing Research.* 2013;22(4):461-474.

152. Lapuk DS. Resident aggression in the long-term care setting: concerns and meanings from the perspectives of other residents. Published online 2007.

153. Zeltzer BB. Roommate-pairing: a nonpharmacologic therapy for treating depression in early to mid stages of Alzheimer's disease and dementia. *American Journal of Alzheimer's Disease and Other Dementias.* 2001;16(2):71-72.

154. Tyrrell J, Genin N, Myslinsky M. Freedom of choice and decision-making in health and social care: views of older patients with early-stage dementia and their carers. *Dementia.* 2006;5(4):479-502.

155. Bourbonnais A, Ducharme F. The meanings of screams in older people living with dementia in a nursing home. *International Psychogeriatrics.* 2010;22(07):1172-1184.

156. Desai AK, McFadden SH. Reducing antipsychotic use in long term care residents: addressing psychological and spiritual needs of residents with dementia Is crucial. *Journal of the American Medical Directors Association.* 2013;14(3):224-225.

157. Centers for Medicare & Medicaid Services. *CMS Manual System. Pub. 100-07 State Operations Provider Certification. Transmittal 22, December 15, 2006.*

158 Cahill P, Zeisel J, Caufield S. *Meet Me at the Movies . . . and Make Memories.* Interactive Film Program. 2011.

159. Zeisel J, Silverstein NM, Hyde J, Levkoff S, Lawton MP, Holmes W. Environmental correlates to behavioral health outcomes in Alzheimer's special care units. *The Gerontologist.* 2003;43(5):697-711.

160. Pear R. Nine of 10 nursing homes in the U.S. lack adequate staff, a government study finds. *The New York Times Health Section.* February 18, 2002.

161. Caspi E. Does self-neglect occur among older adults with dementia when unsupervised in assisted living? An exploratory, observational study. *Journal of Elder Abuse & Neglect.* 2014;26(2):123-149.

162. Robertson C, Mintz T, Ens I. *Baycrest's EATing Program: Eating Assistance Training: Family, Volunteer, & Private Companion Manual.* 1995.

163. Szpiech D. *Mealtime Assistance Program Handbook: A Resource for Volunteers, Families, and Healthcare Professionals.* Bridgepoint Active Healthcare; 2014. https://www.bridgepointhealth.ca/en/what-we-do/resources/BP-8.5x11-MAPHandbook-10-14FinalWeb.pdf

164. Mead R. The sense of an ending: an Arizona nursing home offers new ways to care for people with dementia. *The New Yorker.* May 20, 2013:92-103.

165. Simard J. Making a positive difference in the lives of nursing home residents with Alzheimer disease: the lifestyle approach. *Alzheimer Disease and Associated Disorders.* 1999;13 Suppl 1:S67-S72.

166. Kincaid C. What's so special about special care? Webinar. Assisted Living Consumer Alliance; 2011.

167. Sloane PD, Mitchell CM, Preisser JS, Phillips C, Commander C, Burker E. Environmental correlates of resident agitation in Alzheimer's disease special care units. *Journal of the American Geriatrics Society.* 1998;46(7):862-869.

168. Chen D, Chen M-y, Wactlar H, Gao C, Bharucha A. Video measurement of resident-to-resident physical aggression in nursing homes. In: *Proceedings of the 1st ACM Workshop on Vision Networks for Behavioral Analysis.* Association for Computing Machinery, 2008; 61-68. https://dl.acm.org/doi/abs/10.1145/1461893.1461905

169. Raia P. Avoid resident-to-resident violence in nursing homes. *Alzheimer's Association MA Chapter Newsletter.* 2006;24(1):21-22.

170. Cohen-Mansfield J. Nonpharmacologic interventions for inappropriate behaviors in dementia: A review, summary, and critique. *The American Journal of Geriatric Psychiatry.* 2001;9(4):361-381.

171. Cohen-Mansfield J, Marx MS, Werner P. Observational data on time use and behavior problems in the nursing home. *Journal of Applied Gerontology.* 1992;11(1):111-121.

172. Burgio LD, Scilley K, Hardin JM, et al. Studying disruptive vocalization and contextual factors in the nursing home using computer-assisted real-time observation. *Journal of Gerontology.* 1994;49(5):P230-P239.

173. Casey AN, Low LF, Goodenough B, et al. Computer-assisted direct observation of behavioral agitation, engagement, and affect in long-term care residents. *Journal of the American Medical Directors Association.* 2014;15(7):514-520.
174. Crump A. Promoting self-esteem. *Nursing the Elderly: In Hospital, Homes and the Community.* 1991;3(2):19-21.
175. Donat DC. Altercations among institutionalized psychogeriatric patients. *The Gerontologist.* 1986;26(3):227-228.
176. Holmberg SK. Evaluation of a clinical intervention for wanderers on a geriatric nursing unit. *Archives of Psychiatric Nursing.* 1997;11(1):21-28.
177. Pillemer K. Intervening in resident-to-resident elder mistreatment. In: *1-Day Meeting for Development of Research Agenda on Resident-to-Resident Aggression in Canada.* Hosted by the Institute for Life Course & Aging, University of Toronto. Funded by the Canadian Institutes for Health Research—Institute of Aging; 2014.
178. Lachs M, Teresi JA, Ramirez M. *Documentation of Resident to Resident Elder Mistreatment in Residential Care Facilities.* 2014.
179. Filan SL, Llewellyn-Jones RH. Animal-assisted therapy for dementia: a review of the literature. *International Psychogeriatrics.* 2006;18(4):597.
180. Swaffer K. The power of language. *The Australian Journal of Dementia Care Blog.* February 2015.
181. Phair LG V. *Dementia: A Positive Approach.* Sussex, Chichester, UK: Whurr Publishers Ltd; 1998.
182. Sommer R. Man's proximate environment. *Journal of Social Issues.* 1966;22:59-70.
183. Vittoria AK, Cortland S. "Our own little language": naming and the social construction of Alzheimer's disease. *Symbolic Interaction.* 1999;22(4):361-384.
184. Power GA. *Wandering and Dementia.* 2011. Accessed April 20, 2021. https://www.youtube.com/watch?v=d7LxKTG6B84
185. Marx MS, Werner P, Cohen-Mansfield J. Agitation and touch in the nursing home. *Psychological Reports.* 1989;64(3 Pt 2):1019-1026.
186. HealthCare Interactive®. CARES: Online Dementia Training. *Dementia Basics and Advanced Care.* Module 3: Understanding Behavior as communication. https://hcinteractive.com
187. Mancini M, Pederson K, Ouellet V. "It's a horror movie": Nursing home security footage provides raw picture of resident violence problem. *CBC News Marketplace.* https://www.cbc.ca/news/health/long-term-care-marketplace-1.4501795. Published January 26, 2018.
188. SooToday Staff. Former saultite's abuse featured on W5 (warning: graphic photos). *SooToday.* February 6, 2013.
189. Rinaldo S. Nursing home residents at risk: W5 investigation reveals startling national statistics. *CTV W5.* 2013.
190. Tilly J, Reed P. *Dementia Care Practice Recommendations for Assisted Living Residences and Nursing Homes.* Alzheimer's Association. 2006. https://www.alz.org/media/documents/dementia-care-practice-recommend-assist-living-1-2-b.pdf and https://www.alz.org/media/documents/dementia-care-practice-recommend-assist-living-3-b.pdf.
191. Brawley E. *Designing for Alzheimer's Disease: Strategies for Creating Better Care Environments.* New York: John Wiley & Sons; 1997.
192. Lucero M, Hutchinson S, Leger-Krall S, Wilson HS. Wandering in Alzheimer's dementia patients. *Clinical Nursing Research.* 1993;2(2):160-175.
193. Camp CJ. *Hiding the Stranger in the Mirror: A Detective's Manual for Solving Problems Associated with Alzheimer's Disease and Associated Disorders.* Solon, OH: Center for Applied Research in Dementia; 2008.
194. Fagan LA. Within these walls: creating a safe and supportive environment. In: Radin L, Radin G, eds. *What If It's Not Alzheimer's? A Caregiver's Guide to Dementia.* Amherst, NY: Prometheus Books; 2008:199-210.
195. Namazi KH, Rosner TT, Rechlin L. Long-term memory cuing to reduce visuo-spatial disorientation in Alzheimer's disease patients in a special care unit. *The American Journal of Alzheimer's Care and Related Disorders & Research.* 1991;6(6):10-15.
196. Vigil® Dementia System. Vigil Health Solutions. https://www.vigil.com/vigil-memory-care-system/.
197. Powers BA. The significance of losing things for nursing home residents with dementia and their families. *Journal of Gerontological Nursing.* 2003;29(11):43-52.
198. Snow T. *Understanding Frontotemporal Dementias* (DVD). Sarasota, FL: Pines Education Institute of Southwest Florida; 2014.
199. Ellis JM, Teresi JA, Ramirez M, et al. Managing resident-to-resident elder mistreatment in nursing homes: the SEARCH approach. *Journal of Continuing Education in Nursing.* 2014;45(3):112-121; quiz 122-123.

200. Harris DK, Benson ML. Theft in nursing homes: an overlooked form of elder abuse. *Journal of Elder Abuse & Neglect.* 1999;11(3):73-90.
201. Magan C. Thefts from seniors in assisted living topped 117K, UMN researcher finds. *The Pioneer Press.* https://www.twincities.com/2019/07/01/thefts-from-seniors-in-assisted-living-topped-117k-umn-researcher-finds/. Published July 19, 2019.
202. Kalaria N, Xiangrong S, Abisola M. VA long term care and violence: it isn't easy. *Journal of the American Medical Directors Association.* 2013;14(3):B9.
203. Teresi J. *Resident To Resident Elder Mistreatment (R-REM) Training and Education Guide.* Hebrew Home for the Aged, Riverdale, NY. Published online 2015. http://citra.human.cornell.edu/r-remp
204. Cohen-Mansfield J, Martin LS. Assessment of agitation in older adults. In: Lichtenberg PA, ed. *Handbook of Assessment in Clinical Gerontology.* New York: John Wiley & Sons. 1999:297-330.
205. Brackey J. *Creating Moments of Joy: A Guide for Families and Caregivers.* 5th ed. West Lafayette, IN: Purdue University Press; 2017.
206. Span P. Aggressive neighbors in the nursing home. *The New York Times.* November 25, 2014.
207. Cariaga J, Burgio L, Flynn W, Martin D. A controlled study of disruptive vocalizations among geriatric residents in nursing homes. *Journal of the American Geriatrics Society.* 1991;39(5):501-507.
208. von Gunten A, Alnawaqil AM, Abderhalden C, et al. Vocally disruptive behavior in the elderly: a systematic review. *International Psychogeriatrics.* 2008;20(4):653-672.
209. Cohen-Mansfield J, Marx MS, Werner P. Agitation in elderly persons: an integrative report of findings in a nursing home. *International Psychogeriatrics.* 1992;4 Suppl 2:221-240.
210. Hallberg IR, Norberg A, Ericksson S. Functional impairment and behavioural disturbances in vocally disruptive patients in psychogeriatric wards. *International Journal of Geriatric Psychiatry.* 1990;5:53-61.
211. Hallberg IR, Norberg A, Eriksson S. A comparison between the care of vocally disruptive patients and that of other residents at psychogeriatric wards. *Journal of Advanced Nursing.* 1990;15(4):410-416.
212. Norberg A. Perspective of an institution-based research nurse. *International Psychogeriatrics.* 1996;8 Suppl 3:459-463; discussion 469-73.
213. Sloane PD, Davidson S, Buckwalter K, et al. Management of the patient with disruptive vocalization. *The Gerontologist.* 1997;37(5):675-682.
214. Hallberg IR, Norberg A. Staffs' interpretation of the experience behind vocally disruptive behavior in severely demented patients and their feelings about it. An explorative study. *International Journal of Aging & Human Development.* 1990;31:295-305.
215. Cohen-Mansfield J, Werner P. Verbally disruptive behaviors in elderly persons: a review. Facts and research in gerontology. In: B.J. Vellas, Albaredo JL, Garry PJ, eds. *Dementia and Cognitive Impairment.* Paris, France: Serdi. 1994:73-89.
216. Cohen-Mansfield J, Werner P. Typology of disruptive vocalizations in older persons suffering from dementia. *International Journal of Geriatric Psychiatry.* 1997;12(11):1079-1091.
217. Lindgren C, Hallberg IR, Norberg A. Diagnostic reasoning in the care of a vocally disruptive severely demented patient. A case report. *Scandinavian Journal of Caring Sciences.* 1992;6(2):97-103.
218. Cohen-Mansfield J, Werner P. Management of verbally disruptive behaviors in nursing home residents. *The Journals of Gerontology Series A, Biological Sciences and Medical Sciences.* 1997;52(6):M369-M377.
219. Burgio LD, Flynn W, Martin D. Disruptive vocalizations in institutionalized geriatric patients. *The Gerontologist.* 1988;28:369-371.
220. Cohen-Mansfield J, Werner P, Marx MS. Screaming in nursing home residents. *Journal of the American Geriatrics Society.* 1990;38(7):785-792.
221. Casby JA, Holm MB. The effect of music on repetitive disruptive vocalizations of persons with dementia. *The American Journal of Occupational Therapy.* 1994;48(10):883-889.
222. Burgio L, Scilley K, Hardin JM, Hsu C, Yancey J. Environmental "white noise": an intervention for verbally agitated nursing home residents. *The Journals of Gerontology Series B, Psychological Sciences and Social Sciences.* 1996;51(6):P364-P373.
223. Hantikainen V. Nursing staff perceptions of the behaviour of older nursing home residents and decision making on restraint use: a qualitative and interpretative study. *Journal of Clinical Nursing.* 2001;10(2):246-256.
224. White MK, Kaas MJ, Richie MF. Vocally disruptive behavior. *Journal of Gerontological Nursing.* 1996;22(11):23-29.
225. Enslein J, Tripp-Reimer T, Kelley LS, et al. Evidence-based protocol: interpreter facilitation for persons with limited-English proficiency. In: Titler M, ed. *Series on Evidence-Based Practice for Older Adults.* Iowa City, IA: The University of Iowa College of Nursing Gerontological Nursing Interventions Research Center, Research Dissemination Core. 2001.

226. Sackett V. Landlords are required to protect residents from anti-gay attacks, court says. AARP. https://www.aarp.org/caregiving/financial-legal/info-2018/lgbt-nursing-home-lawsuit.html. Published August 29, 2018.

227. Coon DW, Burleson MH. Working with gay, lesbian, bisexual, and transgender families. In: Yeo G, Gallagher-Thompson, eds. *Ethnicity and the Dementias.* 2nd ed. London, UK: Routledge;343-358.

228. Black S. Tenant comfort trumps LEED status at Orfield Labs. *Minneapolis/St. Paul Business Journal.* February 3, 2012.

229. Smith M, Gerdner LA, Hall GR, Buckwalter KC. History, development, and future of the progressively lowered stress threshold: a conceptual model for dementia care. *Journal of the American Geriatrics Society.* 2004;52(10):1755-1760.

230. Mooney P, Nicell PL. The importance of exterior environment for Alzheimer residents: effective care and risk management. *Healthcare Management Forum / Canadian College of Health Service Executives.* 1992;5(2):23-29.

231. McMinn BG, Hinton L. Confined to barracks: The effects of indoor confinement on aggressive behavior among inpatients of an acute psychogeriatric unit. *American Journal of Alzheimer's Disease & Other Dementias.* 2000;15(1):36-41.

232. Chen C, Sloane P, Dalton T. *Lighting and Circadian Rhythms and Sleep in Older Adults.* 2003.

233. Brawley E, Noell-Waggoner E. *Lighting: Partner in Quality Care Environments.* 2008. https://www.pioneernetwork.net/wp-content/uploads/2016/10/Lighting-A-Partner-in-Quality-Care-Environments-Symposium-Paper-3.pdf

234. Talyaco L. Dignity, longevity, vitality. *The Rogerson Record Newsletter.* 2008;7(4):3.

235. Bell V, Troxel D. *The Best Friends Approach to Alzheimer's Care.* Baltimore, MD: Health Professions Press; 2003.

236. Wapner S, Demick J, Redondo JP. Cherished possessions and adaptation of older people to nursing homes. *International Journal of Aging & Human Development.* 1990;31(3):219-235.

237. Stokes G. Challenging behavior in dementia: a psychological approach. In: Woods RT, ed. *Handbook of Clinical Psychology of Aging.* John Wiley & Sons; 1996:601-628.

238. Kinney JM, Stephens MP, Brockman AM. Personal and environmental correlates of territoriality and use of space. *Long Term Care Services Administration Quarterly.* 1987;3(2):102-110.

239. Nelson MN, Paluck RJ. Territorial markings, self-concept, and mental status of the institutionalized elderly. *The Gerontologist.* 1980;20(1):96-98.

240. Goodman D. Roommate held in killing at Queens nursing home. *The New York Times.* https://www.nytimes.com/2013/10/31/nyregion/resident-is-killed-at-queens-nursing-home.html. Published October 2013.

241. Fleming R, Purandare N. Long-term care for people with dementia: Environmental design guidelines. *International Psychogeriatrics.* 2010;22(7):1084-1096.

242. Garre-Olmo J, Lopez-Pousa S, Turon-Estrada A, et al. Environmental determinants of quality of life in nursing home residents with severe dementia. *Journal of the American Geriatrics Society.* 2012;60(7):1230-1236.

243. La Bey L. Noise, how does it affect you? Dementia Chats webinar presented at the July 9, 2014, Alzheimer's Speaks.

244. Orfield SJ, Brand J. *Better Sound Solutions: Applying Occupant and Building Performance Measurement and Design to Improve Office Acoustics. A Professional Paper.* Washington, DC: American Society of Interior Designers, 2004.

245. Bharathan T, Goldan D, Ramesh A, et al. What do patterns of noise in a teaching hospital and nursing home suggest? *Noise Health.* 2007;9:31-34.

246. Barrick AL, Rader J, Mitchell M. Assessing behaviors. In: Barrick AL, Rader J, Hoeffer B, et al., eds. *Bathing Without a Battle: Person-Directed Care of Individuals with Dementia.* 2nd ed. New York: Springer Publishing Company. 2008:22-34.

247. Ulsperger JS, Knottnerus JD. *Elder Care Catastrophe: Rituals of Abuse in Nursing Homes & What You Can Do About It.* Boulder, CO: Paradigm Publishers. 2011.

248. Nelson J. The influence of environmental factors in incidents of disruptive behavior. *Journal of Gerontological Nursing.* 1995;21(5):19-24.

249. Caspi E. Wayfinding difficulties among elders with dementia in an assisted living residence. *Dementia.* 2014;13(4):429-450.

250. Span P. When aggression follows dementia. *The New York Times.* July 12, 2013.

251. Koenig Coste J. *Learning to Speak Alzheimer's: A Groundbreaking Approach for Everyone Dealing with the Disease.* New York: Houghton Mifflin Company. 2003.

252. Charles J, Greenwood S, Buchanan S. Appendix 3. A guide to optimal use of television/radios/music listening equipment. In: *Responding to Behaviors Due to Dementia)*. 2010. https://sunnybrook.ca/uploads/ABLE_CarePlanningGuide.pdf

253. Cogan DG. Visual disturbances with focal progressive dementing disease. American Journal of Ophthalmology. *American Journal of Ophthalmology*. 1985;100:68-72.

254. Henderson VW, Mack W, Williams BW. Spatial disorientation in Alzheimer's disease. *Archives of Neurology*. 1989;46(4):391-394.

255. Mahoney EK, Volicer L, Hurley AC. *Management of Challenging Behaviors in Dementia*. Baltimore, MD: Health Professions Press; 2000.

256. Passini R, Pigot H, Rainville C, Tetreault MH. Wayfinding in a nursing home for advanced dementia of the Alzheimer's type. *Environment and Behavior*. 2000;32(5):684-710.

257. Orfield SJ, Brand J, Hakkarainen P. *Better Lighting and Daylighting Solutions: Improving Visual Quality in Office Environments. A Professional Paper from the American Society of Interior Designers*. 2006.

258. Faye E, Stappenbeck W. *Changes in the Aging Eye*. New York: Lighthouse Guild; 2000.

259. Orfield SJ. Aging research, design education, and the perceptual limits in seniors housing design: development of a research-based design model for better aging environments. *Seniors Housing & Care Journal*. 2013;21(1):136-144.

260. Calkins M. Lighting for older eyes. *Nursing Home Magazine*. 2003;68:70.

261. Raia P. Habilitation therapy in dementia care. *Age in Action*. 2011;26(4):1-5.

262. Brilliant Image Productions. *Understanding Dementia: The Caregiver's Notebook*. Dementia Care Foundation in collaboration with Lakeview Ranch, Inc; 2007.

263. Collins, J. St. Louis Park nursing home resident dies after tasing. Minnesota Public Radio; August 21, 2013. https://www.mprnews.org/story/2013/08/21/nursing-home-resident-taser-death

264. Serres C. Woman hammers nails into her head; Maplewood assisted-living facility faulted. *The Star Tribune*. https://www.startribune.com/state-faults-maplewood-assisted-living-facility-with-neglect-after-resident-hammers-nails-into-her-head/567281992/. Published January 24, 2020.

265. Orfield SJ. Perception and the elderly—Orfield Labs: Building performance & occupancy research. *Officeinsight*; April 21, 2008. https://officeinsight.com/research/perception-and-the-elderly-orfield-labs-building-performance-occupancy-research/

266. Schwarz B, Chaudhury H, Tofle RB. Effect of design interventions on a dementia care setting. *American Journal of Alzheimer's Disease and Other Dementias*. 2004;19(3):172-176.

267. Rudman D, Bross D, Mattson DE. Clinical indicators derived from the patient assessment instrument in the long-stay residents of 69 VA nursing homes. *Journal of General Internal Medicine*. 1994;9(5):261-267.

268. Morgan DG, Stewart MJ. Multiple occupancy versus private rooms on dementia care units. *Environment and Behavior*. 1998;30(4):487-503.

269. Kovach C, Calkins M. Impacts of a therapeutic environment for dementia care. *American Journal of Alzheimer's Disease*. 1997;12(3):99-110.

270. Heckman GA, Kay K, Morrison A, et al. Proceedings from an International Virtual Townhall. Reflecting on the COVID-19 pandemic: themes from long-term care. *Journal of the American Medical Directors Association*. https://www.jamda.com/article/S1525-8610(21)00338-8/fulltext Published online April 8, 2021.

271. Isaksson U, Astrom S, Sanddman P-O, Karlson S. Factors associated with the prevalence of violent behavior among residents living in nursing homes. *Journal of Clinical Nursing*. 2009;18(7):972-980.

272. Marquardt G, Schmieg P. Dementia-friendly architecture: environments that facilitate wayfinding in nursing homes. *American Journal of Alzheimer's disease and other dementias*. 2009;24(4):333-340.

273. Calkins M, Cassella C. Exploring the cost and value of private versus shared bedrooms in nursing homes. *The Gerontologist*. 2007;47(2):169-183.

274. Lawton MP, Bader J. Wish for privacy for young and old. *Journal of Gerontology*. 1970;25(1):48-54.

275. Goldman B. Tackling nursing home violence. *CBC News*. May 13, 2011.

276. The American Heritage Dictionary. Private. *AHDictionary.com*. Accessed March 2, 2021. https://www.ahdictionary.com/word/search.html?q=private

277. Terakawa Y. The relationship between environment and behavior at the institutional setting for the elderly. In: *Environmental Design Research Association 35th Annual Conference*. 2004.

278. DeLong AJ. The micro-spatial structure of the older person: Some implications for planning the social and spatial environment. In: Pastalan L, Carsen D (eds.), *Spatial Behavior of Older People*. Ann Arbor, MI: Institute of Gerontology. 1970.

279. Calkins MP. *Envisioning Your Future in a Nursing Home.* Letter included in exhibits to modified application to Maryland Health Care Commission. 2019. https://www.pioneernetwork.net/wp-content/uploads/2016/10/Envisioning-Your-Future-in-a-Nursing-Home-The-Importance-of-Private-Rooms-Symposium-Paper.pdf
280. Ministry of Health and Long-Term Care. *Long-Term Care Home Design Manual.* 2009.
281. Passini RC, Rainville, Marchand N, Joanette Y. Wayfinding and dementia: some research findings and a new look at design. *Journal of Architectural and Planning Research.* 1998;15(2-3):133-151.
282. Elmståhl S, Annerstedt L, Ahlund O. How should a group living unit for demented elderly be designed to decrease psychiatric symptoms? *Alzheimer Disease and Associated Disorders.* 1997;11(1):47-52.
283. Sloane P, Mitchell M, Calkins M, Zimmerman S. Lighting and noise levels in Alzheimer's disease special care units. *Research and Practice in Alzheimer's Disease.* 2000;4:241-249.
284. Deremeik J, Broman AT, Friedman D, et al. Low vision rehabilitation in a nursing home population: The SEEING Study. *Journal of Visual Impairment & Blindness.* 2007;101(11):701-714.
285. Alzheimer's Association. Sleep issues and sundowning. https://www.alz.org/help-support/caregiving/stages-behaviors/sleep-issues-sundowning.
286. Brawley EC. *Design Innovations For Aging and Alzheimer's: Creating Caring Environments.* New York: John Wiley & Sons. 2006.
287. Resident care assistant. Certified nursing assistants: the foundation. Presented at the Annual Meeting of the Massachusetts Alzheimer's Association, Marlborough, MA; May 14, 2008.
288. U.S. Department of Health and Human Services, Centers for Medicare & Medicaid Services (CMS). *Medicare and Medicaid Programs: Reform of Requirements for Long-Term Care Facilities (Final Rule).* 2016. https://www.govinfo.gov/content/pkg/FR-2016-10-04/pdf/2016-23503.pdf
289. Boscart VM, Sidani S, Poss J, et al. The associations between staffing hours and quality of care indicators in long-term care. *BMC Health Services Research.* 2018;18:1-7.
290. Harrington C, Mollot R, Edelman TS, Valanejad D. U.S. nursing home violations of international and domestic human rights standards. *International Journal of Health Services.* 2020;50(1):62-72.
291. Bostick JE, Rantz MJ, Fleshner MK, Riggs CJ. Systematic review of studies of staffing and quality in nursing homes. *Journal of the American Medical Directors Association.* 2006;7:366-376.
292. Beck C, Ortigara A, Mercer S, Shue V. Enabling and empowering certified nursing assistants for quality dementia care. *International Journal of Geriatric Psychiatry.* 1999;14(3):197-211.
293. Irvine AB, Bourgeois M, Billow M, Seeley JR. Internet training for nurse aides to prevent resident aggression. *Journal of the American Medical Directors Association.* 2007;8(8):519-526.
294. Schnelle JF, Schroyer LD, Saraf A, Simmons SF. Determining nurse aide staffing requirements to provide care based on resident workload: a discrete event simulation model. *Journal of the American Medical Directors Association.* 2016;17(11):970-977.
295. Long SW. *Caring for People with Challenging Behaviors: Essential Skills and Successful Strategies in Long-Term Care.* Baltimore, MD: Health Professions Press; 2005.
296. Snowdon J. Mental health service delivery in long-term care homes. *International Psychogeriatrics.* 2010;22(7):1063-1071.
297. Allin SJ, Bharucha A, Zimmerman J, et al. Toward the automated assessment of behavioral disturbances of dementia. Paper Presented at the Meeting of the Fifth International Conference on Ubiquitous Computing and the Second International Conference on Ubiquitous Computing for Pervasive Healthcare Applications, Seattle, WA. 2003.
298. Banerjee A, Daly T, Armstrong P, et al. Structural violence in long-term, residential care for older people: comparing Canada and Scandinavia. *Social Science & Medicine.* 2012;74(3):390-398.
299. Robinson KM, Tappen RM. Policy recommendations on the prevention of violence in long-term care facilities. *Journal of Gerontological Nursing.* 2008;34(3):10-14.
300. Rau J. "It's almost like a ghost town." Most nursing homes overstated staffing for years. *The New York Times.* https://www.nytimes.com/2018/07/07/health/nursing-homes-staffing-medicare.html. Published July 7, 2018.
301. Harrington C, Dellefield ME, Halifax E, Bakerjian D. Appropriate nurse staffing levels for U.S. nursing homes. *Health Services Insights.* 2020;13:1-14.
302. Maslach C, Leiter MP. Understanding the burnout experience: recent research and its implications for psychiatry. *World Psychiatry.* 2016;15(2):103-111.
303. Todd SJ, Watts SC. Staff responses to challenging behaviour shown by people with dementia: an application of an attributional-emotional model of helping behaviour. *Aging & Mental Health.* 2005;9(1):71-81.

304. Jenkins H, Allen C. The relationship between staff burnout/distress and interactions with residents in two residential homes for older people. *International Journal of Geriatric Psychiatry*. 1988;13:466-472.

305. McPherson R, Eastley RJ, Richards H, Mian IH. Psychological distress among workers caring for the elderly. *International Journal of Geriatric Psychiatry*. 1994;9:381-386.

306. Chappell NL, Novak M. The role of support in alleviating stress among nursing assistants. *The Gerontologist*. 1992;32(3):351-359.

307. Moniz-Cook E, Woods RT, Richards K. Functional analysis of challenging behaviour in dementia: the role of superstition. *International Journal of Geriatric Psychiatry*. 2001;16(1):45-56.

308. Findorff MJ, McGovern PM, Wall M, et al. Risk factors for work related violence in a health care organization. *Injury Prevention*. 2004;10(5):296-302.

309. Dictionary.cambridge.org. Self-efficacy. In: *Cambridge Dictionary*. Accessed March 8, 2021. https://dictionary.cambridge.org/us/dictionary/english/self-efficacy

310. Duffy B, Oyebode JR, Allen J. Burnout among care staff for older adults with dementia: the role of reciprocity, self-efficacy, and organizational factors. *Dementia*. 2009;8(4):515-541.

311. Mackenzie CS, Peragine G. Measuring and enhancing self-efficacy among professional caregivers of individuals with dementia. *American Journal of Alzheimer's Disease and Other Dementias*. 2003;18(5):291-299.

312. Scales K. *It's Time to Care: A Detailed Profile of America's Direct Care Workforce (Section 1)*. Bronx, NY: Paraprofessional Healthcare Institute; 2020. https://phinational.org/resource/its-time-to-care-a-detailed-profile-of-americas-direct-care-workforce/

313. *U.S. Nursing Assistants Employed in Nursing Homes: Key Facts*. Bronx, NY: Paraprofessional Health Care Institute; 2019. https://phinational.org/resource/u-s-nursing-assistants-employed-in-nursing-homes-key-facts-2019/

314. Cook A. *Paid Family and Medical Leave: How States Should Support Direct Care Workers*. Bronx, NY: Paraprofessional Health Care Institute; 2018. https://phinational.org/resource/paid-family-medical-leave-states-support-direct-care-workers/

315. Maslach C, Jackson SE, Leiter MP. *Maslach Burnout Inventory Manual*. 3rd ed. Palo Alto, CA: Consulting Psychologists Press; 1996.

316. Rasin JH. Taking care of yourself: strategies for caregivers. In: Barrick AL, Rader J, Hoeffer B, et al., eds., *Bathing Without a Battle: Person-Directed Care of Individuals with Dementia*. 2nd ed. New York: Springer Publishing Company; 2008:161-168.

317. Zeller A, Dassen T, Kok G, et al. Factors associated with resident aggression toward caregivers in nursing homes. *Journal of Nursing Scholarship*. 2012;44(3):249-257.

318. Hall J, Karch DL, Crosby A. *Elder Abuse Surveillance: Uniform Definitions and Recommended Core Data Elements. Version 1.0*. https://www.cdc.gov/violenceprevention/pdf/ea_book_revised_2016.pdf; 2016.

319. Skovdahl K, Kihlgren AL, Kihlgren M. Different attitudes when handling aggressive behaviour in dementia: narratives from two caregiver groups. *Aging & Mental Health*. 2003;7(4):277-286.

320. Williams K, Kemper S, Hummert ML. Improving nursing home communication: an intervention to reduce elderspeak. *The Gerontologist*. 2003;43(2):242-247.

321. Williams KN, Herman R, Gajewski B, Wilson K. Elderspeak communication: impact on dementia care. *American Journal of Alzheimer's Disease and Other Dementias*. 2009;24(1):11-20.

322. Kemper S, Harden T. Experimentally disentangling what's beneficial about elderspeak from what's not. *Psychology and Aging*. 1999;14(4):656-670.

323. Brown P, Levinson SC. *Politeness: Some Universals in Language Usage*. Cambridge, UK: Cambridge University Press; 1987.

324. Bonifas RP, Frankel M. Is it bullying? Strategies for assessing and intervening with older adults. Presented at the American Society on Aging Annual Conference, San Francisco, CA; 2011.

325. Castle NG, Decker FH. Top management leadership style and quality of care in nursing homes. *The Gerontologist*. 2011;51(5):630-642.

326. Thomas WH. *What Are Old People For? How Elders Will Save the World*. Acton, MA: VanderWyk & Burnham; 2004.

327. Anderson RA, Toles MP, Corazzini K, et al. Local interaction strategies and capacity for better care in nursing homes: a multiple case study. *BMC Health Services Research*. 2014;14:244.

328. Open minds, open hearts: English Rose Suites' dementia care philosophy. *Provider: Long-Term & Post-Acute Care*. September 2012.

329. Centers for Medicare & Medicaid Services. *Interim Report on the CMS National Partnership to Improve Dementia Care in Nursing Homes: Q4 2011–Q1 2014*; 2014.

330. Paraprofessional Healthcare Institute. *America's Direct-Care Workforce*; 2013. https://phinational. org/wp-content/uploads/2017/07/phi-facts-3.pdf

331. Teresi JA, Ramirez M, Ellis J, et al. A staff intervention targeting resident-to-resident elder mistreatment (R-REM) in long-term care increased staff knowledge, recognition and reporting: results from a cluster randomized trial. *International Journal of Nursing Studies*. 2013;50(5):644-656.

332. Rosen T, Lachs MS, Teresi J, et al. Staff-reported strategies for prevention and management of resident-to-resident elder mistreatment in long-term care facilities. *Journal of Elder Abuse & Neglect*. Published online April 20, 2015:1-14.

333. Gates D, Fitzwater E, Succop P. Reducing assaults against nursing home caregivers. *Nursing Research*. 2005;54(2):119-127.

334. Morgan DG, Crossley MF, Stewart NJ, et al. Taking the hit: focusing on caregiver "error" masks organizational-level risk factors for nursing aide assault. *Qualitative Health Research*. 2008;18(3):334-346.

335. Hirst SP. Defining resident abuse within the culture of long-term care institutions. *Clinical Nursing Research*. 2002;11(3):267-284.

336. Caspi E. Behavioral log: a critical tool for understanding and preventing reactive behaviors among long-term care residents with dementia. Unpublished manuscript, 2013.

337. Cohen-Mansfield J, Werner P, Culpepper WJ, et al. Wandering and aggression. In: Carstensen LL, Edelstein BA, L, eds. *The Practical Handbook of Clinical Gerontology*. Sage Publications; 1996:375-397.

338. Volicer L, Mahoney E. Are nursing home residents with dementia aggressive? *The Gerontologist*. 2002;42(6):875-876.

339. Sue D, Sue DW, Sue S. *Understanding Abnormal Behavior*. 8th ed. Belmont, CA: Wadsworth; 2006.

340. Åkerström M. Slaps, punches, pinches—But not violence. Boundary-work in nursing homes for the elderly. *Symbolic Interaction*. 2002;25(4):515-536.

341. Slone DG, Gleason CE. Behavior management planning for problem behaviors in dementia: A practical model. *Professional Psychology: Research and Practice*. 1999;30(1):27-36.

342. Chiu E. What's in a name—dementia or dysmentia? *International Journal of Geriatric Psychiatry*. 1994;9:1-14.

343. Goffman E. *Asylums: Essays on the Social Situation of Mental Patients and Other Inmates*. New York: Anchor Books; 1961.

344. Ryden MB, Bossenmaier M, McLachlan C. Aggressive behavior in cognitively impaired nursing home residents. *Research in Nursing & Health*. 1991;14(2):87-95.

345. Bridges-Parlet S, Knopman D, Thompson T. A descriptive study of physically aggressive behavior in dementia by direct observation. *Journal of the American Geriatrics Society*. 1994;42(2):192-197.

346. Somboontanont W, Sloane PD, Floyd FJ, et al. Assaultive behavior in Alzheimer's disease: identifying immediate antecedents during bathing. *Journal of Gerontological Nursing*. 2004;30(9):22-29; quiz 55-56.

347. Eller S, Griffin L, Mote C. Clinical assessment and management of agitation in residential settings. In: Hay DP, Klein DT, Hay LK, et al., eds. *Agitation in Patients with Dementia: A Practical Guide to Diagnosis and Management*. Washington, DC: American Psychiatric Publishing; 2003:81-90.

348. Hurley AC, Volicer L, Mahoney EK. Neurologic disorders. In: Tabloski PA, ed. *Nursing Care of the Elderly*. Hoboken, NJ: Prentice Hall; 2005:711-753.

349. Kovach CR, Noonan PE, Schlidt AM, Wells T. A model of consequences of need-driven, dementia-compromised behavior. *Journal of Nursing Scholarship*. 2005;37(2):134-140; discussion 140.

350. Camp CJ, Burant CJ, Graham GC. The InterpreCare System™: overcoming language barriers in long-term care. *The Gerontologist*. 1996;36(6):821-824.

351. Pemberton K. Danger in the dementia care home. *Vancouver Sun*. https://vancouversun.com/news/special-report-danger-in-the-dementia-care-home. Published January 2016.

352. Daly T, Banerjee A, Armstrong P, et al. Lifting the "violence veil": examining working conditions in long-term care facilities using iterative mixed methods. *Canadian Journal on Aging*. 2011;30(02):271-284.

353. Lynn CH. Confronting dementism. ChangingAging. Published January 21, 2015. https://changingaging.org/dementia/confronting-dementism/

354. Bonifas RP. Reducing senior bullying: conversation with bullying expert Robin Bonifas. Published online 2012. http://www.mybetternursinghome.com/senior-bullying-part-3-what-is-the-impact-of-bullying/

355. Burnes D, Syed M, Hsieh J. Process models to understand resident-to-resident aggression among residents with dementia in long-term care. *Journal of Applied Gerontology*. https://journals.sagepub.com/doi/10.1177/0733464820955089. Published online September 10, 2020.

356. MacQueen, K. Old and dangerous: senior violence is getting worse. Maclean's, January 14, 2014. https://www.macleans.ca/society/life/old-and-dangerous/.

357. Paraprofessional Healthcare Institute. *Understanding the Direct Care Workforce*; 2020. https://phi-national.org/policy-research/key-facts-faq/

358. Falk H, Wijk H, Persson L. Frail older persons' experiences of institutional relocation. *Geriatric Nursing*. 2011;32:245-256.

359. Priest L. When seniors turn to violence in their nursing homes. *The Globe and Mail*. November 13, 2004.

360. Kim SC, Berry B, Young L. Aggressive behaviour risk assessment tool for long-term care (ABRAT-L): validation study. *Geriatric Nursing*. 2019;40(3):284-289.

361. Kim SC, Young L, Berry B. Aggressive behavior risk assessment tool for newly admitted residents of long-term care homes. *Journal of Advanced Nursing*. 2017;73(7):1747-1756.

362. Serres C. Left to suffer, part 3. When roommates are the abusers. *The Star Tribune*. November 14, 2017. https://www.startribune.com/surging-resident-on-resident-violence-rarely-investigated/450625693/.

363. Buhr GT, Kuchibhatla M, Clipp EC. Caregivers' reasons for nursing home placement: clues for improving discussions with families prior to the transition. *The Gerontologist*. 2006;46(1):52-61.

364. Seitz D, Purandare N, Conn D. Prevalence of psychiatric disorders among older adults in long-term care homes: A systematic review. *International Psychogeriatrics*. 2010;22(07):1025-1039.

365. Hodgson N, Freeman VA, Granger DA. Biobehavioral correlates of relocation in the frail elderly: Salivary cortisol, affect, and cognitive function. *Journal of the American Geriatric Society*. 2004;52(11):1856-1862.

366. Vernooij-Dassen M, Vasse E, Zuidema S, Cohen-Mansfield J, Moyle W. Psychosocial interventions for dementia patients in long-term care. *International Psychogeriatrics*. 2010;22(7):1121-1128.

367. Brazil K, Maitland J, Walker M, Curtis A. The character of behavioural symptoms on admission to three Canadian long-term care homes. *Aging & Mental Health*. 2013;17(8):1059-1066.

368. The National Consumer Voice for Quality Long-Term Care. *Fact sheet: Resident council rights in nursing homes*. Published online 2017. https://theconsumervoice.org/issues/recipients/nursing-home-residents/resident-council-center

369. Brod M, Stewart AL, Sands L, Walton P. Conceptualization and measurement of quality of life in dementia: The Dementia Quality of Life Instrument (DQoL). *The Gerontologist*. 1999;39(1):25-35.

370. Caspi E. "Why the devil they don't ask us what we're thinking?" The need for residents' council meetings in special care units for persons with dementia in assisted living residences. https://brainxchange.ca/Public/Files/Behaviour/Why-the-devil-they-don-t-ask-us-what-we-re-thinkin.aspx. Published online 2012.

371. Kolanowski A, Cortes, TA, Mueller C. A call to the CMS: mandate adequate professional nurse staffing in nursing homes. *American Journal of Nursing*. 2021;121(3):24-27.

372. O'Hanlon T. Abuse and neglect in nursing homes. Presented at the Long Term Care Community Coalition 2020 Fall virtual symposium Identifying and addressing resident abuse and neglect; November 9, 2020.

373. Lawton MP. Quality of care and quality of life in dementia care units. In: Noelker LS, Harel Z, eds. *Linking Quality of Long Term Care and Quality of Life*. New York: Springer Publishing Company; 2001:136-161.

374. Beck AT, Epstein N, Brown G, Steer RA. An inventory for measuring clinical anxiety: psychometric properties. *Journal of Consulting and Clinical Psychology*. 1988;56:893-897.

375. Lawton MP, van Haitsma, K, Klapper, JA. *Observed Emotion Rating Scale*; 1999. https://abramson-seniorcare.org/research/applications/assessment-instruments/

376. Lawton MP, Rubinstein RL. *Interventions in Dementia Care: Toward Improving Quality of Life*. New York: Springer Publishing Company; 2000.

377. Hurley AC, Volicer BJ, Hanrahan PA, et al. Assessment of discomfort in advanced Alzheimer patients. *Research in Nursing & Health*. 1992;15(5):369-377.

378. Shankar KK, Walker M, Frost D, Orrell MW. The development of a valid and reliable scale for Rating Anxiety in Dementia (RAID). *Aging & Mental Health*. 1999;3(1):39-49.

379. Polisher Research Institute. *Recognizing and Responding to Emotion in Persons with Dementia*. Terra Nova Films; 1998. https://terranova.org/film-catalog/recognizing-and-responding-to-emotion/

380. Buffum MD, Miaskowski C, Sands L, Brod M. A pilot study of the relationship between discomfort and agitation in patients with dementia. *Geriatric Nursing*. 2001;22(2):80-85.

381. Holmes KJ, Gentili A. The message behind the behavior: successful management of scatolia in a resident with dementia. *Journal of the American Medical Directors Association*. 2013;47:235-242.

382. Schuster BG. Constipation in older adults: stepwise approach to keep things moving. *Canadian Family Physician*. 2015;61(2):152-158.

383. Voyer P, Richard S, Doucet L, Carmichael PH. Predisposing factors associated with delirium among demented long-term care residents. *Clinical Nursing Research*. 2009;18(2):153-171.

384. Voyer P, Richard S, Doucet L, et al. Precipitating factors associated with delirium among long-term care residents with dementia. *Applied Nursing Research*. 2011;24(3):171-178.

385. Inouye SK, Bogardus ST, Charpentier PA, et al. A multicomponent intervention to prevent delirium in hospitalized older patients. *The New England Journal of Medicine*. 1999;340(9):669-676.

386 Waszynski CM. *The Confusion Assessment Method (CAM). Try This: Best Practices in Nursing Care to Older Adults*. Hartford Institute for Geriatric Nursing; 2012. https://geriatrictoolkit.missouri.edu/cog/Confusion-Assessment-Method-delirium.pdf

387. Cacchione PZ, Culp K, Laing J, Tripp-Reimer T. Clinical profile of acute confusion in the long-term care setting. *Clinical Nursing Research*. 2003;12(2):145-158.

388. Fick DM, Agostini JV, Inouye SK. Delirium superimposed on dementia: a systematic review. *Journal of the American Geriatrics Society*. 2002;50(10):1723-1732.

389. McCusker J, Cole MG, Voyer P, et al. Prevalence and incidence of delirium in long-term care. *International Journal of Geriatric Psychiatry*. 2011;26(11):1152-1161.

390. Williamson R, Lauricella K, Browning A, et al. Patient factors associated with incidents of aggression in a general inpatient setting. *Journal of Clinical Nursing*. 2014;23(7-8):1144-1152.

391. Clegg A, Siddiqi N, Heaven A, Young J, Holt R. Interventions for preventing delirium in older people in institutional long-term care. *The Cochrane Database of Systematic Reviews*. 2014;1:CD009537-CD009537.

392. Inouye SK, van Dyck CH, Alessi CA, Balkin S, et al. Clarifying confusion: the confusion assessment method. A new method for detection of delirium. *Annals of Internal Medicine*. 1990;113(12):941-948.

393. Wei LA, Fearing MA, Sternberg EJ, Inouye SK. The Confusion Assessment Method: a systematic review of current usage. *Journal of the American Geriatrics Society*. 2008;56(5):823-830.

394. McCusker J, Cole MG, Voyer P, et al. Environmental factors predict the severity of delirium symptoms in long-term care residents with and without delirium. *Journal of the American Geriatrics Society*. 2013;61(4):502-511.

395. Horgas AL, Tsai PF. Analgesic drug prescription and use in cognitively impaired nursing home residents. *Nursing Research*. 1998;47(4):235-242.

396. Wasserman C. Pain: the fifth vital sign. The challenge of assessment in dementia patients. *The Newsletter of the Alzheimer's Association*. 2004;22(1):4-5.

397. Ahn H, Garvan C, Lyon D. Pain and aggression in nursing home residents with dementia: Minimum Data Set 3.0 analysis. *Nursing Research*. 2015;64(4):256-263.

398. Campbell JN. American Pain Society 1995 Presidential Address, Pain Forum. 1996;5:85-88.

399. Cohen-Mansfield J. Pain Assessment in Noncommunicative Elderly persons--PAINE. *The Clinical Journal of Pain*. 2006;22(6):569-575.

400. Hadjistavropoulos T, Fitzgerald TD, Marchildon GP. Practice guidelines for assessing pain in older persons with dementia residing in long-term care facilities. *Physiotherapy Canada*. 2010;62(2):104-113.

401. Dementia Care Foundation. *Understanding Dementia: The Caregiver's Notebook*; 2007. https://terranova.org/film-catalog/understanding-dementia-the-caregivers-notebook/

402. Whitehouse PJ, George D. *The Myth of Alzheimer's Disease: What You Aren't Being Told about Today's Most Dreaded Diagnosis*. New York: St. Martin's Griffin; 2008.

403. Fox N, Norton L, Rashap AW, et al. Well-Being: Beyond Quality of Life [White Paper]. Available as "The Eden Alternative Domains of Well-Being: Revolutionizing the Experience of Home by Bringing Well-Being to Life". https://www.edenalt.org/about-the-eden-alternative/the-eden-alternative-domains-of-well-being/; 2005.

404. Power GA. Well-being: a strength-based approach to dementia. *Australian Journal of Dementia Care*,. 2015;10(1). https://journalofdementiacare.com/well-being-a-strengths-based-approach-to-dementia/

405. NY State Department of Health. *Individual Resident Crisis Prevention Plan Coping with Physically Aggressive Behavior*. https://www.health.ny.gov/diseases/conditions/dementia/edge/forms/disruptive_behaviors_forms_individual_crisis_plan.pdf

406. Caspi E. Early-life events and current reactive behaviors among elders with dementia. Unpublished manuscript. 2011.

407. Snellgrove S, Beck C, Green A, McSweeney JC. Putting residents first: Strategies developed by CNAs to prevent and manage resident-to-resident violence in nursing homes. *The Gerontologist*. 2015;55(S1):S99-S107.

408. Alzheimer's Society. *This Is Me* (leaflet). https://www.alzheimers.org.uk/get-support/publications-factsheets/this-is-me; 2012.

409. Mast BT. *Whole Person Dementia Assessment.* Baltimore, MD: Health Professions Press; 2011.

410. Chaudhury H. Place-Biosketch as a tool in caring for residents with dementia. *Alzheimer's Care Quarterly.* 2002;3(1):42-45.

411. Flannery RB. Addressing psychological trauma in dementia sufferers. *American Journal of Alzheimer's disease and Other Dementias.* 2002;17(5):281-285.

412. Kitwood T. Towards a theory of dementia care: the interpersonal process. *Ageing & Society.* 1993;13(1):51-67.

413. Talerico KA, Evans LK. Making sense of aggressive/protective behaviors in persons with dementia. *Alzheimer's Care Quarterly.* 2000;1(4):77-88.

414. Kane RL, West JA. *It Shouldn't Be This Way: The Failure of Long-Term Care.* Nashville, TN: Vanderbilt University Press; 2005.

415. Castle N, Harris JA. Consistent assignment: an update on the quality impact. *Innovation in Aging.* 2019;3(Suppl 1):S802.

416. Castle NG. The Influence of Consistent Assignment on Nursing Home Deficiency Citations. *The Gerontologist.* 2011;51(6):750-760.

417. Davis R, Davis B. *My Journey into Alzheimer's Disease: Helpful Insights for Family and Friends.* Carol Stream, IL: Tyndale House Publishers; 1989.

418. Camp C. Engaging persons with dementia to maximize their potential: use of Montessori-based activities in a variety of settings. In: Massachusetts Alzheimer's Association Annual Conference—Map Through The Maze; 2009.

419. Paige H, Bonifas R. Organizational processes matter: addressing resident-to-resident aggression in nursing homes. Poster abstract. *Journal of the American Medical Directors Association*; 2013.

420. Bonifas RP. Resident-to-resident aggression in nursing homes: social workers involvement and collaboration with nursing colleagues. *Health & Social Work.* 2015;40(3):e101-e109.

421. DeMarco CE. The abusive resident: can activities help? *Activities, Adaptation & Aging.* 1996;21(1):13-21.

422. Temkin-Greener H, Gross D, Kunitz S, Mukamel D. Measuring interdisciplinary team performance in a long-term care setting. *Medical Care.* 2004;42(5):472-481.

423. Bureau of Labor Statistics. *Violence in the Workplace Comes under Closer Scrutiny*; 1994.

424. Bureau of Labor Statistics. *Violence in the Workplace, Patterns of Fatal Workplace Assaults Differ from Those of Nonfatal Ones*; 1995.

425. TJA Protect-Systems International. Train the Trainer Certification Course: Non-Violent Self-Protection for Healthcare Trainers. https://tjapsi.com/hcpnvsp.htm

426. Kutzik DM, Glasscock AP, Lundberg L, York J. Technological tools of the future. In: *The Assisted Living Residence: A Vision for the Future.* Baltimore, MD: The Johns Hopkins University Press; 2008:223-247.

427. Bharucha AJ, Anand V, Forlizzi J, et al. Intelligent assistive technology applications to dementia care: current Capabilities, limitations, and future challenges. *The American Journal of Geriatric Psychiatry.* 2009;17(2):88-104.

428. Freedman VA, Calkins M, DeRosier R, Van Haitsma K. *Barriers to Implementing Technology in Residential Long-Term Care Settings.* U.S. Department of Health and Human Services, Polisher Research Institute; December 10, 2005.

429. Berry J. *Dementia Care Training Manual.* 2012. Unpublished manuscript.

430. Zeller A, Dassen T, Kok G et al. Nursing home caregivers' explanations for and coping strategies with residents' aggression: a qualitative study. *Journal of Clinical Nursing.* 2011;20(17-18):2469-2478.

431. Knettel D. Entering the world of dementia with Validation: a holistic approach of care. (Webinar). Volunteers of America; 2013.

432. Mayo Clinic. Dry macular degeneration. Definition. https://www.mayoclinic.org/diseases-conditions/dry-macular-degeneration/symptoms-causes/syc-20350375

433. Merriam-Webster.com. Respect. In: *Merriam-Webster.* Accessed April 27, 2021. https://www.merriam-webster.com/dictionary/respect

434. Volicer L, Hurley AC. Management of behavioral symptoms in progressive degenerative dementias. *The Journals of Gerontology Series A, Biological Sciences and Medical Sciences.* 2003;58(9):M837-M845.

435. Gold MF. Creating harmony from discord: Strategies for calming residents with dementia. *Provider.* 1996;22(3):66-71.

436. Gallo P. *Resident-to-Resident Elder Mistreatment Training Video.* Research Division of the Hebrew Home at Riverdale; 2009. http://citra.human.cornell.edu/r-remp

437. Sturm VE, Yokoyama JS, Seeley WW, et al. Heightened emotional contagion in mild cognitive impairment and Alzheimer's disease is associated with temporal lobe degeneration. *Proceedings of the National Academy of Sciences.* 2013;110(24):9944-9949.

438. Pinkowitz J, Love K. *Living Fully with Dementia: Words Matter.* Dementia Action Alliance. https://daanow.org/wp-content/uploads/2015/01/Living-Fully-with-Dementia-Words-Matter_9.9.2015.pdf; 2015.

439. Lunde A. Emotional memory affects behavior of persons with Alzheimer's. *Alzheimer's disease expert blog.* Mayo Clinic, September 2013.

440. Feil N, Altman R. Validation theory and the myth of the therapeutic lie. *American Journal of Alzheimer's Disease and Other Dementias.* 2004;19(2):77-78.

441. Mehrabian A. *Silent Messages: Implicit Communication of Emotions and Attitudes.* 2nd ed. Belmont, CA: Wadsworth; 1981.

442. Bucks RS, Radford SA. Emotion processing in Alzheimer's disease. *Aging & Mental Health.* 2004;8(3):222-232.

443. Cheston R. Commentary on the chapter Improving care: the next step forward. In: Kitwood T. *Dementia Reconsidered, Revisited: The Person Still Comes First.* 2nd ed (edited by Dawn Brooker). London, UK: Open University Press; 2019:119-122.

444. Acton GJ, Mayhew PA, Hopkins BA, Yauk S. Communicating with individuals with dementia. The impaired person's perspective. *Journal of Gerontological Nursing.* 1999;25(2):6-13.

445. Goffman E. On face work. In: Goffman E, ed. *Interaction Ritual: Essays on Face-to-Face Behavior.* New York: Anchor Books; 1967:5-45.

446. Yeo G, Gallagher-Thompson D, eds. *Ethnicity and the Dementias.* 2nd ed. London, UK: Routledge; 2006.

447. Tran JN, Tran CGU, Hilton L. Working with Vietnamese American families. In: Yeo G, Gallagher-Thompson D, eds. *Ethnicity and the Dementias.* 2nd ed. London, UK: Routledge; 2006:262-283.

448. Snow T. *Accepting the Challenge: Providing the Best Care for People with Dementia* (DVD); https://dementianc.org/education/accepting-the-challenge/; 2003.

449. Mentes JC, Ferrario J. Calming aggressive reactions: a preventive program. *Journal of Gerontological Nursing.* 1989;15(2):22-27.

450. Hart BD, Wells DL. The effects of language used by caregivers on agitation in residents with dementia. *Clinical Nurse Specialist.* 1997;11(1):20-23.

451. Heilman KM, Doty L, Stewart JT, et al. *Helping People with Progressive Memory Disorders: A Guide for You and Your Family.* 2nd ed. University of Florida, Health Science Center; 1999.

452. Ferman TJ, Smith GE, Melom B. *Understanding Behavioral Changes in Dementia*; Lilburn, GA: Lewy Body Dementia Association; 2015.

453. CNN. *World's Untold Stories: Dementia Village*; 2013. http://www.youtube.com/watch?v=LwiOBlyWpko

454. Husband HJ. Diagnostic disclosure in dementia: an opportunity for intervention? *International Journal of Geriatric Psychiatry.* 2000;15(6):544-547.

455. Kemper BJ. Therapeutic listening: developing the concept. *Journal of Psychosocial Nursing and Mental Health Services.* 1992;30(7):21-23.

456. Sheafor BW, Horejsi CR. *Techniques and Guidelines for Social Work Practice.* 7th ed. Boston, MA: Allyn & Bacon; 2006.

457. Frankel M, Freed G, Isenberg L, et al. *Tips and Techniques for Supporting Residents with Mental Illness: A Guide for Staff in Housing for Older Adults.*; Boston, MA: Jewish Community Housing for the Elderly (JCHE) and Jewish Family & Children's Service (JF&CS); http://www.jfcsboston.org/Portals/0/Uploads/Documents/Mental_Health__guide_compressed.pdf; 2012.

458. Baker AS, Wheeler C, Vozzella S. The true meaning of non-pharmacologic management of behavioral symptoms in older adults with cognitive impairment. Webinar, American Medical Directors Association; December 13, 2011.

459. Haight BK, Haight BS. *The Handbook of Structured Life Review.* Baltimore, MD: Health Professions Press; 2007.

460. Hellen C, Sternberg P. *Dealing with Physical Aggression in Caregiving: Physical and Non-Physical Interventions.* Terra Nova Films; 1999. https://terranova.org/film-catalog/dealing-with-physical-aggression-in-caregiving-non-physical-and-physical-interventions/

461. Abel D, Ellement JR. In nursing home slaying, only questions. *The Boston Globe.* http://archive.boston.com/news/local/massachusetts/articles/2009/10/09/in_nursing_home_slaying_only_questions/. Published October 9, 2009.

462. Corkery M, Silver-Greenberg J. Pivotal nursing home suit raises a simple question: who signed the contract? *The New York Times.* https://www.nytimes.com/2016/02/22/business/dealbook/pivotal-

nursing-home-suit-raises-a-simple-question-who-signed-the-contract.html. Published February 21, 2016.

463. Curran K. Nursing home found not negligent in murder of 100-year-old woman. WBZ-TV; March 9, 2012. https://boston.cbslocal.com/2012/03/09/family-of-100-year-old-murder-victim-files-suit-against-nursing-home/

464. Hurley AC, Gauthier MA, Horvath KJ, et al. Promoting safer home environments for persons with Alzheimer's disease. The Home Safety/Injury Model. *Journal of Gerontological Nursing.* 2004;30(6):43-51.

465. Zillmann D. Cognitive-excitation interdependencies in aggressive behavior. *Aggressive Behavior.* 1998;14:51-56.

466. Judy Berry. Two-hour special on frontotemporal dementia. https://www.blogtalkradio.com/alzheimersspeaks/2015/02/24/two-hour-special-on-frontotemporal-dementia-on-alzheimers-speaks-radio. Published online February 24, 2015.

467. Snow T. Understanding the different forms of dementia. Webinar. Dementia Care Academy; 2011.

468. Mapes D. Mean old girls: Seniors who bully. NBC News; *https://www.nbcnews.com/health/health-news/mean-old-girls-seniors-who-bully-flna1c9465919* February 2011.

469. Rosen A, Lachs MS, Pillemer K, Teresi J. Staff responses to resident-to-resident elder mistreatment in nursing homes. Results of a multi-site survey. *Journal of the American Geriatrics Society.* 2012;60(Suppl 4):S166-S166.

470. U.S. General Accounting Office. *VA Community Living Centers. Actions Needed to Better Manage Risks to Veterans' Quality of Life and Care.* Report to the Ranking Member, Committee on Veterans' Affairs, U.S. Senate; 2011. https://www.gao.gov/products/gao-12-11

471. Snow T. *Improving Emergency Services for Dementia Patients.* DVD. Sarasota, FL: Pines Education Institute of Southwest Florida; 2012.

472. DeBaggio T. *Losing My Mind: An Intimate Look at Life with Alzheimer's Disease.* The Free Press; 2002.

473. Lanza ML, Zeiss RA, Rierdan J. Multiple perspectives on assault: The 360-degree interview. *Journal of the American Psychiatric Nurses Association.* 2009;14(6):413-420.

474. Serres C. Despite deadly toll, Minnesota nursing home residents with COVID-19 still sharing rooms. *The Star Tribune.* https://www.startribune.com/despite-deadly-toll-minnesota-nursing-home-residents-with-covid-19-still-sharing-rooms/570738212/. Published May 24, 2020.

475. Serres C, Howatt G. "Death was everywhere." How a Minnesota nursing home fell into a COVID-19 black hole. *The Star Tribune.* https://www.startribune.com/desperate-at-death-ridge-minnesota-nursing-home-descended-into-covid-19-coronavirus-black-hole/573141421/. Published December 13, 2020.

476. Osborne J. Restraints in memory loss: are they appropriate? Presented at the Caring for a Person with Memory Loss Conference, University of Minnesota School of Nursing, Minneapolis, MN; 2014.

477. Malcolm J. Minnesota Department of Health's Assisted Living Licensure Work Group. Saint Paul, MN; November 5, 2018.

478. Justice in Aging. Involuntary transfer and discharge: a closer look at the revised nursing home regulations. Issue Brief. http://justiceinaging.org/wp-content/uploads/2017/01/Revised-Nursing-Facility-Regulations_Involuntary-Transfer-and-Discharge.pdf

479. The National Consumer Voice for Quality Long Term Care. Nursing home discharges: You've been told to leave . . . now what? Fact sheet. Published online 2018. https://theconsumervoice.org/nursing-home-discharges

480. The National Consumer Voice for Quality Long-Term Care. COVID-19 emergency declaration blanket waivers for health care providers: summary of CMS waivers for nursing homes. Published online 2020. https://theconsumervoice.org/uploads/files/actions-and-news-updates/Summary_of_CMS_Waived_Regulations_-_COVID-19_4-6-20.pdf

481. Carlson E, Edelman T, Grant R, Smetanka L. A deeper dive into the revised Federal nursing home regulations: Part 1. Webinar, National Consumer Voice for Quality Long-Term Care, February 15, 2017. https://www.youtube.com/watch?v=0ZmfLDx1UuA.

Index

Page numbers followed by "f" and "t" indicate figures and tables.